Outbreak Investigations Around the World: Case Studies in Infectious Disease Field Epidemiology

Editor

Mark S. Dworkin, MD, MPH&TM, FACP

Associate Professor
Division of Epidemiology and Biostatistics
University of Illinois at Chicago
School of Public Health
Chicago, Illinois

JONES AND BARTLETT PUBLISHERS
Sudbury, Massachusetts
BOSTON   TORONTO   LONDON   SINGAPORE

World Headquarters
Jones and Bartlett Publishers
40 Tall Pine Drive
Sudbury, MA 01776
978-443-5000
info@jbpub.com
www.jbpub.com

Jones and Bartlett Publishers
Canada
6339 Ormindale Way
Mississauga, Ontario L5V 1J2
Canada

Jones and Bartlett Publishers
International
Barb House, Barb Mews
London W6 7PA
United Kingdom

Jones and Bartlett's books and products are available through most bookstores and online booksellers. To contact Jones and Bartlett Publishers directly, call 800-832-0034, fax 978-443-8000, or visit our website, www.jbpub.com.

Substantial discounts on bulk quantities of Jones and Bartlett's publications are available to corporations, professional associations, and other qualified organizations. For details and specific discount information, contact the special sales department at Jones and Bartlett via the above contact information or send an email to specialsales@jbpub.com.

This publication is designed to provide accurate and authoritative information in regard to the Subject Matter covered. It is sold with the understanding that the publisher is not engaged in rendering legal, accounting, or other professional service. If legal advice or other expert assistance is required, the service of a competent professional person should be sought.

Production Credits
Publisher: Michael Brown
Production Director: Amy Rose
Associate Editor: Katey Birtcher
Editorial Assistant: Catie Heverling
Senior Production Editor: Tracey Chapman
Marketing Manager: Sophie Fleck
Associate Marketing Manager: Jessica Cormier
Manufacturing and Inventory Control Supervisor: Amy Bacus
Composition: Publishers' Design and Production Services, Inc.
Cover Design: Scott Moden
Cover Image: © Tischenko Irina/ShutterStock, Inc.; © brem stocker/ShutterStock, Inc.
Printing and Binding: Malloy, Inc.
Cover Printing: Malloy, Inc.

Library of Congress Cataloging-in-Publication Data

Outbreak investigations around the world : case studies in infectious disease field epidemiology / editor, Mark S. Dworkin.
    p. ; cm.
  Includes bibliographical references and index.
  ISBN-13: 978-0-7637-5143-2 (pbk.)
  ISBN-10: 0-7637-5143-X (pbk.)
  1. Epidemiology—Case studies.   I. Dworkin, Mark S.
  [DNLM: 1. Disease Outbreaks—Personal Narratives.   2. Epidemiologic Methods—Personal Narratives.
WA 105 O94 2009]
  RA652.4.O98 2009
  614.4—dc22

                                                                        2008051156

6048

Printed in the United States of America
13   12   11   10   09   10   9   8   7   6   5   4   3   2   1

Dedication

This book is dedicated to my wife, Renee, and daughters, Josie and Julieanne, whose love and support have made it possible for me to pursue the unusual infectious diseases career that has been my life for the past 16 years. I also dedicate it to my parents, Edward and Una Dworkin, who nurtured my curiosity and sacrificed to ensure that I would have the best education that they could provide.

Acknowledgments

I wish to recognize the chapter authors who graciously donated their time to contribute to this book. They each have a strong commitment to public health education. I know that they are all very busy (or even retired), and thus, taking on writing a chapter about an outbreak that in some cases occurred decades ago was a true labor of love. They are really special people who have spent most or all of their careers in public health, and I feel honored to have had them accept my request for their contribution. I also appreciate the review of the preface and Chapter 1 by Frank Sorvillo and Bill Keane, respectively. Additionally, there have been many persons who have directly and indirectly helped me to develop an understanding of outbreak investigation, including teachers, supervisors, co-workers, colleagues, public health personnel, infection control practitioners, microbiologists, and the many others with whom I have interacted during and after these events. Finally, I acknowledge the students, fellows, and EIS officers whom I have had the privilege to instruct and the many students and public health workers for whom I hope this book will become a useful complement to the study and practice of epidemiology.

Contents

Preface

An outbreak (or epidemic) is a unique public health event and poses many challenges and opportunities to those tasked with the response. It occurs when more cases of a disease are recognized than would normally be expected at a given time among a specific group of people, whether it is a dozen persons with gastroenteritis that attended a church supper (where the term outbreak is most suitable) or the occurrence of a marked rise in cases of a disease among the population of an entire country (where the term epidemic may be better applied). Unlike a research experiment in which you try to control many things such as precisely how the study subjects are exposed to some health-related variable, the responder to an outbreak has had no control over the exposure and may not even know what the exposure was. Rather, the focus is on investigating and describing this natural experiment that nature or man (intentionally or unintentionally) has caused. The investigator might only be confronted with a syndrome (such as an outbreak of diarrheal illness) without even knowing which agent has specifically caused this outbreak. They may even be challenged with the cause of the outbreak being a novel organism that has not previously been described. In the case of the many thousands of public health employees working in local or state health departments in units or sections that are responsible for more than one disease (such as those dealing with communicable or immunization preventable diseases), they never know what will be the next outbreak and are challenged to master the information about each of what can be 40, 60, or more reportable conditions. Regardless of whether the disease is named on the list of reportable conditions, usually if it causes an outbreak, it is automatically reportable.

In an outbreak, there is typically an urgent need to control the public health outcome and minimize its impact especially through prevention of further cases. One of the first things that is needed by the public health responder is some familiarity with what is already known about how to deal with the problem. For example, when one is confronted with a Salmonella outbreak, it is useful to have had experience investigating previous outbreaks of salmonellosis and to have read the literature of Salmonella outbreaks to gain familiarity with methods of investigation and issues that can arise. The scientific literature has many publications of outbreak investigations. Some of these are descriptive and others focus on one or more aspects of the outbreak, such as laboratory issues or infection control. These publications are wonderful resources but may be less accessible to those not trained in epidemiology, the laboratory science, or biostatistics. Such reports are also limited by journal word count and scientific writing requirements that may make them less accessible to some public health employees and students.

Outbreaks are fascinating stories. They are real-life events that sometimes weave together all of the drama any Hollywood producer could wish for in a blockbuster. The baker vomiting in the kitchen sink and then resuming his work duties, a casual or even celebratory meal out at a restaurant followed days later by hospitalization and death only because the deceased decided that he would have the Caesar salad with the entrée for a small additional price, or perhaps a family reunion at a hotel followed by a family cluster of illnesses with fever because the whirlpool they enjoyed may have been aerosolizing Legionella species. Some outbreaks, including several in this book, are even more dramatic, making national headlines when previously unrecognized organisms hospitalize and kill, massively large numbers of persons are sickened, or a relatively small number of persons are sickened or killed but an entire nation is fearful for their own safety. An outbreak might be heartbreaking when it ruins a family business as its reputation is tainted by a *Salmonella*-contaminated chicken or egg-containing dish or is responsible for the death of a student from an immunization preventable disease such as measles.

A pessimist who studies outbreaks finds reason not to drink, swim, relax in, or even shower in water and not to eat shellfish, meat, chicken, pork, fried rice, home-canned vegetables, fresh spinach, tomatoes, alfalfa sprouts, peanut butter, apple cider, and even pasteurized milk! Beware hotels, any banquet especially at a wedding, any catered meal, and don't even think of flying on an airplane or taking a cruise. Heaven forbid that your child goes to a daycare, plays on an athletic team, visits a petting zoo, or just plain goes to school at all. Just when you thought it might be good to get away, you had better avoid the beaver dams and rivers, caves, well water, and rustic cabins where ticks are hiding to bite you and your friends or family painlessly in the night. Don't get sick with anything so that you can avoid the hospitals and surgicenters, and don't even think of having sex!

The optimist recognizes, however, the incredible potential to learn and apply public health skills while performing useful and rewarding work. It is no coincidence that some of the most important outbreak investigations have had lead investigators who lacked subspecialty knowledge of the disease that they were investigating (before they began the investigation); however, the reason that they were suitable for the investigation was due in large part to their epidemiologic skill set. They brought their "epidemiologic tool kit" with them to the outbreak and, in the midst of investigating, attempted to master relevant knowledge of the disease and, whenever possible, to partner with others who had disease-specific knowledge. I have seen many successful epidemiologists move their careers from one area of study to a seemingly unrelated area of study. How can someone who worked on AIDS for 8 years transfer to work on cancer or air pollution or smoking cessation, and then some years later transfer to work on influenza? Why do such programs hire that person? The answer is that these individuals have a highly valuable "epidemiology tool kit," and those that hire them understand its value. A well-rounded epidemiologist has been involved in a diversity of epidemiologic analyses; a great way to develop and polish these epidemiologic skills is through outbreak investigation.

This book attempts to reach out to the experienced and the less experienced outbreak investigator, as well as anyone interested in the study of epidemics, by presenting extraordinary and illustrative outbreaks. It is the hope of the editor and the chapter authors that these outbreak descriptions will clarify what was involved in the outbreak investigation beyond what is found in published scientific articles and illustrate the kind of issues that can arise. The first person style of these chapters is intended to create a reader-friendly format that is more like a story in that it can entertain while instructing. They also provide a context for the outbreaks by introducing the reader to where the author was in his or her career at the time, with whom he or she was working, as well as the real world conditions that he or she had to face while practicing field epidemiology. In an article written for the *New York Times*, Lawrence K. Altman recalled the Legionnaires' disease outbreak of 1976. He described an interview with a patient that left the epidemiologic team unable to explain why that patient developed the disease but not four other Legionnaires with whom he spent a great deal of time. He goes on to recognize that dead ends such as these in epidemiologic investigations are not what scientific journals publish. The concise and focused scientific article that becomes what most persons know of the outbreak investigation (along with other factors) "creates a false impression that investigations and discoveries are simpler than they really are" (*New York Times*, August 1, 2006). These investigations are typically very complex and bring together many challenges, including recalling and applying epidemiologic knowledge, making numerous decisions quickly and under stressful conditions, working as a team including team members with whom one has never worked before, working in an environment away from the office where most of one's resources are located, and many more.

A special feature of this book is that it includes some of the most historically important outbreaks of the past 40 years, including an outbreak of cholera in Portugal, an outbreak of toxic shock syndrome linked to tampons, the outbreak of Legionnaires' diseases that led to the discovery of the bacterium *Legionella pneumophila*, the early investigation of what would become recognized as a global AIDS epidemic, the massive outbreak of cryptosporidiosis in Milwaukee, and the New York City experience with the intentional outbreak of anthrax. Other outbreaks presented here illustrate a variety of problems, modes of transmission, populations, and control measures, including Ebola virus in Gabon, hepatitis A among injection drug users in Iowa, hepatitis B among Israeli hospital patients, community outbreaks of shigellosis and whooping cough, and syphilis among men who have sex with men after meeting in Internet chat rooms. Importantly, there is also a chapter illustrating the discovery of a pseudo-outbreak.

Each of the authors was asked to describe his or her personal experience within an outbreak investigation while describing the methods that were employed. As a result, the chapters are not uniform in their presentation, and one chapter actually has more than one perspective. This informality with style was intentional, and it is hoped that it makes these investigations more accessible to some readers.

An outbreak is both a negative public health event and an opportunity. Although people are ill, there are many benefits to outbreak investigation.

Outbreak investigations identify populations at risk for a disease, allow for modes of disease transmission to be characterized, and provide information that can be used to control the outbreak (thus preventing further disease transmission), as well as prevent similar occurrences in the future. Outbreak investigations also provide the opportunity to evaluate public health programs or policy (such as a requirement for universal immunization against a particular disease) and whether they have been effective. In the course of an outbreak investigation, laboratory methods might reveal whether there is something new about the causative organism (such as a strain that is novel and not well covered by the current vaccine) or whether the strain is usual and therefore immunity from the vaccine may be less long lasting than hoped or believed. These investigations allow for the evaluation of new control measures that might be introduced in the course of the outbreak and are derived from the data analysis. They also allow for an improved understanding of the disease, especially when the disease is relatively uncommon. Whereas a disease might occur only sporadically throughout the country and get reported occasionally as a case report, the outbreak creates a series of cases under the thoughtful observation of an investigator or team of investigators who may recognize epidemiological, clinical, or laboratory features not previously observed. The outbreak also generates what can be relatively large numbers of samples (such as stool or blood) or isolates of an organism that can allow for advancement of the scientific knowledge related to that disease or organism.

Outbreak investigations are also an opportunity for public health staff training. It is common for outbreaks to occur where staff have little to no experience dealing with them (such as outside of a city or county with a very large population). As a result, the administrative staff may wisely request assistance from the state or federal health department. The arrival of experienced staff under real-world conditions can lead to training that advances the skills of the staff in the jurisdiction requesting the help and also the individual(s) who provide assistance to them. The Centers for Disease Control and Prevention's (CDC) Epidemic Intelligence Service (EIS) is a wonderful example of this benefit. There have been numerous deployments of the EIS officers into outbreaks of all kinds throughout the United States, its territories, and to other countries. Many of the chapters in this book derive from EIS officer experiences. I have heard numerous former EIS officers describe their time in the EIS as the best 2 years of their career. In certain countries such as Kenya, India, and Thailand, the CDC has created the Field Epidemiology Training Program (FETP) to provide a similar EIS-like experience in collaboration with the country's ministry of health.

Outbreak investigations also allow for the fulfillment of legal obligations and duty of care for the public. State legislatures have passed rules and regulations establishing what should happen under certain circumstances such as the reporting of a disease or outbreak. These outbreaks allow for the fulfillment of these legally mandated control measures such as removing a food handler from food preparation activities while they have diarrheal illness or are shedding *Salmonella* species in their stool despite recovery from diarrhea. Other legislative mandates such as the authority to close down a business (such as a restaurant) or to isolate or quarantine a patient may be fulfilled as the public health authority responding to the outbreak carries out its control efforts.

An outbreak investigation offers a unique opportunity to educate the public about disease prevention. Although the media is sometimes an investigative watchdog and can be overzealous or less than scientific in their approach to a public health problem, they can also be a terrific partner of the health department with the mutual goal of informing the public of what they need to know. As a result, although information about hand washing, covering your cough, receiving immunizations, or cooking meat or chicken to a certain temperature might not be news on any given day, during an outbreak, it might be a critical control measure and can even become front page news. Contact with the media can also be very useful for calming fears, combating rumors, directing the public to where it can access special assistance (such as antibiotics, immunizations, or information), and promoting the single overriding communication objective. The single overriding communication objective is very important because although a thoughtful investigator can talk about many features of the outbreak that may be of interest, the journalist is limited by the space and focus of his or her article; therefore, it is helpful to be concise and focused with what is being shared with the journalist, even to the point of being redundant: "We really want to emphasize that thorough hand washing after using the bathroom is an essential way to prevent the spread of this disease." "Parents need to help their children wash their hands thoroughly to minimize risk of spread of this disease." "The public does not need to be afraid of this disease. Something as simple as hand washing can protect them and others from getting it."

Public health departments often go unnoticed by many in the community. They might be aware of influenza or other immunization services offered by them, but a lot of the very important functions of the local public health department are performed quietly, without fanfare. As a result, when there is an outbreak investigation, it is an opportunity for the public health department to improve and promote its credibility in dealing with a health emergency. As mentioned previously, although not every health department can take an active lead in such an investigation due to the heterogeneous distribution of epidemiologic skills from health department to health department, even inexperienced staff members can provide vital support roles to those invited in to take the lead. A public health department can be praised for calling in needed assistance, just as it can be condemned for not realizing when it has delayed getting help to the detriment of the community. It is a difficult balance that should be kept in mind as it impacts on the credibility of the health department to its stakeholders including the community it serves.

An outbreak also provides an opportunity to intelligently direct laboratory resources. I have heard laboratory workers on more than one occasion in my career recoil or ridicule the outbreak investigator who, when asked "what do you want us to test for" about food or environmental samples, replied "test for everything." Although testing for everything might eventually find the pathogen, it is an unrealistic use of laboratory personnel and financial resources, and can create a great deal of unfocussed busy work for the laboratory. Laboratory testing should ideally follow epidemiologic information and test a hypothesis.

Finally, an outbreak is an opportunity for sharing of information with other health professionals, scientists, the public, and many others (such as our elected leaders). In addition to a written report that might sit for years in a file drawer, some outbreaks are published. These published outbreaks may be disseminated worldwide as their journals circulate to subscribers, including libraries where many persons gain access to them. With the Internet, some of these outbreak investigations are available for study without any subscription through free access or access granted through academic institutions. There is great value in many of these publications as they can provide useful information on background information about the disease, summaries of methods used to perform part or all of the investigation, ways to display and interpret the results, and references to other publications that might be useful to future outbreak investigators.

Outbreak investigation would be considered beneficial if only one or two of the previously mentioned reasons applied; however, the benefits of outbreak investigation are many and substantial. Outbreak investigation is a vital public health duty and, as this book demonstrates, can also be a fascinating and instructive drama.

Mark S. Dworkin, MD, MPH&TM, FACP

About the Author

Dr. Mark S. Dworkin is a medical epidemiologist and is board certified in internal medicine and infectious diseases. After receiving his medical degree from Rush Medical College (Chicago), he trained in Internal Medicine at Rush Presbyterian St. Luke's Medical Center and in Infectious Diseases at Tulane University Medical Center, he also obtained a Master's Degree in Public Health and Tropical Medicine from the Tulane University School of Tropical Medicine and Public Health in New Orleans. He then served for 2 years in the Centers for Disease Control and Prevention's (CDC) Epidemic Intelligence Service stationed at the Washington State Department of Health where he investigated many outbreaks including those due to pertussis, Salmonella, Cryptosporidium, Trichinella, and measles. Dr. Dworkin worked at the CDC in Atlanta for 4 years in the Division of HIV/AIDS Prevention and performed many epidemiologic analyses related to opportunistic infections. During 2000 to 2006, he was the Illinois Department of Public Health State Epidemiologist in the Division of Infectious Diseases and team leader for the rapid response team (an outbreak investigation team). He is now an associate professor in the Division of Epidemiology and Biostatistics at the University of Illinois at Chicago School of Public Health and an attending physician at the HIV outpatient Core Center of the John H. Stroger Jr. Hospital of Cook County (formerly Cook County Hospital) and provides on-call coverage to a private practice infectious disease group in the Chicago area. Dr. Dworkin lectures at Northwestern University and the University of Chicago. He has authored or co-authored many scientific publications on various topics including outbreak investigations, surveillance, HIV/AIDS opportunistic infections, salmonellosis, tick-borne illnesses, and vaccine-preventable infections. He has been awarded both the Commendation Medal and the Achievement Medal by the United States Public Health Service.

Contributor List

Mary E. Bartlett, BA
Division of Parasitic Diseases
National Center For Zoonotic,
    Vectorborne and Enteric
    Diseases
Centers for Disease Control and
    Prevention
Atlanta, GA

**Daniel G. Bausch, MD,
MPH&TM**
Associate Professor
Tulane School of Public Health
    and Tropical Medicine
New Orleans, LA

Paul A. Blake, MD, MPH
Salem, OR

Thomas M. Carney
President
Carney Consulting, LLC
Johnston, IA

Ken W. Carter
Adjunct Instructor
Des Moines Area Community
    College
Des Moines, IA

Jeffrey P. Davis, MD
Chief Medical Officer and State
    Epidemiologist for
    Communicable Diseases
Wisconsin Division of Public
    Health
Madison, WI

Ronald C. Hershow, MD, MPH
Associate Professor of
    Epidemiology
Clinical Associate Professor of
    Medicine
University of Illinois-Chicago
    School of Public Health
Chicago, IL

Gregory Huhn, MD, MPH&TM
Assistant Professor
Section of Infectious Diseases
John H. Stroger Jr. Hospital of
    Cook County
Chicago, IL
Rush University Medical Center
Chicago, IL

Yvan J.F. Hutin, MD
Medical Officer, Field
  Epidemiology Training
  Programme
WHO India country office
New Delhi, India

**Harold W. Jaffe, MD, MA,
  FFPH**
Department of Public Health
University of Oxford
Oxford, England

Charles E. Jennings
CEO
Inject-Safe Bandages, LLC
Jacksonville, IL

Jeffrey D. Klausner, MD, MPH
Deputy Health Officer
Director, STD Prevention and
  Control Services
San Francisco Department of
  Health
Associate Clinical Professor of
  Medicine
Divisions of AIDS and Infectious
  Diseases
Department of Medicine
University of California
San Francisco, CA

Marci Layton, MD
Assistant Commissioner, Bureau of
  Communicable Disease
The City of New York
  Department of Health and
  Mental Hygiene
New York, NY

Janet Mohle-Boetani, MD, MPH
Chief Medical Officer
Public Health Unit
California Prison Health Care
  Services
Sacramento, CA

Kenrad E. Nelson, MD, PhD
Department of Epidemiology
Bloomsburg School of Hygiene
  and Public Health
Johns Hopkins University
Baltimore, MD

Peter M. Schantz, VMD, PhD
Department of Global Health
Rollins School of Public Health
Emory University
Atlanta, GA

Frank Sorvillo, PhD
Associate Professor in Residence
University of California Los
  Angeles
School of Public Health
Los Angeles, CA

Patricia Quinlisk, MD, MPH
Medical Director and the State
  Epidemiologist
Iowa Department of Public Health
Adjunct Professor
College of Public Health
The University of Iowa
Iowa City, IA

Kevin Teale, MA
Senior Communications
  Consultant
Media Relations

Wellmark Blue Cross and Blue
  Shield
Des Moines, IA

Stephen B. Thacker, MD, MSc
RADM (Ret.), USPHS
Director
Office of Workforce and Career
  Development
Centers for Disease Control and
  Prevention
Atlanta, GA

J. Todd Weber, MD
CDC Liaison
European Centre for Disease
  Prevention and Control
Stockholm, Sweden

U.S. Department of Health and
  Human Services
Centers for Disease Control and
  Prevention
Atlanta, GA

Don Weiss, MD, MPH
Director of Surveillance
Bureau of Communicable Disease
New York City Department of
  Health and Mental Hygiene
New York, NY

CHAPTER 1

How an Outbreak is Investigated

Mark S. Dworkin, MD, MPH&TM

INTRODUCTION

It is worth summarizing and elaborating briefly on the steps (or activities) of outbreak investigation (Exhibit 1-1). Although the steps may not always occur in exactly this order, this is the general pattern of events. It is not unusual for more than one step to be occurring at the same time. Not all lists of outbreak investigation steps are identical, as some steps may be combined into one overarching step or may not be listed as a step but included in a discussion of outbreak methods. It is important to recognize that a list of outbreak investigation steps is less of a recipe to be followed precisely than it is guidance. Also, as the investigation progresses, knowing where one is at within the outbreak investigation steps can make it easier to stay organized and plan ahead for what may need to occur next. (The reader is also encouraged to examine other good reviews of outbreak investigation referenced at the end of this chapter.)[1–3]

VERIFY THAT AN OUTBREAK IS OCCURRING

Often a telephone call reports the suspicion of an outbreak. Someone has noticed something out of the ordinary, such as an unexpectedly high number of cases of a disease or syndrome. The call might come from someone who attended a group function, like a wedding, and now they and others

---

Exhibit 1-1   The Steps of an Outbreak Investigation

---

1. Verify that an outbreak is occurring.
2. Confirm the diagnosis.
3. Assemble an investigation team.
4. Create a tentative case definition.
5. Count cases.
6. Perform epidemiologic analysis.
7. Perform supplemental laboratory or environmental investigation (if indicated).
8. Develop hypotheses.
9. Introduce preliminary control measures.
10. Decide whether observation or additional studies are indicated.
11. Perform additional analyses or plan and perform additional study.
12. Perform new (investigation derived) control measures, and/or ensure the compliance of existing control measures.
13. Communicate prevention information and findings.
14. Monitor surveillance data.

---

they know are ill. It might come from a hospital infection-control nurse or hospital microbiologist who notices that they have more than typical numbers of a particular bacterial isolate in the laboratory or infectious disease among the patients. It could arise, however, from a thoughtful review of surveillance data (perhaps from a public health laboratory) demonstrating an unexpected rise. Whether the recognition arises from a community member, a health professional, or an astute public health employee, the first step of an outbreak investigation is to verify that there is indeed an outbreak occurring. This is the first, but not the only, time during an outbreak investigation that one must be careful not to assume anything and to have a healthy skepticism about the information that they are receiving.

A common method of verifying that an outbreak exists is to examine surveillance data (if that condition is a reportable disease). One of the important uses of surveillance data is outbreak detection. It can quickly be determined whether the suspicion of a high number of case reports of salmonellosis, shigellosis, or pertussis bears out as accurate by comparing the report to a median number of reported cases during a similar time period historically. In some cases, the disease is not known but the outbreak is initially recognized as a sudden rise in the onset of a sign or symptom such as rash or diarrhea. A report might be that someone attended a group event where food was served and that many persons are ill; however, until it has been confirmed that more than one person is truly ill with a similar illness and that they consumed food in common, it is premature to declare that a foodborne outbreak has occurred.

CONFIRM THE DIAGNOSIS

Another early step of the investigation is to confirm the diagnosis. A classic example of this would be when a hospital laboratory might report that they have several isolates of an uncommon bacteria or virus. Because the isolate is unusual, the laboratory might not have substantial expertise in identifying it; therefore, it is necessary to confirm the diagnosis by forwarding the isolates to a reference laboratory such as at the state health department or Centers for Disease Control and Prevention (CDC). In such reference laboratories, it can be determined, for example, whether the *Salmonella* outbreak is really five isolates of *Salmonella* (and which serotype is involved) or actually one or even no *Salmonella* at all.

ASSEMBLE AN INVESTIGATION TEAM

Depending on the outbreak and the public health jurisdiction(s) involved, an investigation team may need to be assembled. This is especially likely if it is of a remarkable size or complexity that it needs a more formal group to work on it. Sometimes the investigation is conducted by an individual for whom this is an occasional duty and there isn't a team per se, but individuals who react to the reports coming in and deal with them as needed (in other words, not every outbreak receives a full formal investigation). In some settings, a team already is assembled and on call for the next outbreak whenever it may occur. In that case, this step was actually the first step as that public health jurisdiction recognizes that outbreaks occur with a great enough frequency to have planned ahead; however, more commonly, outbreak teams are assembled based on the unique issues surrounding the outbreak.

Considerations in assembling the team include determining a team leader. This is based on experience and expertise of the team leader, and therefore, it might be a communicable disease section chief if there was an outbreak of salmonellosis, whereas it might be an immunization section chief for an outbreak of measles. Alternatively, there could be a program staff level individual (ideally with epidemiologic training) who is well suited to this task, or an epidemiologist might be invited in from a higher level jurisdiction (such as state or federal government) when necessary skills are lacking locally or when an investigation was attempted but was unsuccessful and still needs resolution. A higher profile investigation or one involving multiple jurisdictions might be led by a state epidemiologist or other senior epidemiology personnel. The team leader may not always be an epidemiologist but may be a skilled administrator or environmental health worker. The most important thing is that it should make sense that someone in the lead belongs there as there is much to be gained with a well run outbreak investigation and much to be lost when it is poorly run.

Team members should be considered based on their experience, abilities, and availability. A team is best comprised of one or more members with experience, as the activities are likely to proceed much more smoothly with fewer misunderstandings or errors along the way; however, some team members may be inexperienced but need on-the-job training, or they may be needed to ensure that certain activities (such as interviewing) are adequately staffed to gather quickly the data needed for analysis. If they have the needed abilities (such as interviewing, data entry, or analysis skills), they can become useful contributing members once provided the appropriate guidance or training. However, providing guidance or training in the setting of an urgent outbreak investigation can pose quite a challenge with many priorities competing for one's time.

If medical record abstraction or other clinical-related work is needed as part of an investigation, a healthcare provider such as someone with nursing or medical training may be essential.

Given that outbreaks don't schedule themselves when it is convenient to staff them, however, an additional consideration is who can be available for the duration needed. Personnel are typically diverted off their routine duties (which may also be essential and can only be delayed briefly). They may need to travel, including staying overnight for several days or longer. It is best to staff an outbreak with personnel who can remain with their outbreak duties without interruption, although this may just not be possible at times.

CREATE A TENTATIVE CASE DEFINITION

Once convinced that an outbreak is really occurring and having confirmed the diagnosis (or syndrome) that is involved, a tentative case definition is needed to begin to determine the extent of the outbreak in a systematic way. Essentially, this is a surveillance system that one is creating within the outbreak investigation. If it is a reportable disease that is responsible for the outbreak, much of the outbreak definition may already be available. The case definition should involve elements of person, place, and time. Routine reporting of a reportable disease would not include the wedding, church supper, or other cohort information, nor would it necessarily include any geographic boundaries that might be needed to define the outbreak; therefore, a reportable disease case definition is often adapted but not just used without any modification at all in an outbreak setting.

This case definition is tentative because as additional information is learned then there may be a need to modify it so that it is most accurate and useful for analysis. It is important that when communicating with the media and others such as administrators who may not have epidemiologic training that the preliminary information is just that—preliminary. An outbreak investigation needs to remain flexible, including the possibility of revising the case definition to achieve its goals of disease control and prevention.

The creation of a case definition may involve a thoughtful discussion of sensitivity and specificity. In an attempt to identify every case of a disease that might lead to death or severe morbidity, a highly sensitive case definition might be needed; however, when performing data analysis of reported cases, a more specific case definition is desired to limit the influence that inclusion of those without the disease of interest that happen to meet the case definition may have on the analysis results. As an illustrative but extreme example, if an investigation wanted to identify nearly every case of influenza, the case definition might include anyone with fever; however, such a definition also captures cases of numerous other illnesses and thus lacks the specificity needed to trust any data analysis intended to be specific to the control of influenza. Alternatively, if the case definition required the isolation of the influenza virus, there would be a high degree of certainty about the cases reported, but because most persons with influenza do not have laboratory procedures performed that lead to isolation of the virus, relatively few cases would be reported. A case definition should avoid including any potential risk factors within it, as that would prevent the analysis of determining whether those risk factors are statistically associated with the exposure.

A case definition often has more than one category within it, such as confirmed versus probable or primary versus secondary. Confirmed cases typically represent cases that have been laboratory confirmed. It is important to make this distinction of "laboratory confirmed" versus just saying "confirmed" because some surveillance systems, such as the one used for pertussis in the United States, include cases without laboratory confirmation as confirmed cases if they are epidemiologically linked to a laboratory confirmed case. Probable cases usually refer to cases that have not met the relatively specific criteria of laboratory diagnostic testing but have other information that makes their likelihood of being true cases high.

The case definition is for the investigator's benefit. It is intended to assist the investigator with counting the cases and best determining the associated factors and source. This can madden the media, who are following some of these investigations and even public health officials who don't understand why the case count is changing, but keep in mind that its usefulness is in helping the investigator to provide a sound explanation for what has happened and why. The case definition in this setting is not designed to count most accurately exactly how many people got that disease. That number is likely to get underestimated in the race to solve and control the outbreak.

Primary cases are the cases that were exposed to the implicated source, whereas secondary cases usually arise from their contact with an infectious primary case. For example, a restaurant may be implicated in an outbreak. The cases that ate a *Salmonella*-contaminated food develop gastroenteritis and are called primary cases. They will shed the organism in their stool, and if they do not practice good hand hygiene after using the bathroom, they may transfer the organism to a family member or friend (such as if they prepared sandwiches for them). These new cases of salmonellosis may never have been to the implicated restaurant and are secondary cases. Unfortunately, sometimes you can have cases in the same household where the second case in the household could have been exposed to the implicated source but had a long enough delay after the first household case to be caused by secondary transmission as well. This needs to be kept in mind when designing the case definition.

When later performing analysis of the cases ascertained through outbreak investigation, it is important to exclude the secondary cases from the analysis of risk factors, especially when the goal is to identify the primary source of the outbreak. In addition, if there are sufficient numbers of laboratory-confirmed cases, probable cases may be excluded to increase the likelihood that an association is real and to avoid the possibility of bias against a true association if probable cases include some persons who met the case definition but do not (unknown to the investigation staff) have the outbreak disease. Thus, while chasing down laboratory specimens (sputum, vomit, feces, blood, or others) from many of the cases can involve a lot of work, it can pay off if it yields a big enough number of cases that you are confident really are cases.

CASE COUNTS

After a case definition has been created, the work of identifying as many cases as is feasible follows. In some situations, like a commercial product outbreak or one that has substantial morbidity or mortality and is not readily being solved, that means trying to get all of the cases reported often by announcing the outbreak through a variety of means, including electronic, fax, and press release, although there may be situations where the outbreak is so massive that efforts are eventually best directed toward prevention and control. In this uncommon situation where an outbreak is massive, an estimate of the case burden may be performed. It is a judgment call whether resources are to be expended on reporting tens of thousands of cases versus allowing passive reporting to decline naturally without active and persistent efforts. Broadcasting the existence of an outbreak may be indicated when there is a good prevention intervention (like an effective vaccine or immunoglobulin), and thus, raising awareness could help exposed persons prevent the onset of illness (such as in the case of hepatitis A exposure).

PERFORM EPIDEMIOLOGIC ANALYSIS

After there are cases to analyze and those data are entered into a computer database, it is time to perform descriptive epidemiology. This allows for many basic questions to be answered, especially when the number of cases on the initial "line list" where the first reports were summarized on paper or in spread sheet has become numerous. The initial analysis might include frequencies of all the variables, thus demonstrating basic patterns of the outbreak such as age, gender, racial, occupational, clinical manifestations, and exposure information. Cases may be examined for their geographical distribution, and the results may lead to a hypothesis regarding a suspected exposure site. If an onset of illness date and an exposure date are known, a mean or median incubation period might be calculated that can be compared with what is already known for certain suspected pathogens (most useful when the pathogen is unknown). Depending on the type of outbreak (such as respiratory or foodborne) and whether the number of persons who have been exposed is known, preliminary overall or food-specific attack rates can be determined. Several computer statistical software packages are available for analyzing outbreak data, but one of the more commonly used and freely accessible epidemiological software packages is Epi Info (available for free download from the CDC at http://www.cdc.gov/epiinfo/). Epi Info is particularly convenient for investigators with limited epidemiologic and analysis skills because it has many functions that do not involve writing any programming code.

PERFORM SUPPLEMENTAL LABORATORY OR ENVIRONMENTAL INVESTIGATION

Environmental or laboratory studies may be recognized as potentially useful early in some outbreak investigations. For example, in foodborne outbreak investigation where a food establishment such as a restaurant is implicated by several of the cases, a restaurant inspection by the local health authority is a routine response. This would typically occur even if that food establishment had received a routine inspection some time in the recent past. The inspection could reveal useful clues that may help with use or interpretation of the epidemiologic data (such as learning of ill food handlers or discovery that there was a recent plumbing problem). It may simply reveal sooner (rather than after data are entered and analyzed) that there are violations of required food sanitation practices that must be remedied for that business to stay in business. In other words, a control measure such as closing down a restaurant should not have to wait until epidemiologic analysis if an onsite inspection of an implicated site reveals the need for such actions. Alternatively, an implicated site may not be recognized as in need of inspection until epidemiologic analysis provides the hypothesis of such a site. This might be the case for an outbreak of sporadic cases of a disease (such as travel-associated Legionnaire's disease) where cases are not becoming recognized all at one time and the outbreak is picked up by a central repository of cases such as a national or international surveillance system.[4] Alternatively, the sporadic cases may become linked by a laboratory surveillance system that identifies identical bacterial strains referred from cases in disparate locations reported to different health jurisdictions.[5]

DEVELOP HYPOTHESES

The development of a hypothesis usually is a very early step in outbreak investigation. The first hypothesis may even come from a case, and it's possible that it could be correct ("My husband, daughter, and I are all sick and so is my sister's family. We both attended my cousin's wedding and I'm sure it was the chicken because it wasn't fully cooked.") Alternatively, a hypothesis may be difficult to develop as the information may not be revealing enough. This might occur when the questions that are needed to be asked simply have not been asked yet; however, enough is known of many diseases that cause outbreaks to lead experienced investigators to at least some hypothesis to explore with the descriptive data. For example, there have been many outbreaks of diarrheal disease attributed to *E. coli* O157:H7, and among the potential sources, undercooked ground meat is a well recognized source; therefore, it is common for cases of this disease to be asked whether ground meat was consumed. An examination of the frequency of having eaten ground meat among the cases is helpful because when many of the cases have this exposure it leads to a biologically plausible hypothesis that ground meat was the source of the outbreak. Although it is reasonable to consider ground meat in every *E. coli* O157:H7 outbreak (and therefore to inquire about it), the absence of a majority of the cases with such an exposure should raise the issue of alternative hypotheses; however, recall of an exposure can be poor, whether early or late in an investigation, leading to the response to a question about the true exposure that caused the outbreak not reaching 50% with a yes answer (William Keene, PhD, personal communication). Efficiency in solving outbreaks comes with increasing familiarity with the most common pathogens that cause them and the emerging information about these pathogens.

INTRODUCE PRELIMINARY CONTROL MEASURES

As early as possible, preliminary control measures should be introduced. Some of these control measures may be already established and incorporated into legislated rules and regulations for a reportable disease. In the case of botulism, removing any suspected product (such as a batch of a suspected home canned vegetable) might be performed immediately on the recognition of this source before any data analysis has occurred and possibly before any data have even been entered into a database. Similarly, there need not be an outbreak of meningococcal meningitis for the control measure of providing prophylactic antibiotics to close contacts of a case to occur. When more than one person with gastroenteritis implicates having eaten at the same restaurant and becoming ill within a biologically plausible time period, an inspection of that restaurant by the local health department is reasonable, although it is uncertain whether that restaurant is the source at this early time; therefore, a restaurant inspection is a reasonable preliminary control measure, but closing the restaurant might be premature.

This brings up the important issue of when to pursue an extreme control measure such as closure of a business where the economic implications could be substantial for the business and are being weighed against the public health implications of delaying such an action. Each decision should be made on a case-by-case basis. If the decision is made to take the extreme action and it is wrong, there is risk for litigation and loss of credibility. If the decision is made not to take the extreme action and it is wrong, again there is risk for litigation and loss of credibility. Thus, with such a dilemma, what is one to do? Essentially, the basis for this decision should be made by weighing factors such as the severity of the illness, the vulnerability of the population exposed, and whether the suspected exposure is ongoing. An illness that is killing its victims is certainly worthy of a heavier hand than one that causes an inconvenient gastroenteritis with very rare mortality. If the exposure is threatening persons at higher risk for clinically severe manifestations such as infants, older individuals, or immunocompromised persons, it increases the weight of considering a more extreme measure (at least temporarily until more evidence comes in). If the exposure is a food and the product has been discarded or its preparation has been discontinued, then closure of a restaurant with the aim of controlling the outbreak would be of little benefit after this activity has already occurred. In the case of a business, it may be possible to reason with the owner or manager to lead to his or her enacting the control measure of closure on a voluntary basis. It may be decided that they have less to lose by closing voluntarily and appearing cooperative than by being closed involuntarily or announced in a press release from the health department.

Other preliminary control measures might involve public education about the mode of transmission and prevention methods that are recognized about the outbreak disease from previous experience. Alternatively, a more expensive or difficult outbreak control measure such as mass vaccination may need to wait for clear evidence from additional studies or supplemental laboratory testing that demonstrates whether the vaccination is appropriate. For example, in an outbreak of invasive meningococcal disease, the vaccine covers four of the five most common serotypes of the organism (types A, C, Y, and W135 of *Neisseria meningitidis*); therefore, if the laboratory investigation determines that the outbreak is due to serotype B, mass vaccination with the quadrivalent vaccine would not be expected to impact on the outbreak.

Finally, political considerations can trump everything as a decision may be made by a high-level administrator who has determined that there is a right side and a wrong side of this issue to be on and they have decided to get on what they consider to be the right side. At a minimum, the investigators can offer wise counsel to the administrator based on the evidence and any other information, but sometimes these decisions are out of the investigators hands.

DECIDE WHETHER OBSERVATION OR ADDITIONAL STUDIES ARE INDICATED

Before launching into additional studies such as case control or cohort studies to test hypotheses, a decision should be made whether further studies are warranted. Sometimes these additional studies may be done with the existing data depending on the question. In some situations, an outbreak has "burnt out." No further cases are being reported and it seems that whatever the exposure was, it may have all been consumed. The pursuit of additional study at this time may be of little public health use compared with the resources needed to carry it out. Sometimes a case control study may be possible as with an *E. coli* O157:H7 outbreak where one or two dozen cases have been reported over a few months in a geographic area where that is unexpected. Preexisting outbreak investigation questionnaires are available from the Internet (an example can be found at http://www .oregon.gov/DHS/ph/acd/keene.shtml). It may be tempting to pursue a case control study because there are well-recognized risk factors and asking these questions of controls is feasible; however, in the absence of a sound hypothesis, there is little chance for success with such an approach compared with the likelihood of wasting personnel resources.

One of the authors of a chapter in this book, Dr. Paul Blake, was formerly the head of the Foodborne and Diarrheal Diseases Branch at the CDC in Atlanta. Back in 1984, he authored a memorandum that provided guidance at the CDC on this issue. He emphasized the importance of interviewing the initial cases and that if such interviews did not lead to a hypothesis about the exposure that it would be best to have a more experienced interviewer reinterview them. If that still did not lead to a hypothesis, rather than pursue a study not based on a sound hypothesis, one could try to bring the cases together (with their consent either in person or perhaps by conference call) to discuss possible exposures that could weave a common thread among them. Their interaction with each other could lead to information that an interviewer might not think to have asked.

The in-depth and open-ended hypothesis-generating interview can be very useful to lead to the discovery of unexpected vehicles for disease. A single investigator would be best to perform each of these hypothesis-generating interviews. The interviews should be performed as soon as possible after the report of the case because recall may diminish with time. Recalling one Louisiana outbreak of cholera that Dr. Blake investigated, he said this:

> It was not until I interviewed the fourth case and he mentioned eating cooked crabs which the first three had also mentioned, that a chill went up my spine and I thought, "Cooked crabs could be the cause of this outbreak." We would never have otherwise included cooked crabs on a case control questionnaire because we did not consider cooked crabs to be a possible vehicle for cholera because they were cooked.[6]

PERFORM ADDITIONAL ANALYSES OR PLAN AND PERFORM ADDITIONAL STUDY

If a sound hypothesis exists, additional analysis may be performed such as a cohort or case control study. Entire books can be written on these study methods. The cohort study gets its name from the convenience of having the entire population exposed clearly defined as with a church supper, catered banquet, or persons who share the same well for their drinking water. In the latter example, it can be difficult to demonstrate an association because everyone may have had the exposure, and thus, you do not know whether the well water drinkers are ill because they drank the well water or because they have some other common exposure. In this type of situation, it can be helpful if a dose-response relationship can be demonstrated. The more well water those exposed drank, the more likely they became ill. In the case of a heavily contaminated vehicle, this may be more difficult to show.[7]

Multiple studies may be needed to get to final conclusions. In the case of an Illinois outbreak caused by the parasite Cryptosporidium, the first study performed was a community case control study to determine whether a popular water park was the exposure site. Other possibilities considered included other recreational water exposure such as a lake, contact with animals, and drinking a possibly contaminated beverage. After exposure to the water park was strongly associated with having cryptosporidiosis, a cohort study was performed among water park attendees to determine the exposure within the water park. This study demonstrated the importance of ingesting the pool water. Finally, supplemental laboratory investigation involving testing of the water filter system for the presence of the parasite was also performed.[8] These studies taken together made a strong case for the source being the water at the water park.

Selecting controls for a case control study can be a challenge. Controls should not have had the outbreak disease but should have had a similar likelihood of having been exposed as the cases (as best one can establish this). This may be handled by picking controls that live in the same neighborhood as the cases or are referred by controls (friends and family). They may be matched to cases by age group or gender to control for behavioral differences that are influenced by these factors, some of which may be unknown to the investigator. After a control is identified and the interviewing has begun, it should be established right away whether the control could meet the case definition completely or even partially (perhaps qualifying as a probable or suspect case). Exclusion criteria should be established to ensure that any controls could not actually be cases. Although this might ideally be done with laboratory testing, this is often not realistic, and thus, screening them with questions that determine whether they satisfy the case definition is more feasible. Controls that may meet the case definition should be investigated further and reclassified as cases as needed.

A variety of biases could be introduced when selecting cases and controls for further study.[7] These include sampling bias if there is a need to select among the cases as when there are a very large number but a large number of interviews are not feasible or statistically necessary to evaluate a hypotheses (an uncommon fortuitous situation to be in). Diagnostic suspicion bias may occur if the cases are well aware of the suspected vehicle, perhaps from widespread media attention. Diagnostic access bias may interfere with selection of controls because cases may have (by definition) had access to diagnostic tests and thus been recognized as cases while controls may include persons who, for reasons that could be relevant to the analysis, were less likely to access such diagnostic testing. Misclassification bias can be dealt with by the screening of controls for any similar illness to cases as stated previously here. Other biases such as recall bias or interviewer bias must also be considered. A good outbreak investigation will consider these biases and interpret the results with them in mind.

Several factors may support a decision to perform additional analytic studies even when the outbreak appears to be over when it is first recognized. These include a high morbidity or mortality of the disease, high visibility of the outbreak as with substantial media attention, enthusiasm by those affected by the outbreak (where their cooperation and/or their desire for an answer to what happened is high), and the novelty of the pathogen, its mode of transmission, or its clinical manifestations such that it provides an opportunity to learn something new about the organism or disease. Another important factor is the availability of personnel and financial resources to continue with the investigation.

Sometimes outbreak investigation studies are referred to as "quick and dirty" because biases are not substantially dealt with in the study design and the number of cases and controls is not derived from any power calculations based on the hypothesis and assumptions. This is a reality of outbreak investigation because, as they are essentially experiments of nature, there is no control over how many cases will have occurred. The best one can do is pursue case ascertainment aggressively to attempt to populate the database with as many cases as may be needed to lead to statistically significant findings. It should also be recognized that even statistically significant findings are not the same thing as cause and effect, or simply stated, if it is 95% likely that an association did not occur by chance, it is still 5% likely that it could have; therefore, for any results from these studies, there should be biologic plausibility. Also, the finding (or association) should account for most of the cases if the source of the outbreak will be attributed to that finding and be of a sufficiently high magnitude to be relevant.

Outbreak investigators should also be familiar with the binomial probability method. When enough information is available, this method can allow for estimation of the probability that a particular exposure was present among cases by chance alone. Without performing a case control study, the results of such a study can be estimated. For example, in an outbreak caused by *Salmonella enterica* serotype enteritidis, routine food exposure interviews had not indicated a common exposure. A much expanded questionnaire was then used, and it led to a hypothesis concerning consumption of raw almonds. Using the binomial probability method, the rate of consumption of almonds (and other foods) was compared with the background rates of consumption of these foods based on available Oregon survey results. It was helpful that background information on the expected rate of consumption of almonds was available for the Oregon population. In that survey, 9% of 921 Oregon residents had consumed raw almonds in the preceding week; however, all five of the sporadic cases had consumed raw almonds in the week before illness. These and other data from this investigation contributed to a recall of 13 million pounds of almonds![9] Additional information on this method can be found on the Internet (http://www.oregon.gov/DHS/ph/acd/outbreak/binomial.xls and http://faculty.vassar.edu/lowry/binomialX.html), and "A Population Survey Atlas of Exposures" is available from the CDC (http://www.cdc.gov/foodnet/reports.htm).

PERFORM NEW CONTROL MEASURES AND/OR ENSURE THE COMPLIANCE OF EXISTING CONTROL MEASURES

Depending on the outbreak, new control measures may derive from the investigation results. If identification of an exposure such as a food item or activity like swimming is revealed as the source of the outbreak only after additional studies were performed, a food may need to be recalled and product embargoed, or perhaps a swimming pool or lake may need to be closed to the public. New environmental and laboratory investigations may follow as an attempt is made to explain more fully the origin of the outbreak. In the case of a foodborne outbreak, a trace back might help to explain where an imported product became contaminated. Alternatively, when monkeypox was imported to the United States, a trace back determined that the outbreak likely began from giant Gambian rats imported from Ghana that later mixed with highly susceptible United States prairie dogs sold (unknowingly infected) to lovers of "pocket pets."[10]

It is an important practical matter to ensure that control measures put into place are being carried out. This is usually not an issue unless the persons who are directly responsible for carrying out the control measure (such as closing a restaurant or catering business) fail to accept that the control measure is sound or perhaps if they do not trust the source of the prevention information. If a publicly accessible area is restricted, such as when a beach is closed because it is a risk, it should be a routine matter that someone is assessing that there are no swimmers and that the sign(s) posted is readily visible and posted in the appropriate languages to make sure that the message is readily understood.

COMMUNICATION OF PREVENTION INFORMATION AND FINDINGS

Communication is a key issue from the beginning to the end of the outbreak. Within the outbreak investigation team, information such as telephone and fax numbers and e-mail addresses are all basic information to be exchanged. Regularly, the team should be meeting either in person or by conference call to update each other, and it is beneficial to summarize the update in a written format such as an e-mail circulated internally among those with responsibility directly or indirectly for the investigation such as high-level administrators. It is especially important for no assumptions to be made related to communication. In other words, it can be an unwise gamble to assume that someone else is sharing important information with the team leader or an administrative person in a central office if that is not known with certainty. Redundancy of communication may be inefficient, but it is far less of a sin than lack of communication.

The public and other stakeholders of the outbreak are important communication targets as well. These may include hospital staff such as emergency room physicians or infection control workers, day care workers, school principals or teachers, parents, and the media. Depending on what information is being released, those responsible at the site of the outbreak (such as a restaurant or hotel manager or hospital administrator) should be made aware of basic developments, as their level of anxiety can be very high and their cooperation may be linked to the trust that can come from good communication. Partnering organizations, such as the U.S. Department of Agriculture or the Food and Drug Administration as well as state or local equivalents, should also be updated. Those who need to be informed and what they need to be told may vary based on the specifics of the outbreak investigation.

What is said in oral versus written communication is also worth considering because written word typically becomes part of a permanent record. It may be read or reread, sometimes with unintended negative intonation. E-mails may be sent to one party and forwarded to another. Written communication may be released to attorneys if legal action follows. It is a practical matter for any investigator to be open and honest in all of their communication but to be concise and clear without unneeded unbalanced accusation or risk of breeching confidentiality by recording names unnecessarily. An example of this could be when the investigation staff might name a person or restaurant they are investigating in an e-mail that is forwarded to someone outside of the investigation team who then reveals this name prematurely perhaps to the media. The person to whom this e-mail was forwarded may have had too little information about the details of the outbreak or too little experience with these situations. The use of terms "Hotel X," "Product A," "Nurse B," or Restaurant Y" arose to help protect the unnecessary release of identities where that information could be damaging and would not benefit public health. Alternatively, if protection of public health warrants it, communication broadly of the name of a person, institution, or other exposure source is warranted. Investigators should be aware of legal requirements in their jurisdictions concerning matters that involve confidentiality.

Communicating the prevention message of the outbreak and the findings through internal report or scientific publication is also important. In the case of the latter, agreement early on concerning who will be assigned the lead authorship is very important to avoid conflict or resentment later on. This is especially important when more than one person on the team might be qualified to lead the investigation or to undertake the writing of a scientific article describing it. It is also especially important when multiple public health jurisdictions are involved, including when federal assistance is performed at the state or local level.

MONITOR SURVEILLANCE DATA

Finally, it is important to continue to monitor surveillance data as the outbreak ends. This may reveal that the control measures were inadequate and that new hypotheses and new investigation may be needed. Also, secondary outbreaks may arise. For example, after the massive cryptosporidiosis outbreak in Wisconsin (described in this book), additional smaller outbreaks were recognized as the parasite was shed by persons with cryptosporidiosis in a variety of settings such as a swimming pool.[11]

CONCLUSION

The steps of outbreak investigation are extremely useful to keep in mind during an outbreak to help provide some order to what can be a stressful and fast moving or complicated process. Outbreak work is reactive. Although some outbreaks are actually over when they are recognized, many are in progress and have an urgency to them. The hours can be long but some of an epidemiologist's best work actually is performed in this intense setting. The examples in this book will hopefully provide the reader with an illustration of how some of these steps have played out in real outbreaks of infectious diseases. Keep in mind, however, that sometimes not all of the steps need to get done before a press release comes out to announce the concern. There is an art to making the decision of how far to go with an investigation, and that comes with much experience. Nonetheless, it is a gamble every time.

REFERENCES

1. Reingold AL. Outbreak investigations: a perspective. *Emerg Infect Dis* 1998;4:21–27.
2. Gregg MB. Conducting a field investigation. In Gregg MB, ed. *Field Epidemiology*, 2nd ed. New York: Oxford University Press, 2002:62–77.
3. Magnus M. Outbreak investigations. In *Essentials of Infectious Disease Epidemiology*. Sudbury: Jones and Bartlett, 2008:43–61.
4. Ricketts KD, Yadav R, Joseph CA. European Working Group for Legionella Infections. Travel-associated Legionnaires disease in Europe: 2006. *Euro Surveill* 2008;13:18930.
5. Jones TF, Scallan E, Angulo FJ. FoodNet: overview of a decade of achievement. *Foodborne Pathog Dis* 2007;4:60–66.
6. Yoder J, Ritger K, Dworkin MS. Foodborne outbreak investigation: how do I find the implicated food when I have few cases and no good hypothesis? Illinois Infectious Disease Report (Volume 3, Spring 2006). Retrieved June 25, 2008, from www.idph.state.il.us/health/infect/ID_Report_Spring06.pdf.
7. Palmer SR. Epidemiology in search of infectious diseases: methods in outbreak investigation. *J Epidemiol Com Health* 1989;43:311–314.
8. Causer LM, Handzel T, Welch P, et al. An outbreak of Cryptosporidium hominis infection at an Illinois recreational waterpark. *Epidemiol Infect* 2006;134:147–156.
9. Keady S, Briggs G, Farrar J, et al. Outbreak of *Salmonella* serotype enteritidis infections associated with raw almonds: United States and Canada, 2003–2004. *MMWR* 2004;53:484–487.
10. Reed KD, Melski JW, Graham MB, et al. The detection of monkeypox in humans in the Western Hemisphere. *N Engl J Med* 2004;350:342–350.
11. Mac Kenzie WR, Kazmierczak JJ, Davis JP. An outbreak of cryptosporidiosis associated with a resort swimming pool. *Epidemiol Infect* 1995;115:545–553.

CHAPTER 2

Leptospirosis at the Bubbles

Kenrad E. Nelson, MD

INTRODUCTION

After completing a rotating internship and Internal Medicine residency at Cook County Hospital in Chicago, I joined the Epidemic Intelligence Service (EIS) at the Centers for Disease Control (CDC) in Atlanta in 1963. The EIS provides a 2-year experience in applied public health and field epidemiology for health professionals who have recently completed their training. Most EIS officers were physicians, who like me had just completed residency training, but the EIS program also included other health professionals, such as veterinarians, nurses, dentists, biostatisticians, and public health specialists.

I became interested in the EIS program during my year as chief resident in Internal Medicine at Cook County Hospital. When I was on the pulmonary rotation, I had cared for many patients with tuberculosis (TB), a very common disease in the 1960s at Cook County. Although some patients with TB responded well to therapy, it was very frustrating that many did not. It was common in those days for TB patients to leave the hospital against medical advice after having received a week or two of anti-TB drugs, especially if they were asked to undergo bronchoscopy, which was done then using a rigid bronchoscope. Unfortunately, the director of the chest surgery service in the hospital viewed training surgery residents to do bronchoscopy on TB patients as his most important teaching responsibility. Patients who left the hospital were often readmitted several months later with more advanced, active TB after having stopped their treatment as soon as they became afebrile or felt better.

When I did a follow-up study of the outcome of TB treatment of about 120 patients with positive cultures 2 years earlier, the results were very discouraging. Only about a third of these patients were cured of their TB and still alive. About a third had died, often with active TB because they had discontinued their therapy and resumed drinking alcohol or injecting drugs or were just lost to follow-up by the Chicago TB clinics. This was long before directly observed treatment became the standard of care in Chicago.

The results of this study peaked my interest in public health and epidemiology. When I visited CDC before joining the EIS I became interested in public health and epidemiology because of its more comprehensive and inclusive analysis of the sociocultural and environmental determinants, as well as the biological factors, related to disease and health problems. Also, the investigation of outbreaks of disease was a fascinating and important responsibility of an epidemiologist in the EIS program, and this interested me as well.

When I joined EIS in 1963, I was assigned to the Washington State Health Department. The position included reviewing and analyzing the reports of diseases submitted by the county health departments, communicating with the public and health professionals about public health issues and prevention programs, and performing field epidemiology whenever an outbreak or cluster of illness was reported. There were many opportunities for evaluating possible outbreaks because the state epidemiologist was very competent and had established a good working relationship with most of the local health officers and practicing physicians in the state. Consequently, I investigated outbreaks of foodborne illnesses (i.e. salmonellosis, *Clostridium perfringens*, and botulism), measles, vaccine-associated polio, influenza, diphtheria, and other diseases. One of the more memorable and interesting outbreak investigations is described here.

THE BUBBLES OUTBREAK

In August 1964, I received a call from the director of the Benton-Franklin County Health Department in southeastern Washington asking for assistance in investing a cluster of cases of a febrile illness in adolescents. Several local physicians had cared for teenaged children who had become ill with a fever, headache, and muscle aches that seemed to be clinically similar. Several of these patients had been hospitalized. Some patients had a stiff neck, but respiratory or gastrointestinal symptoms or a skin rash was uncommon.

I agreed to come and help with the investigation. I was aware that several arboviruses that cause encephalitis and meningitis, including Western equine and St. Louis Encephalitis viruses, had been frequently isolated from patients with central nervous system infections living in central and eastern Washington in the past. No horse deaths had been reported, however. All of the ill persons seemed to have recovered, and these patients seemed to be somewhat older than most reported arbovirus encephalitis cases in the past. Another possible consideration could have been a systemic fungal infection; however, central Washington was north of the area of endemicity of coccidioidomycosis (Valley Fever). Another consideration was an enterovirus infection, as these viruses are common in the summer and may cause aseptic meningitis, sometimes as outbreaks. Another, less likely possibility was amebic encephalitis. Thus, I packed my copy of Benenson's *Infectious Diseases of Man* (a public health book that has been essential to communicable disease investigators in health departments for decades, although its editor has changed over the years) and flew to eastern Washington.

When I arrived, I met with the director of the health department, and together we outlined a plan to investigate the outbreak. By that time, about 35 to 40 cases had been reported. Although we did not know which diagnosis we were dealing with, we believed an outbreak was occurring because this was a much higher number of similar illnesses in the adolescent population than any of the local practitioners or the health department routinely recognized. An initial look at the descriptive epidemiology of the cases revealed that the dates of illness onset extended back a couple of months to the middle of June. Since then, several cases had been reported each week, without obvious temporal clustering; therefore, it didn't appear to be a single exposure, common source outbreak, but perhaps an ongoing epidemic of an arbovirus or enterovirus infection should be considered. Another curious feature was that most of the cases (about 80%) were in boys. This appeared to be evidence against the outbreak being an arbovirus or an enterovirus because we were unaware of any gender predilection for illnesses caused by those viruses.

My first step after reviewing the data available at the health department was to go to the local hospital and review the charts of several typical cases who had been hospitalized. This was long before the HIPPA legislation had been enacted, which might have complicated this approach. I took the list of names of the reported cases to the hospital and asked the record librarian to pull the charts for me. I discovered that a typical illness characteristically included fever, myalgia, headache, and shaking chills with a stiff neck reported in about half the cases (Tables 2-1 and 2-2). The illness lasted about 5 to 7 days, and respiratory symptoms, diarrhea, and rash were uncommon. Some patients had a recurrence of their symptoms a few days after they had recovered. Lumbar punctures had been done in four cases; three were normal, but one had 798 white blood cells/mm^3, of which 53% were polymorphonuclear cells and 47% were mononuclear cells. In this patient, the protein was elevated at 130 per 100 ml, and the sugar was normal (50 mg/100 ml). The normal glucose was evidence against TB or fungal meningitis. All cultures of blood, urine, and cerebrospinal fluid were sterile. There was a modest increase in the peripheral white blood cell count. Urinalysis performed on 26 patients revealed that 22 had more than five white blood cells per high-power field with a slight proteinuria (1 to 2+) in 10 cases. These clinical data were peculiar and unexpected for any common seasonal infection in a presumably healthy adolescent population.

I decided that the next step should be to interview a few typical cases as a way toward generating a hypothesis of what was going on. My colleagues at the health department said this could be arranged. Thus, I met with several recently reported cases and a couple of those who had become ill in

Table 2-1   Symptoms of 61 Children with Leptospirosis

Symptom	No.	Percentage
Fever	61	100.0
Myalgia	60	98.4
Headache	58	95.1
Shaking Chills	56	91.8
Nausea	55	90.2
Vomiting	33	54.1
Arthralgia	19	31.1
Diarrhea	7	11.5

Reprinted with permission from Nelson KE, et al. *Am J Epidemiol* 1973;98:336–347.

Table 2-2   Abnormal Physical Findings in 46 Leptospirosis Patients
Seen by a Physician

Finding	Number Affected	Percentage
Fever	46	100.0
Stiff neck	23	50.0
Throat injection	14	30.4
Biphasic course	10	21.7
Adenopathy	8	17.4
Flank tenderness	5	10.9
Conjunctivitis	5	10.9
Splenomegaly	1	2.2

Reprinted with permission from Nelson KE, et al. *Am J Epidemiol* 1973;98:336–347.

June. These cases didn't report any common meals, gatherings, or special associations or common exposures with other children who had been ill; however, they usually knew several other children who had experienced similar illnesses. Finally, one of them said, "Doc, you should check out 'the Bubbles,'" after which I asked what and where were the Bubbles? He offered to take me there.

The next day we went to the Bubbles. It was a concrete block structure a few miles out in the country in the field between the three surrounding towns of Kennewick, Pasco, and Richland (Figure 2-1). Connected to the small concrete structure at the Bubbles were two concrete walls about 5 feet high. These walls extended out about 7 feet. The Bubbles was a part of the irrigation system that divided the stream of irrigation water into two directions with a pump, which created bubbles when the water was pumped forcefully from below the surface. The structure was known by irrigation specialists as a "bifurcator." It was used to distribute the water in two directions and keep it flowing downstream. We were told that about 800 gallons of water passed through the bifurcator every 1 to 2 seconds. This caused the water to bubble and churn forcefully when the bifurcator was operating at full speed.

To the junior and senior high school students, however, the Bubbles was a great place to go swimming during the summer. During that summer, as was not uncommon in southeastern Washington, the temperature often exceeded 95°F to 100°F. The local swimming pool was often closed and

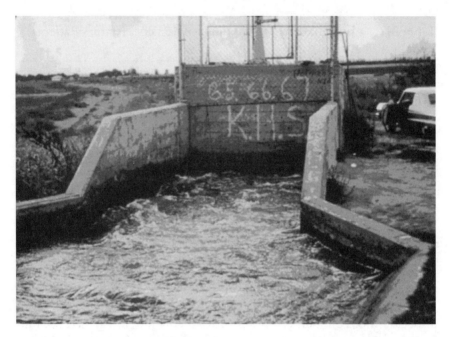

FIGURE 2-1 "The bubbles." The depth of the water at this point was 2.1 meters, the walls rose 1.1 meter above the water and were 3 meters apart. The churning of the water was caused by subsurface feeding.

Reprinted with permission from: Nelson KE et al. *Am J Epidemiol* 1973;98:336–347.

very crowded when it was open. Thus, the Bubbles was a great and special place to swim for teenagers. Students could stand on the concrete wall and jump into the bubbling water to be swirled around and often careen into the walls of the structure. Swimming at the Bubbles combined the joy of a swimming pool with the thrill of a ride at an amusement park. Swimming at the Bubbles often caused small skin abrasions, but it was described as "fun" and "exciting."

After learning about the Bubbles, I contacted several adolescents that I had decided were typical "cases" of the mysterious illness based on their reported symptoms of fever, headaches, myalgia, and stiff neck. Interestingly, all of the typical cases reported swimming at the Bubbles before they became ill. It then became clear to me that swimming at the Bubbles was a very important exposure that occurred before the onset of this febrile illness. The water at the Bubbles appeared clean, although it wasn't potable but used only for irrigation. The ultimate source was the Columbia River, which was very nearby. We found later that the water at the Bubbles had a very high coliform count (>240,000 colonies per ml) and was alkaline (pH, 8.3).

We then decided to explore the irrigation canal upstream from the Bubbles for potential sources of contamination. The most effective way to do this was to hire a small plane that was used for crop dusting and fly over the irrigation canal, as there were no roads running parallel to the canal. This was an exciting trip, which resembled a roller coaster ride, as the plane was flying quite low and at slow speeds so that we could observe the canal and take pictures. This trip was quite revealing in that about 300 yards upstream from the Bubbles we noticed a herd of cattle, some of whom were also using the irrigation ditch as a watering hole to cool off (Figure 2-2). These were the only animals that we found to have direct access to the irrigation canal between the Bubbles and the origin of the canal a couple of miles upstream at the Yakima River. Thus, after the plane landed

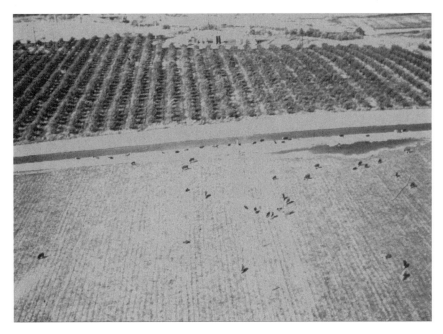

FIGURE 2-2 Aerial view of site of epidemic of leptospirosis among swimmers in irrigation canal. Note numerous cattle upstream from irrigation canal site used for swimming.

Reprinted with permission from: Nelson KE et al. *Am J Epidemiol* 1973;98:336–347.

we decided to investigate the herd further. By then, we had decided that it was likely that the outbreak was due to leptospirosis. The exposure of cases to water that may have been contaminated by cattle and the clinical epidemiology made this diagnosis biologically plausible. This was confirmed when we obtained blood specimens from several of the typical cases and sent them to the CDC laboratory in Atlanta for testing.

There are very few laboratories in the United States or worldwide that test for leptospirosis. The assays are not commercially available, nor are they included in the standard screening panel for meningoencephalitis screening. (Because of the limited availability of laboratory confirmation of suspect cases and the protean clinical manifestations, the disease was removed from the list of officially reportable diseases by the Council of State and Territorial Epidemiologists in 1995.) The definitive serological assay is the Microscopic Agglutination Test (MAT). In this assay, various serogroups of pathogenic leptospiral organisms are incubated with dilutions of sera from persons or animals with suspected infection, and the maximal dilution of sera that will cause 50% of the organisms to agglutinate when viewed under the microscope is reported to be the MAT titer. The MAT titers are read using serial dilutions of sera and live or formalinized organisms from several different leptospiral organisms, that is, serovars, to make the diagnosis and to estimate which organism might have caused the infection. The need for live or formalin treated antigens from several leptospiral organisms explains why so few laboratories test for infection. There is a significant risk of infection among laboratory workers when the organisms are subcultured. Nevertheless, the definitive serological assay for leptospirosis and the specific organism responsible for the infection are reported as the MAT titer.

In our study, MAT antibodies against leptospires from 18 serovars were evaluated, and the titers against *Leptospira pomona* were generally highest. This was consistent with the literature, as *L. pomona* and *L. hardjo* serovars from the *L. pomona* serogroup have been reported to be the predominant organisms infecting cattle and among persons who had acquired their infection from cattle worldwide. Since we now had evidence that the leptospirosis infections were acquired by swimming at the Bubbles, we needed to take action to prevent further infections; therefore, we posted warnings and publicly advised persons against swimming in the water at the Bubbles or other areas of the irrigation canal, especially downstream from the cattle herd. Also, the cattle were screened off to prevent them having direct access to the irrigation canal.

We also wanted to evaluate the cattle and the environment further; therefore, we collected water samples for culture from the irrigation canal and from water standing in the field where the cattle were herded. We cultured the blood samples from the children who had been ill, although all of the children had recovered from their illness before we obtained a blood specimen. *L. pomona* was recovered by guinea pig inoculation from water standing in the cattle pasture at three sites; however, cultures of water from the irrigation canal and sera from the students who had been ill were all negative (Figure 2-3).

Culturing blood and urine from the cattle was also a priority. We clearly needed assistance from a veterinarian to obtain these cultures. Fortunately, my colleague Dr. Everett (Ted) Baker, DVM, also an EIS officer, was

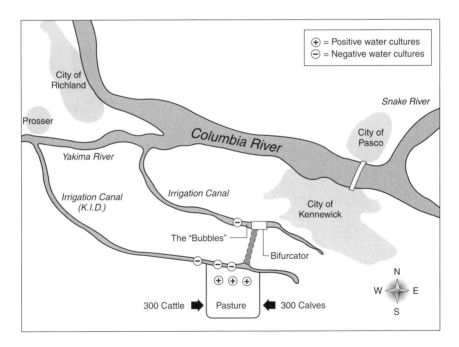

FIGURE 2-3 Schematic of the area in which outbreak of leptospirosis occurred during the summer of 1964.

Reprinted with permission from: Nelson KE et al. *Am J Epidemiol* 1973;98:336–347.

available to help obtain these specimens for culture. I was not experienced with the methods for getting a urine specimen from a cow! I knew I couldn't be successful if I just asked the animal to provide it, which is how I usually got a urine sample from my patients. I was told that often urine appeared after you massaged the cows under belly. If this failed you could poke or push the area firmly, but I don't know how Ted eventually managed to obtain the samples from the cattle.

Eventually, we found that 9 of 43 cattle (21%) were shedding *L. pomona* in their urine in September, about a month after the last human case, and 21 of 25 sera (84%) from the cattle herd were seropositive in the MAT test with the highest titers to *L. pomona*. The herd of 300 cattle had been purchased locally in the spring before the outbreak. There had been no reports of illness or unexpected deaths in the cattle and no abortions, which have commonly been reported as a consequence of animal leptospirosis. The animals had not been vaccinated for leptospirosis. We obtained blood specimens from 305 additional cattle entering two local sales yards between August 31 and October 31; 26 of these sera (8.5%) were positive for leptospiral antibodies.

In addition to warning the students and the public about the dangers of swimming or other exposures to the irrigation canal, we recognized the need for other public health measures to prevent additional cases. These included restricting the cattle from direct access to the canal and stopping the process of rill (flooding) irrigation of the pasture where the cattle were located. This could lead to contamination of the standing water with cattle urine, which could then be washed back into the irrigation canal when it rained. Leptospires can survive for considerable periods, especially in an alkaline environment. As mentioned previously, we had isolated *L. pomona* from the standing alkaline water in the pasture by guinea pig inoculation.

We made an effort to locate all of the cases in order to further define the risk exposures. Although this swimming hole was quite small, it clearly was a major site of exposure. There was also a possibility of infections occurring from exposures to the irrigation water at other areas, as the canal was several miles long winding between the fields. In order to detect additional (unreported) cases, we asked all of the known cases the names of everyone they knew who visited the Bubbles or who had swum elsewhere in the irrigation canal that summer. Another source of possible exposed persons was the signatures on the concrete wall of the Bubbles. We made certain that we interviewed each of the persons who had left their name on the wall of the Bubbles (i.e., had "signed in" at the site).

We decided to do a larger survey after the schools reopened in September. We designed a questionnaire that included questions about having had a compatible illness during the summer, swimming anywhere in the irrigation canal during the summer, and swimming at the Bubbles during the summer. This questionnaire was distributed to the 6,062 students attending the three high schools and two junior high schools in the three neighboring towns of Kennewick, Pasco, and Richland. We found that 594 of the students (9.8%) in these five schools reported swimming at the Bubbles, and 60 had an illness confirmed serologically to be leptospirosis, for an attack rate of 10.1% among Bubbles swimmers (Table 2-3). We used a clinical definition of "suspected cases" (compatible illness), which included the reported symptoms of fever, myalgia, and headache, that were reported by over 95% of the serologically confirmed cases for our epidemiological survey. We also put notices in the local newspaper, and our interest in locating additional cases was mentioned by the local news media. We supplemented the request for reporting illnesses by reviewing local hospital and clinic records of febrile illnesses. When our case-finding efforts had been completed, we had identified 61 serologically confirmed cases (Table 2-4). All were between the ages of 12 and 19 years; 53 were

Table 2-3   Number of Students Who Swam at the Bubbles During the Summer of 1964 and Leptospirosis Attack Rates by School

	Enrollment	Swam at "Bubbles" Number (%)	Leptospirosis Cases	Swimmers' Attack Rate (%)
Kennewick High School	1,420	184 (13.0)	31	16.8
Park Jr. High School	994	54 (5.4)	6	11.1
Highland Jr. High School	746	58 (7.8)	6	10.3
Pasco High School	1,284	100 (7.8)	7	7.0
Columbia High School	1,618	198 (12.2)	10	5.1
Total	6,062	594 (9.8)	60*	10.1

* One of the 61 cases occurred in a nonstudent.
Reprinted with permission from Nelson KE, et al. *Am J Epidemiol* 1973;98:336–347.

Table 2-4   Distribution of 61 Patients with Leptospirosis by Age and Gender

Age (Years)	Male	Female	Total
12	2	0	2
13	2	1	3
14	6	0	6
15	8	1	9
16	14	3	17
17	18	2	20
18	3	0	3
19	0	1	1
Total	53	8	61

Reprinted with permission from Nelson KE, et al. *Am J Epidemiol* 1973;98:336–347.

male (86.9%) and 8 were female (13.1%). The numbers of cases increased with increasing age between 12 and 17 years (Table 2-4). In our school surveys, we found that 594 students (10.3%) reported swimming at the Bubbles during the summer; 16.0% of boys and 4.3% of girls reported swimming at the Bubbles. The proportion who reported swimming at the Bubbles also increased with age between 12 and 18 years; the distribution of those who reported swimming was similar to the age and gender distribution of the cases (Table 2-5).

The highest attack rate of leptospirosis (16.8%) was experienced by the students attending Kennewick High School. Students at Kennewick High School and Columbia High School in Richland had the highest rates of exposure to the Bubbles, 13.0% and 12.2%, respectively (Table 2-3); however, because the Bubbles was located closer to Kennewick, we believe that exposures were more frequent among students living in Kennewick than those from Richland or Pasco, but we didn't collect data on the frequency or specific dates that students swam at the Bubbles.

We did not detect any laboratory-confirmed cases of leptospirosis in those who had not swum at the Bubbles; however, a few children with leptospirosis reported swimming elsewhere in the irrigation canal in addition to the Bubbles. Nevertheless, several features of exposure to water when swimming at the Bubbles may have been important in increasing the risk of leptospirosis among these swimmers. First the churning, swirling water

Table 2-5 Students' History of Swimming at the Bubbles by Age and Gender, Summer 1964*

Age (Years)	Male Total	Male Swam	Male % Swam	Female Total	Female Swam	Female % Swam	Both Genders Total	Both Genders Swam	Both Genders Swam
< 11	1	0		0	0		1	0	
11	21	2	9.5	20	1	5.0	41	3	7.3
12	224	14	6.3	278	3	1.1	502	17	3.4
13	278	24	8.6	265	15	5.7	543	39	7.2
14	320	36	11.3	302	4	1.3	622	40	6.4
15	646	84	13.0	637	22	3.5	1,283	106	8.3
16	716	122	17.0	646	38	5.9	1,362	160	11.7
17	650	161	24.8	598	33	5.5	1,248	194	15.5
18	101	30	29.7	36	4	11.1	137	34	24.8
> 18	8	0		6	0		14	0	
Unknown	3	1	33.3	2	0		5	1	20.0
Total	2,968	474	16.0	2,790	120	4.3	5,758	594	10.3

* Based on questionnaires answered by 5,758 students.
Reprinted with permission from Nelson KE, et al. *Am J Epidemiol* 1973;98:336–347.

at the Bubbles often resulted in abrasions when the swimmers were thrown against the concrete walls of the structure, providing a source of entry for *L. pomona* organisms. Second, diving into the water usually resulted in immersion of the swimmers head, exposing the conjunctiva as a site of entry of the organisms. Cases often reported recurring exposure; only three of the confirmed cases reported swimming at the Bubbles only once during the summer. Their illnesses had onset 7 to 10 days after their exposure. In addition, the number of cases increased about 10 days after the warmest day in June, when the ambient temperature reached 97°F and a similar period after the temperatures exceeded 100°F between July 10 and July 14 (Figure 2-4). We also learned that the water flow was slowed on July 13 and July 14 to facilitate repairs to the Bubbles. We suspect that the number of students exposed to the Bubbles was high during these very warm days and that the risk of infection among swimmers may have increased when the rate of water flow decreased, but we could not confirm this level of detail in our interviews.

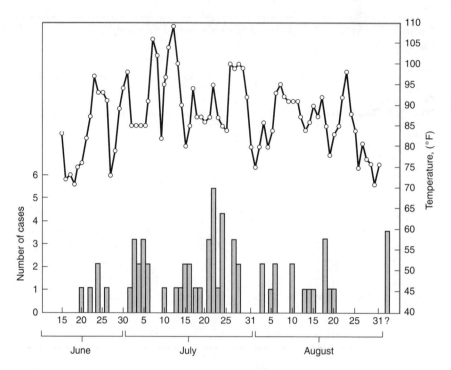

FIGURE 2-4 Cases of leptospirosis by date of onset of symptoms and daily maximum temperature, June 15–August 31, 1964.

Reprinted with permission from: Nelson KE et al. *Am J Epidemiol* 1973;98:336–347.

LABORATORY STUDIES OF THE OUTBREAK

We were very fortunate to have access to the excellent Leptospirosis Reference Laboratory at the CDC in the investigation of this outbreak. Many suspected outbreaks of leptospirosis have not had laboratory confirmation of the cases or the animal reservoir as detection of the organisms or the serological response to leptospiral infection is highly specialized and available in only a few reference laboratories.

Recovery of leptospiral organisms in culture requires special media and often very long incubation times. Primary cultures are retained for up to 13 weeks before being discarded, if there is no growth. When there is growth, it usually occurs within 10 to 14 days in liquid media.[1] Growth of contaminants is inhibited by adding 5-fluorouracil to the media.

Serologic investigation of cases also requires specialized laboratories. The traditional gold-standard method of detecting a specific antibody response is the MAT, which has been described previously here. Several other genus-specific serological diagnostic assays have been described, but they are not well standardized or widely available.

In this outbreak the Leptospirosis Reference Laboratory at the CDC performed the MAT test on all suspect cases that resulted in the 61 laboratory-confirmed cases mentioned previously here. The CDC laboratory also tested the sera with a microscopic slide test, which is a less sensitive test than the MAT but is easier to perform in the laboratory and sometimes used as a screening assay. Among the 61 students that were positive on the MAT, only 48 were positive on the microscopic slide test. The highest titers and most frequent reactions were to *L. pomona* antigens. We did follow-up testing of 45 ill students 200 to 264 days after the outbreak. At this time, only 10 sera were MAT positive for antibodies to *L. pomona*. This decline of reactivity in the MAT test was evidence against chronic infection or re-exposure.

LEPTOSPIROSIS HISTORY, EPIDEMIOLOGY, AND CAUSATIVE ORGANISMS

The clinical features of leptospirosis in humans have been known since 1886 when Adolph Weil reported cases of febrile jaundice among sewer workers in Heidelberg, Germany.[2] Although there were other earlier reports of this syndrome,[3] the clinical disease became known as "Weil's Disease." A spirochetal organism, identified in the kidney tubules of a patient with the disease by silver staining, was reported by Stimson in 1909.[4] The spirochetes had hooked ends and Stimson called them Spirochete interrogans because of their resemblance to a question mark. The importance of rats as a carrier of the organism, which was excreted chronically in their urine, was recognized and reported by Japanese investigators in 1917.[5] After these seminal discoveries, Weil's disease came to be known as an occupational disease of sewer workers throughout the world, especially in Europe. The disease also occurred frequently among persons harvesting rice in China and other countries in Asia. The Japanese called the disease "Akiyami," or Autumnal fever. Spirochetes were detected by injecting guinea pigs with blood from infected patients by German investigators.[6] Leptospirosis in livestock was recognized several decades later.[7]

In the last couple of decades, it has been recognized that leptospirosis is a very common disease globally. The clinical picture and epidemiology of leptospirosis in humans is quite variable. The disease is quite common in the tropics and has been estimated to be one of the most common zoonotic infectious diseases of humans globally.[8] Leptospirosis has been reported not only as an occupational disease but among other populations as well. Human infections have been acquired by occupational or recreational exposures to a wide range of infected animals or their urine. A wide range of exposures have been reported to transmit the organisms. High-risk groups include miners, veterinarians, farmers, abattoir workers, sugar cane cutters, fish workers, soldiers, and other occupations having direct or indirect exposures to animals. During World War II, an outbreak of a febrile illness with a pretibial rash and splenomegaly occurred among troops at Fort Bragg, North Carolina, which became known as "Fort Bragg fever" or pretibial fever. This illness was later found to be leptospirosis caused by the *L. autumnalis* infection.[9]

In addition, several outbreaks of leptospirosis among swimmers after exposure to contaminated water have been reported. A recent comprehensive review found 26 reported water-borne outbreaks among swimmers or rafters that have occurred between 1931 and 1998.[10] Most of these outbreaks were small; however five, including this one, involved more than 60 cases. In over half of the outbreaks, the source of infection was unknown, and the serogroup of the infecting organism was estimated based on serologic evidence. The water had been contaminated by urine from cattle, pigs, dogs, or rodents in most of these outbreaks.

Human leptospirosis is acquired by direct contact with infectious material, generally water contaminated with urine from an infected animal; however, subculturing the organism in the laboratory can cause infection among laboratory personnel by direct contact or possibly by aerosol. The organism is thought to enter the body through abrasions in the skin or through the conjunctiva; however, drinking of contaminated water also has been reported to transmit infection.[10]

The protean clinical features of leptospirosis in humans include clinical Weil's disease manifested by jaundice, sepsis, and renal failure, but also aseptic meningitis, as in this outbreak, pulmonary disease, cardiac involvement, and ocular disease. In addition, animals and also humans may have abortions if the infections occur during pregnancy. Cattle can develop mastitis, and ocular disease has been seen in animals.[10]

Recently, international interest in leptospirosis has been generated by several large clusters of cases that have occurred in South and Central America after flooding from storms.[10,11] It has been recognized in the past decade that human exposures to animals have caused the emergence and re-emergence of many infectious diseases, including SARS (severe acute respiratory syndrome), hantavirus, monkeypox, HIV/AIDS, avian influenza, and many others. In fact, cross-species transmission of infectious agents may be the most significant of the many factors leading to the emergence of important infections in humans in recent times. In reality, our experience in investigating the Bubble's outbreak of leptospirosis could have been viewed as a "seminal" experience of newly emerging infections on the horizon.

LESSONS FROM THIS OUTBREAK

1. Although the most common reported infectious etiology of aseptic meningitis cases and outbreaks in the summer time are enteroviruses and arboviruses, other organisms contribute, such as leptospires, whose importance may be underappreciated because of the hurdles of laboratory diagnosis.
2. Zoonotic infections appear to have become increasingly important in the emergence of new infectious diseases in humans.
3. It is often an excellent idea to determine which exposures the infected patients believe might have caused their illness and then follow-up on their suggestion(s). Epidemiologists should "listen to their patients."
4. Recreational activities, such as swimming, hiking, and rafting, may expose persons to a wide variety of infectious risks.
5. Outbreak investigation is interesting and challenging but often requires support from several disciplines, including laboratory scientists, veterinarians, and other professionals with special skills, such as irrigation experts as in the case of this outbreak.
6. We learned several months after this outbreak had been investigated and controlled that a spill of radioactive waste into the Columbia River from the Hanford Nuclear Energy facility had occurred just before this outbreak. There was some concern among officials at the facility and the Department of Energy that the epidemic might have been related to the spill.

REFERENCES

1. Nelson KE, Ager EA, Galton MM, Gillespie RW, Sulzer CR. An outbreak of leptospirosis in Washington State. *Am J Epidemiol* 1973;98:336–347.
2. Weil A. Ueber eine eigentümliche, mit Milztumor, Icterus und Nephritis einhergehende akute Infektionskrankheit. *Dtsche Arch Klin Med* 1886;39:209–232.
3. Landouzy LT. Typhus hépatique. *Gaz Hospital* 1883;56:913.
4. Stimson AM. Note on an organism found in yellow-fever tissue. *Public Health Rep* 1907;22:541.
5. Ido Y, Hoki R, Ito H, Wani H. The rat as a carrier of *Spirochaeta icterohaemorrhagiae*, the causative agent of Weil's disease (spirochetosis icterohaemorrhagiae). *J Exp Med* 1917;26:341–353.
6. Huebner EA, Reiter K. *Dtsche Med Wochenschr* 1915;41:1275–277.
7. Alston JM, Broom JC. *Leptospirosis.* Edinburgh, UK: Livingston Ltd., 1958.
8. Bhort AR, Nally JE, Ricaki JN, et al. Leptospirosis: a zoonotic disease of global importance. *Lancet Infect Dis* 2003;3:757–771.
9. Gochenour WS, Smadel JE, Jackson EB, Evans LB, Yager RH. Leptospiral etiology of Fort Bragg fever. *Public Health Rep* 1952;67:811–812.
10. Levett PN. Leptospirosis. *Clin Micro Rev* 2001;34:296–326.
11. Epstein PR, Pena OC, Racedo JB. Climate and disease in Colombia. *Lancet* 1995;346:1243–1244.
12. Ko AI, Galvao Reis M, Ribeiro Dourado CM, Johnson WD, Riley LW, the Salvador Leptospirosis Study Group. Urban epidemic of severe leptospirosis in Brazil. *Lancet* 1999;354:820–825.

CHAPTER 3

Cholera for a Dime
Paul A. Blake, MD, MPH

INTRODUCTION

Listening to the radio late one night in Boston in May, 1974 while taking a break from studying for my master's degree in public health finals from the Harvard School of Public Health, I was riveted by the news that cholera had broken out in Portugal. Might I be sent to Portugal? I would soon be an epidemiologist in the enteric diseases branch of the Centers for Disease Control (CDC) and would be an obvious candidate for an investigation in Portugal because I could speak Portuguese, having lived as a child in a Portuguese colony, Angola. On the other hand, my epidemiologic skills were weak. I had joined the Epidemic Intelligence Service (EIS) at the CDC because of my international public health interests and to avoid military service in Vietnam* and had been sent to Puerto Rico. My 2 years there had been rich in public health experience but devoid of on-the-job supervision in traditional CDC "shoe-leather epidemiology." In those days, communication with my supervisors at the CDC in Atlanta required hours, even days, of struggles with the much-loathed Federal Telecommunications System. I was buffing up my fledgling epidemiologic expertise with a master's in public health, but I still felt inadequate. Within days, however, the CDC called to ask whether I was interested in going to Portugal, and I was indeed. My wife, who would be left with two small boys in a new neighborhood in Atlanta, was less enthused.

---

* We occasionally referred to ourselves as the "Yellow Berets" (in contrast to the Green Berets, elite troops who fought in Vietnam), although in truth our work could be dangerous, and one of my classmates died in the line of duty when his plane crashed in Africa.

Cholera is a diarrheal disease caused by toxigenic *Vibrio cholerae* O-group 1 or O-group 139. The infection is often mild or subclinical, but in the worst cases, severe diarrhea and vomiting can cause death within 24 hours. The incubation period ranges from a few hours to 5 days. In the Northern Hemisphere, cholera usually peaks in August to September. The main source of infection is human feces. The infectious dose is very high, requiring about 1 million organisms in food and even more in water. The organisms are very sensitive to acid, and persons with low gastric acid are at greater risk for cholera. Back in 1974, few analytic studies of cholera transmission had been performed. The disease was thought to be caused largely by polluted drinking water, with food playing a minor role. Fish and shellfish had been reported to cause cholera, but the evidence was circumstantial until 1973, when studies in Italy showed that cholera was associated with eating mussels thought to be contaminated after harvest by "freshening" with polluted harbor water.[1]

Portugal had been free of cholera for many decades until 1971, when it reported 89 cases caused by *V. cholerae* O-group 1 serotype Ogawa, mostly in the Lisbon area. Neither the source of introduction nor the vehicles of transmission were determined; however, the outbreak ended, and no cases were detected in 1972 and 1973.

Throughout the summer of 1974 I was kept on alert, and the epidemic grew while the CDC worked with officials in Washington, DC to secure an invitation from Portugal. Most countries understandably are reluctant to have foreigners document their public health failures, and few invitations materialize. The situation was complicated by uncertainty after Portugal's virtually bloodless leftist military coup (the "Carnation Revolution") in April 1974 against the right-wing dictatorship of President Américo Thomaz and Prime Minister Marcelo Caetano, successor to António Salazar. There was ongoing infighting in the government and military. Remarkably, an invitation arrived on Friday, September 6, perhaps prompted by the escalating epidemic, which peaked in late August. My departure was delayed until Monday so that I could fly to Washington to be briefed on Portuguese politics at the State Department's "Portugal Desk"; however, the briefer was taking a 3-hour lunch break, and I proceeded unbriefed.

My CDC supervisors had instructed me thoroughly on cholera, and I was crammed with advice and laden with reference material. Most useful was Bill Baine's CDC report on his investigation of cholera in Italy the year before,[1] when his matched-pair case control studies incriminated ingestion of raw shellfish. The matched-pair case control technique had been used in chronic disease investigations, but to our knowledge, Bill was the first to use it in an infectious disease investigation outside of a hospital. It was particularly useful in investigating scattered, apparently unrelated cases because each case was matched to an age- and gender-matched neighborhood control subject (rather than a hospital control—Bill's innovation), and the matching was maintained in the analysis; thus, the results would not be distorted by age, gender, or socioeconomic (as reflected by neighborhood) status. My supervisors expected me to have a study of new Lisbon cases using Bill's technique underway by the end of the week. My objectives were to learn how cholera transmission was occurring to guide prevention and control measures in Portugal and to gain a better understanding of cholera transmission that would help cholera control worldwide.

FIRST INVESTIGATION—LISBON

I arrived in Lisbon at dawn on Tuesday, September 10, with little sleep, a headache, and no luggage (it arrived 36 hours later), but fearing the worst, I had my papers in a carry-on bag. Black and green taxis drumming along cobblestone streets, streetcars, double-decker buses, red tile roofs, colorfully tiled facades, palm trees, cascading bougainvilleas, Portuguese voices, and the smell of grilling sardines and diesel exhaust in the air—despite my fatigue, it was exhilarating to be in Lisbon! I checked into my hotel and hurried to the U.S. Embassy; immediately, however, I faced the first of many delays as I discovered that not everyone shared my sense of urgency. I had to wait all day to see the deputy ambassador and used the time to work with consular officials to get statistics for Portugal, newspaper clippings on the cholera epidemic, a desk, and access to a mimeograph machine and a massive mechanical calculator that used metal parts rather than electronics to add and subtract (these were the olden days). For division and multiplication, I had a slide rule.

The embassy arranged for me to meet with three national Portuguese officials, including Portugal's director general of health and the national epidemiologist, on Wednesday afternoon. They had only descriptive information. The first known cholera case had onset of illness on April 24 in Tavira on Portugal's southern coast. The 33-year-old man had diarrhea and dehydration so severe that he suffered a cardiac arrest, and the national laboratory isolated *V. cholerae* O-group 1 biotype El Tor serotype Inaba from his stool. The disease spread 300 km to Lisbon within 16 days and 600 km to Porto in the far north within 20 days and eventually was reported from 17 of 18 districts (Figure 3-1). When I arrived in Portugal in early September, approximately 2,000 laboratory-confirmed cases and

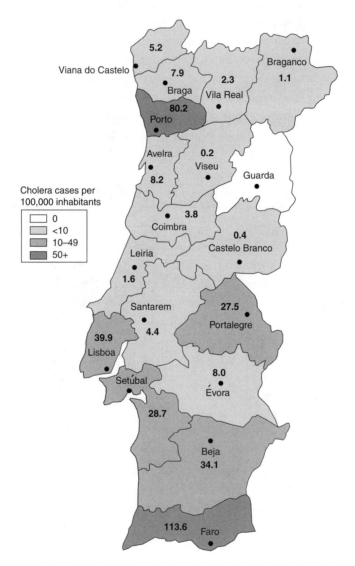

FIGURE 3-1 Hospitalized cholera patients in Portugal, by district of residence, April–October, 1974.

Reprinted with permission from Blake P et al. Cholera in Portugal 1974. II Transmission by bottled mineral water. *Am J Epidemiol* 1977;105:344–348.

several dozen deaths had been reported. The epidemic had peaked the last week in August and was now declining rapidly (Figure 3-2), but a few new widely scattered cases were still occurring in Lisbon. I began to worry that while an investigation of cases that were part of the peak of the epidemic might incriminate one or more important vehicles that caused the bulk of the cases, the last few scattered cases at the tail end of the epidemic might be caused by many different exposures (e.g., food contaminated by an infected household member), making successful incrimination of any one vehicle unlikely; however, I had arrived primed to concentrate on new cases and did not yet have the self-confidence or experience to deviate from the plan.

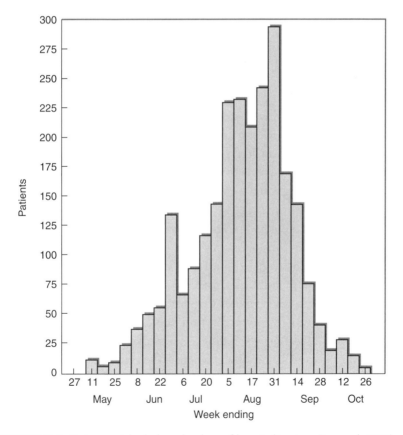

FIGURE 3-2 Patients with cholera, by date of hospitalization, Portugal, 1974.

Reprinted with permission from Blake P et al. Cholera in Portugal 1974. II Transmission by bottled mineral water. *Am J Epidemiol* 1977;105:344–348.

From anecdotes, cultures of food and the environment, and educated guesses, the Portuguese officials suspected several vehicles—cooked snails collected from sewage-contaminated gullies, lettuce irrigated with human sewage during the dry summer, watercress, Lupini beans sold by street vendors, raw shellfish, and well water. Later I learned that spring water and commercially bottled mineral water were also suspected, but were not mentioned initially because they involved an important company and thus were politically sensitive.

The national officials made it clear that they were too understaffed and overburdened to find staff to work with me, but they referred me to the Lisbon District Health Department. I went there Thursday morning; the Director was on vacation until Friday, but I met with an elderly physician who specialized in waterborne disease.* While waiting to meet the Director, I worked on a draft questionnaire and included the suspect foods, other plausible foods, and various sources of water, as well as possible risk factors such as gastric surgery and the use of antacids. I planned to ask the cases about exposures during the 5 days before onset and to ask age- and gender-matched neighbor controls about the 5 days before interview. The Portuguese had been doing a good job of culturing suspect cases, and in this and all subsequent investigations, we were able to define cases as persons with *V. cholerae* O1 isolated from their stools. In this investigation, we defined our cases as any culture-confirmed case from Lisbon or the adjacent city of Oeiras diagnosed on or after September 13.

Writing the questionnaires was doubly difficult because although I could speak Portuguese, I had never learned to read or write the language; I had to write the questions phonetically and get help from Portuguese staff in the embassy. I then struggled until nearly midnight to type stencils and mimeograph questionnaires. I returned to my hotel with inky hands and clothes but enough questionnaires to get started.

The next morning the director told me about the Lisbon District cholera activities. Eight nurses in four teams worked on cholera. One team interviewed new cases in hospitals, whereas the other three visited recent cases and their families. World Health Organization (WHO) epidemiolo-

---

* Dr. Leopoldo de Figueiredo gave me his publications on water and sewer systems in Portugal. My mother later told me (and he confirmed) that he was our family doctor in 1947 when I was 4 and my parents were in Lisbon learning Portuguese—a small world!

gists had visited Portugal several months earlier. At their recommendation, the Lisbon District had begun to complete a new cholera case-investigation form for all cholera patients in July. It included questions about exposures, including recent travel and sources of drinking water. The questionnaires lay unanalyzed in stacks destined, as is so often the case, for the archives rather than for analysis and use in disease control. They were to prove useful, however, in the weeks ahead.

I went out with a team the same day and completed questionnaires on three cases and two controls. On Saturday, the work went more smoothly as the nurses (and I) gained experience and our team interviewed three case control pairs in 6 hours. Being naturally diffident, it was stressful for me to knock on the doors of complete strangers, try to explain why I was there, and ask them personal questions in a language that I had hardly used in 17 years. Each interview was easier than the last, however, and the experience of going into private homes all over Lisbon was vastly more interesting than being a tourist. The case and control subjects were cooperative, and I enjoyed talking with them. One woman control looked at me quizzically as I stumbled through questions in my rusty Portuguese and finally said, "Ah! You are from Mozambique!" She recognized the African colonial accent but had the wrong colony.

Despite the seemingly interminable delays, the case control study was underway on schedule. Over the weekend I revised the questionnaires to fix problems turned up by the interviews and retyped and mimeographed them. I decided that the same person should interview both subjects in each case control pair so that the questions would be asked similarly. I worried that we needed more rigorous methods to select neighbor controls because investigators might unknowingly introduce bias if left to their own devices. Thus, I improved on the Italian studies, which selected neighbor controls from passers-by or other conveniently accessible neighbors, by adapting methods learned in a chronic disease course to create a scheme that I used in all subsequent investigations. The investigators would start at the case's house and go door to door following a printed schematic map (go right until the corner, then return to the case's house and go left until the corner, etc.) until they located a person of the same gender and within the same age range. After I amended the schematic map to include apartments, it failed only once, when the patient was a railroad crossing operator who lived in a hut by the rails—his residence was not part of a block.

I intended to train and enlist all three field teams, but although most of the nurses quickly learned proper techniques, one was overenthusiastic; she pressed patients to admit that they had eaten suspect foods and suggested to controls that they had *not* eaten those foods. Also, her suicidal driving caused a minor crash, and thus, we dropped her team from the investigation.

These were politically turbulent times in Portugal. Early one Sunday morning as I was walking up an empty cobblestone street, President (and General) António Spínola swept past in a small white car surrounded by National Republican Guards—impressive solidly built, middle-aged men on eerily quiet motorcycles. Shortly afterward, there were mass demonstrations in Lisbon and an attempted coup, and President Spínola was forced to resign on September 30. Despite the unrest, I never felt threatened, even though an American consular official chilled me by saying that as a Portuguese-speaking American I would be suspected of being a Central Intelligence Agency operative.

Each week brought fewer new cases in Lisbon; they were widely scattered and difficult to locate in the labyrinthine streets. We visited the addresses of many subjects repeatedly and at odd hours before we caught them at home. Over 3 weeks our strenuous efforts interviewed just 34 case control pairs, 59% of the 58 reported new cases. On analysis of the data, I had my worst fears realized. My effort for almost 4 weeks had failed to associate cholera with any exposure. My CDC supervisors were dissatisfied. Portuguese officials were losing interest, and some nurses returned to their precholera duties. I was dejected and wanted to go home; however, I was learning how to operate in Portugal. My Portuguese was improving daily, and I was learning the limitations of case control studies. I wanted to try again with cases that had occurred earlier in the epidemic when single vehicles might have been important.

On September 20, in the midst of the Lisbon investigation, I was joined by Mark Rosenberg, an Afro-coifed, Earth Shoe-shod, first-year EIS officer from my branch (this was the 1970s, after all—I sported a bushy C. Everett Koop beard) (Figure 3-3). We quickly adapted to each other's work styles, and although he did not know Portuguese, he could communicate with many Portuguese professionals in French. He plunged into the work but helped the most by being an epidemiologist with whom I could discuss the details of our investigations face to face; he was the quintessential devil's advocate, sometimes to a fault.

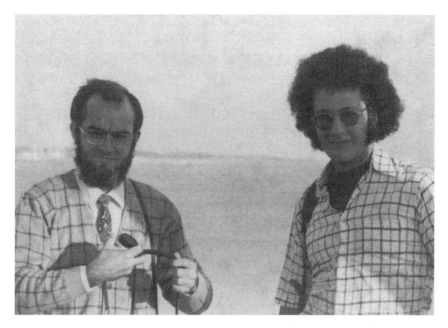

FIGURE 3-3 Paul Blake and Mark Rosenberg in the Algarve, October 1974.

As the Lisbon case control study of current cases limped to a close, Mark and I explored possibilities for other studies. The Lisbon cholera nurses told us in late September that back in August they began to see cases in the upper and upper-middle classes for the first time. Many of these patients reported recent travel to Vimeiro Thermal Springs, a spa in Lisbon District but 50 km north of Lisbon in Torres Vedras County, and others had drunk Agua do Vimeiro, commercially bottled water from the same springs. At about the same time, prompted by two cholera cases in a nearby village, a sanitarian cultured water from the springs as part of a sanitation inspection of the area. On August 22, *V. cholerae* was isolated from the spring water samples. On the 23rd, the springs and the bottling plant were closed, and the bottled water was recalled. A press release was issued on August 24.

We painstakingly reviewed the Lisbon government cholera question-naires for August; there was no bottled water question, but the nurses asked about it on their own initiative (smart nurses!) after they learned of the potential problem. Torres Vedras County had 16 cases in persons who worked at (4), visited (1), or lived near (11) the springs within 5 days before onset. In Lisbon District, excluding Torres Vedras County, 29 of 418 cases reported visiting the springs, and at least 81 reported drinking Vimeiro bottled water within 5 days before onset. The peak number of cases appeared in all three groups (Torres Vedras county residents, spa visitors, and Vimeiro water drinkers) at about the same time—the last 2 weeks of August.

Our interest was piqued. We asked the Lisbon Health Director for a car and a sanitarian to visit the Vimeiro springs and bottling plant. He agreed, but for several days, there was one delay after another—car trouble, illness, and so forth. Finally, the light dawned—because a large business was involved, the situation was politically sensitive, and they did not want us to visit the springs but did not want to tell us that directly. We had been careful not to rock the political boat, but we decided it was time to take risks. Accordingly, I told the authorities that we understood how difficult it was to free up a car and a sanitarian for a day and that Mark and I would just hire a taxi and visit the plant without a health department escort. I feared that they might forbid it, but suddenly they found a car and a sanitarian to take us. Sr. João Florencia, the wiry, chain-smoking, espresso-fueled sanitarian who had collected the Vimeiro water samples, drove us sedately to the springs, giving us no hint of the driving style that he would exhibit on the ride back to Lisbon; in retrospect, he was still sizing us up.

The spa's owner gave us some statistics. In 1973, the previous year, about 20,000 people visited the spa during August, and about 70% of these were from Lisbon District. Approximately half of the bottled water was carbonated, and half was untreated. Usually about 10.5 million liters of water were bottled annually, but in 1974, production increased about 50%, apparently because people turned to bottled water for fear of cholera. The uncarbonated water was distributed in 5-gallon jugs and in smaller capped bottles (Figure 3-4) that sold for 3 escudos (10 cents). In August, the month of greatest demand, bottles could be on Lisbon store shelves within 4 hours after production. Approximately 42% of the bottled water was distributed outside of Lisbon District.

We visited the two springs, the spa, and the bottling plant. Most interesting was the Fonte Santa Isabel (Santa Isabel Spring), the source of most of the water. The Fonte lay less than 50 feet from a small river, the Ribeira de Alcabrichel, which carried sewage from upstream towns; cultures of river water samples collected on August 13 and August 26 yielded *V. cholerae* O1. The Fonte originally welled up spontaneously from the underlying limestone rocks, but subsequently, a large chamber was dug

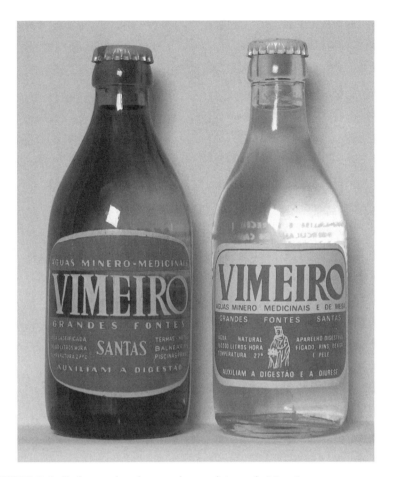

FIGURE 3-4 Carbonated and noncarbonated Agua do Vimeiro.

into the limestone and covered with concrete, creating an underground reservoir. Untreated water was pumped from this reservoir to the baths, drinking water spigots (Figure 3-5), a swimming pool, and the bottling plant. Limestone aquifers are infamous for having underground fissures and channels through which water can flow rapidly. Five of six water samples collected from the Fonte on August 13, 22, 26, and 28 yielded *V. cholerae*. The springs were closed to the public on August 23 and were still closed when we were there.

In the midst of our tour, we had soft drinks, but the spa's bartender said he had been ordered not to charge us. We insisted that we could not appear

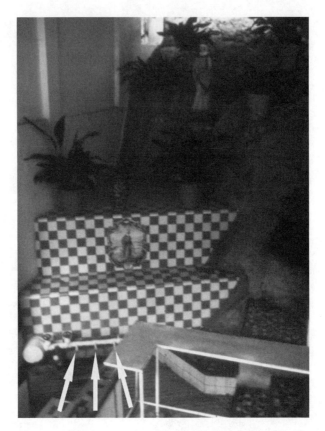

FIGURE 3-5 Termos do Vimeiro grotto with drinking water outlets (bottom).

to be "bought," but he looked shaken and resisted. Finally we just left money on the bar.

We finished late and had a wild ride back to Lisbon through the gathering night. João careened the VW beetle at up to 90 km/h through town and country on the narrow winding roads, flashing the high beams and passing on curves. He compensated for the car's anemic acceleration by not slowing for anything other than certain catastrophe. He said he had been a paratrooper until recently and didn't know the meaning of fear, but we certainly did. Fortunately, I was in the back seat (my invariable choice), but Mark sat in the front passenger seat which, João told him with relish, the Portuguese refer to as "o lugar do morto" (the place of the dead). João stopped half a block short of our hotel—to let us out, or so we thought. Instead, we were out of gas. We pushed the car to a gas station.

We planned a case control study in Lisbon to find out whether Agua do Vimeiro was associated with cholera, but our CDC supervisors vetoed it, pointing out that bottled water was a highly unlikely vehicle because it had never been shown to cause cholera or any other disease. They directed us toward Faro District (the Algarve), Portugal's southern coast where the epidemic had begun and the incidence was highest to see whether we could implicate shellfish. Mark left for Faro on October 8 to see whether studies there were feasible, and I followed 2 days later after tying up loose ends.

My calls to Atlanta to brief and consult with my supervisors were always challenges. Public telephones were invariably in noisy public places where I found it difficult to hear and to think, and I had to watch what I said in public. At the CDC end, a crowd would gather on a bad speaker phone, making the acoustics even worse, and interruptions were frequent, breaking trains of thought. Our study's progress was slow, and I was asked by someone at CDC, "Are you working nights and weekends?" This implied that I was loafing—I could barely contain my rage. I couldn't explain all of the details and subtleties by telephone, and I was plied with advice that I thought was misguided; however, I couldn't say that to my new bosses. I felt at a great disadvantage because I was new to the branch and had no significant publications from my EIS experience, although the branch was one of the most "academic," prestigious, and publication-oriented units at the CDC. I was afraid that I would return to the CDC a failure and would have no future in the branch. Thus, I was noncommittal on the phone and once off did what I thought was best. I wrote this to my wife: "I'm going to avoid calling Atlanta—they are trying to solve the problems without understanding the situation, and I can't explain it all to them at $2 a minute ($8 in today's dollars) standing in the embassy lobby surrounded by a dozen noisy people, shouting into the telephone, and barely able to hear. It takes me a couple of hours to calm down after every call. When Bill Baine investigated cholera in Italy he called them once in 2 months, and that sounds about right to me!" Nevertheless, I kept on calling as instructed.

SECOND INVESTIGATION— TAVIRA, FARO DISTRICT

We had a warm welcome in Faro, the capital of Faro District, although we had to "waste" a lot of time building relationships by enduring well-meant distractions—for example, a 7-hour tour of the district's many hotels and seemingly endless irrelevant (although entertaining) stories. The district health director gave us a key to the health department for after-hours access and found nurses to help us.

We discussed the cholera epidemic with local health officials and pored over their lists of cases to chart the course of the epidemic in the various municipalities. The first case had been detected in Tavira, a coastal town in Faro District near the Spanish border. Founded by the Phoenicians over 2,700 years ago, Tavira is known for its "Roman" bridge (actually Moorish from the 12th century) over the Gilão River. The river flows through the town into the Ria de Faro, a coastal strip of mud flats and islands 50 km long and up to 5 km wide that separates Tavira and Faro from the open sea and supplied most shellfish consumed in Portugal. Raw sewage from coastal towns emptied into the Ria, where water and shellfish had been known to have high coliform bacteria counts for at least a decade. After anecdotal reports of shellfish causing cholera, the Maritime Biology Institute in Faro isolated *V. cholerae* from 24% of seawater and 42% of shellfish samples from the Ria between May and August 1974.

We went to Tavira to try to find out how the epidemic began. Local health officials pointed out elements that might have contributed to the outbreak—raw sewage flowing into the tidal river, people gathering shellfish near the sewage outlets ('where the cockles are fattest"), sewage and water lines under repair, and two closed springs. Although chlorinated, Tavira's municipal water supply was suspect because the water lines were old, ruptured frequently, and ran beside leaking sewage lines. Water and sewer system renovation began in 1973, and we found excavated streets and wooden plugs in exposed pipes. We were told that when cholera first occurred heavy rain filled the excavations with sewage-contaminated water, enhancing the potential for sewage to contaminate potable water. Two suspect springs within the town were closed on May 10 and May 11.

The first detected case in Tavira (this was also the first case detected in Portugal, as described previously) had onset of illness on April 24. No other cases were identified for 13 days, but then a cluster of 14 cases in Tavira had onset between May 6 and May 15, followed by other clusters within the town over the succeeding months. Review of Tavira hospitalization records revealed an increase in diarrheal illnesses the second half of April; thus, there may have been some undetected cholera in April, and there may have been cases before the first detected case. We decided to focus on the first 15 culture-proven cases in Tavira, hoping that our findings would help us to understand how the Portuguese epidemic began.

In planning an investigation, we worried that recall of specific exposures 6 months before would be difficult for cases and worse for control subjects who had no illness as a reference point; however, we guessed (correctly, as we found out) that subjects would be able to recall their usual practices and unusual experiences like travel. Our questionnaire asked about demographic data; travel; frequency of eating raw vegetables, fruits, and seven varieties of shellfish; shellfish cooking methods; and drinking water sources. We asked all subjects about exposures during April and May and also asked the cholera patients about exposures during the 5 days before the onset.

Working with two nurses, we located and interviewed 14 of the 15 initial cases and matched controls in 2 days (October 14 and 15). The work went quickly because of short distances and relative ease in locating the patients. Our excitement mounted as case after case said that they liked the flavor of the water from one of the two local springs, the Fonte do Bispo, so much that they regularly walked across town to fill their jugs. Furthermore, they were angry that it was closed because decades of drinking that water had never made them sick. Eleven of 14 cases and none of 14 control subjects recalled drinking water from the Fonte do Bispo. We constructed a table that shows how matched-pair case control data are analyzed (Table 3-1). It maintains the matching, and the numbers refer to case control pairs of individuals rather than just to individuals. The probability that the result of our interviews occurred by chance is calculated using just two cells: pairs in which the case drank but the control did not

Table 3-1 Distribution of 14 Case Control Pairs by History of Drinking Fonte do Bispo Water During April and May, 1974, Tavira, Portugal

Case	Control		Total Pairs
	Drank	Did Not Drink	
Drank	0	11	11
Did not drink	0	3	3
Total pairs	0	14	14

The other local spring was not implicated.

(11) and pairs in which the control drank but the case did not (0). The two-tailed exact test for matched pairs testing our hypothesis that having cholera was associated with drinking water from the Fonte do Bispo yielded a P value of 0.001, and the relative risk (11/0) was infinite. More than a month after arriving in Portugal, we had a significant P value!

Our epidemiologic analysis failed to explain the index case in which the person did not drink water from the Fonte do Bispo or travel outside Portugal in 1974. Although our analysis had not demonstrated that having cholera was statistically associated with eating raw or partially cooked shellfish, the story from the index case suggested that they played a role. Three days before onset of illness, he gathered cockles from the Ria near the mouth of the Gilão and heated them only until they opened, and then he and two others ate them. Only the patient, who took antacids, developed diarrhea. There was no suggestion that any cases were related to drinking municipal water, and thus, the broken pipes appeared to be a red herring.

How might *V. cholerae* O1 El Tor serotype Inaba, the epidemic strain, have been introduced into Portugal? Soldiers traveled back and forth from a military training base 120 meters uphill from the Fonte do Bispo to the wars in Portugal's three African colonies—Angola, Mozambique, and Portuguese Guinea—where El Tor Inaba cholera was endemic. Sewage from the base emptied into the Gilão and flowed to the Ria. Thus, vibrios from an infected soldier could be taken up by filter-feeding shellfish in the Gilão and the Ria. Then people infected by eating contaminated shellfish would discharge more vibrios down the river, and the epidemic would be underway. Even though they were thousands of miles away, the African colonies were a much more likely source than nearby North Africa, where only El Tor Ogawa cholera was being reported. Subsequently, phage typing, a more sensitive method than serotyping to detect differences between cholera strains, showed that the 1974 Portuguese Inaba strains were indistinguishable from Angolan Inaba strains. Angola is a south-central African country that was a Portuguese colony until 1975.

Health officials had suspected that the Fonte do Bispo (a pipe emerging from the side of a hill through a concrete wall on a street corner) (Figure 3-6) caused a typhoid outbreak long before the advent of cholera; however, the public would not let them close it because they did not believe that it had caused the outbreak and they liked the flavor of the water. The officials said the spring produced clear water until September 1973, when, after construction blasting of the rock behind the spring followed by a

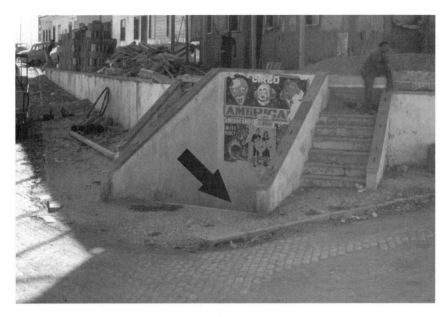

FIGURE 3-6 Fonte do Bispo, Tavira, Portugal, October 1974.

heavy rain, the emerging water was muddy for a few days. A sewer line running down the hill beside the spring could have been damaged during the blasting. The sewer line was renovated in 1973, but it was unclear whether that occurred before or after the blasting. Perhaps damage from the blasting allowed sewage from persons infected by shellfish or from troops up the hill to pollute the spring. Unfortunately, dye testing was not politically feasible.

THIRD INVESTIGATION—FARO

There is nothing like a significant *P* value to raise epidemiologists' spirits. Now that we knew how the epidemic began, we wanted to examine the vehicles of transmission during the rest of the epidemic. We decided to try to continue our investigations in Faro District because we had good working relationships there and it had the highest incidence of cholera in Portugal. We immersed ourselves in analyses of Faro District data to pick our next target. We chose as our subjects the 59 cases identified in the city of Faro during the 5 months of May through September. Only eight cases occurred during May through July, but there were 51 cases during August through September. Compelling anecdotes pointing to shellfish abounded. In one instance, four small boys found a pile of cockles by the shore, heated them on a flattened tin can over a small fire until they opened, and ate them. All four developed diarrhea, and stool from one was cultured and yielded *V. cholerae*. Our questionnaire asked cases and individually matched controls about exposures during a 2-month period—the month of onset of illness and the nearest adjacent month. On October 18, as the study began, Mark was recalled to the CDC because the branch was so shorthanded that our supervisors feared (horrors!) that they would have to investigate the next outbreak themselves. Two nurses and I interviewed and matched 53 cases over the next several days and showed that eating raw or semicooked cockles was significantly associated with cholera. I was ecstatic. These findings added credence to the theory that distribution of contaminated live shellfish from the Ria throughout Portugal could explain the rapid spread of cholera nationwide (Figure 3-7).

Now I had been in Portugal for over 6 weeks, and I ached to go home; however, on my next call to Atlanta (the worst yet, from a bar packed with rowdy tourists), my supervisors changed their minds about the plausibility of bottled water as a vehicle for cholera. Now, after Mark briefed them

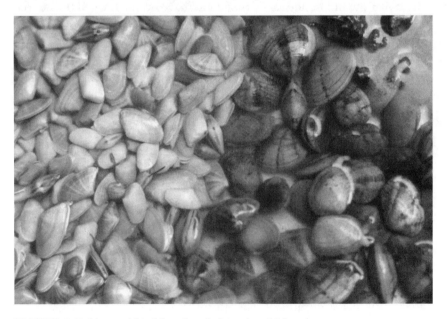

FIGURE 3-7 Live cockles (above) and clams in a Lisbon bar.

in person, they wanted me to conduct a case control study of Agua do Vimeiro in Lisbon. I finished up in Faro, flew back to Lisbon on October 26, and plunged into planning the investigation.

FOURTH INVESTIGATION— BOTTLED WATER

I was able to use the available data from the Lisbon Health Department's cholera case investigation forms in a retrospective cohort approach to show that visiting the springs was associated with cholera. During August, 36 (2.57/1,000) of the estimated 14,000 visitors to the springs from Lisbon District, excluding Torres Vedras County, had cholera, but only 382 (0.25/1,000) of 1,530,831 who did not visit the springs had cholera. The cholera risk was 10.3 times greater for visitors than for nonvisitors. The big question, however, was whether bottled Agua do Vimeiro had caused cholera.

I decided to study Lisbon District cases with onset during the week ending August 24 for several reasons: The government's cholera questionnaires showed the number of new cases in persons who recalled drinking Agua do Vimeiro in the 5 days before onset peaked during that week; it was the last week when bottled Agua do Vimeiro was available in stores (it was recalled on August 23). A news release on August 24 said that the bottled water was suspect, and thus, after that date, the public would be less likely to drink bottled water they bought before the recall. Also, water collected from the Fonte Santa Isabel on August 22 was positive for *V. cholerae* O1. When I reviewed the government's cholera case investigation forms more carefully to identify the cases for study, I found that some cases had date of positive culture but not date of onset. Allowing for delay between onset and positive culture, I included cases with no recorded onset date if the patient's positive culture was between August 22 and 28. That gave me 47 symptomatic cases. I then excluded six who visited the springs (they might have been infected by drinking the water directly from the springs), three less than 10 years of age (their recall might be inaccurate), one who was not the first case of cholera in the family (cholera can spread through multiple vehicles within households), and two nonresidents who were ill before arriving in Lisbon (they were not infected in Lisbon District), leaving 35 for the investigation. Planning the study was the easy part, however; now I had to get help.

When I approached the Lisbon District Health Director, it was clear that I had worn out my welcome. Lisbon had been cholera-free for 8 days, and cholera was old news. Even though 4 days earlier he had told me by telephone that he would provide nurses to investigate Agua do Vimeiro, he now said rather brusquely that he could not. I didn't know if he really could not, if he just wanted to get rid of me, or if cholera from bottled water was so politically sensitive that he had been told to not let me touch it. I suspected the last. One official told me confidentially that under the dictatorship, before the Carnation Revolution, the public would never have known about the contamination at Termos do Vimeiro because it was a big business—it would have been hushed up. Although the revolutionary government had recalled the water and issued a press release in late August, now more than 2 months had passed, and there was reluctance to bring fresh attention to the problem through an epidemiologic investigation by a foreigner.

I visited the national epidemiologist with all of the results to date and made the case for the investigation. I told him that all I needed was a car and driver—no nurses—so that I could track down cases nights and weekends when they were most likely to be home and that when it was done I would stop bothering him and go back to Atlanta. Somehow he was able to get me the best help possible—the sanitarian João Florencia and a car. We began the study the next day.

Investigating cases with João was a revelation. With no previous experience in epidemiology, he quickly grasped the investigation's logic and techniques and worked enthusiastically far into the night, over the weekend, and on All Saints Day even though he was not paid for overtime. Finding cases in Lisbon was often exceedingly difficult. Addresses were incomplete. There were multiple streets with the same name, and some streets were only a few houses long; however, with the aid of a detailed street guide in tiny print and his experience as a sanitarian, João found almost all of them. He also proved to be an excellent interviewer, maintaining rapport and eliciting information without "leading" the interviewees. Throughout my career, I was to find that one of the pleasures of working in the field with local coworkers was serendipitous encounters with extraordinary people.

Interviewing cases at night led to awkward situations. At 10:30 one night we sat in our VW on a dark street waiting for a 17-year-old schoolgirl to return home. A person with high thick-heeled shoes, long hair, and bell-bottoms came clopping down the street and approached the door with a young man, so I got out to interview her. At the door I asked, "Are you Constância Engrácia?" Unfortunately, the person was a young man, and I asked the question while looking him full in the face. His friend exploded with laughter while I tried to blame the darkness.

Another night we traced an older woman with cholera to a palatial mansion and were interrogated on the marble steps politely but suspiciously by the patient's son, an admiral. Apparently he checked us out with the authorities because the next day the national epidemiologist said with a knowing smile, "So you have been visiting admirals late at night?"

We tracked down 32 of the 35 patients (91%) and found neighborhood control subjects matched by age (within 5 years), gender, ethnic group, and approximate socioeconomic status. The cases and controls were asked whether, during August, they drank carbonated or uncarbonated bottled Agua do Vimeiro or visited the springs. As the investigation progressed, it became increasingly obvious that bottled water would be associated with cholera, and I worked in an advanced state of euphoria.

My fear of failure was gone. I knew that I would be going home soon, and I reveled in the opportunity to immerse myself in Lisbon and all things Portuguese. It was a privilege to talk with people at every social level in their homes and in their language. I found places that I dimly remembered from having lived in Lisbon for 8 months in 1947–1948 when I was 4 years old—our basement apartment at 22 Abaracamento de Peniche, a small park with a spreading tree under which I had played, and the botanical garden. I savored Portuguese food and music; I had café com leite and superbly crusty and chewy pães pequenos for breakfast, bife a Portuguesa for lunch, and concoctions of potato, onion, tomato, and fish with olive oil for dinner. I drank one brand of orange soft drink almost exclusively and then learned at the end from João that it had the worst coliform counts among the soft drinks. I continued, however, to add iodine to my drinking water, didn't have a salad in 9 weeks, and stayed well.

The results were clear-cut: 13 cholera patients, but only two control subjects had consumed bottled non-carbonated Agua do Vimeiro ($P = 0.003$) (relative risk = 12). Interestingly, cholera was not associated with drinking carbonated Agua do Vimeiro, which made sense because carbonated water is acidic and *V. cholerae* cannot tolerate a low pH. The bottled water had infected all levels of society from an admiral's mother living in a mansion to someone living under metal roofing leaning against a wall. As I pored over the national data, I began to suspect that Agua do Vimeiro caused many cases all over Portugal because the epidemic peaked in the north (Porto), middle (Lisbon), and south (Faro) and in some other districts during the last 2 weeks of August, coinciding with contamination of the bottled water. Although 42% of the bottled water was distributed outside of Lisbon District, I wondered if vibrios could survive being trucked long distances at ambient temperature. It was too late to do more investigations, but I returned to our incompletely analyzed Faro case control data and discovered that we had implicated Agua do Vimeiro in Faro without realizing it! In Faro, nine cases and two control subjects reported having drunk Agua do Vimeiro ($P = 0.046$), and the association remained significant ($P = 0.031$) when controlling for eating cockles. Because the spa and the bottled water plant were closed on August 23 but the spring remained culture positive until at least August 28, stopping access to the spring water clearly prevented many cases of cholera. The Portuguese government did not allow the bottled water plant to reopen until the water source was changed to a deep well drilled in the same area as the Fonte Santa Isabel; however, at a higher altitude, the well water was shown to contain no pathogenic bacteria, and the plant began to treat the water with ultraviolet light before bottling.

WRAP-UP

I prepared a report for my exit interviews with Portuguese officials, and after 9 weeks, my work in Portugal was finally done. I felt, however, that I had barely scratched the surface of the possibilities that the cholera epidemic in Portugal presented for understanding cholera transmission. Once *V. cholerae* O1 is widely distributed by a vehicle of transmission (in Portugal raw shellfish), each infected person excretes enormous numbers of vibrios that can then contaminate foods (where they can multiply) and water and cause other outbreaks. Thus, the epidemic curve describing the course of an epidemic may represent the combined effects of many outbreaks, large and small, caused by a variety of vehicles, with only the largest outbreaks (such as the bottled water outbreak) having enough cases to cause marked distortion of the overall epidemic curve. Bits and pieces of information from across Portugal suggested that further investigations could have been fruitful. I mourned the lost opportunities—among others, a large inland outbreak attributed to a contaminated well in Portalegre, a sharp and massive outbreak in Porto affecting all age groups equally that may have been caused by public water, and a daycare center outbreak in

Portimão that may have been caused by the diaper washer reconstituting powdered milk.

I returned to Atlanta through Geneva at the request of the WHO. Epidemiologists often feel that the value of outbreak investigations is self-evident; however, that is not true, and it was certainly not the case at the WHO in the early 1970s. Our data, however, impressed the WHO officials, and they asked me to write a simple description of how to perform matched-pair case control studies to determine vehicles of transmission for use and publication by the WHO. Subsequently I complied, thinking it would help the WHO provide critical assistance to countries with epidemics, but in fact, it was buried in an appendix of a WHO monograph on shellfish hygiene.[2] Sic transit gloria mundi (thus passes the glory of the world). Nevertheless, at the WHO, the successful cholera investigations in Portugal and Italy lent credibility to CDC investigations and may have helped ease the way for future requests from the WHO for CDC epidemiologists to investigate outbreaks worldwide.

On November 29, 1974, Portugal was declared free of cholera. In all, 2,467 culture-confirmed cases and 48 deaths were reported to the WHO. The case-fatality ratio was 1.9%, remarkably low considering that only the more severe cases were likely to be culture confirmed. Cholera did not reappear the following year. In 1974, five European countries reported 10 cases of cholera imported from Portugal. By writing to a case's physician in England, I learned that the patient visited Vimeiro Thermal Springs in mid August and drank spring water there.

Back in Atlanta, I struggled to find time to complete the analyses and write up the results, and I quickly discovered that my work had just begun and that the "fun" part was over. Over the years, I have seen many exquisite investigations (some of them, sadly, my own) that failed to achieve their potential public health impact and faded from memory because the investigators lacked the self-discipline to publish them. I had little experience in scientific writing, and organizing the results from our multiple studies in Portugal was particularly difficult. Now any resentment I harbored against my supervisors from our difficult communications in Portugal faded as they provided superb mentoring one on one. With help from my supervisors and coworkers, I eventually produced two papers (with five Portuguese coauthors) that we thought were ready for publication, and in September 1975, I sent them to the Portuguese director general of health for approval.

Two months dragged by with no response from Portugal, and thus, I sent the papers again stating that we planned to submit them to a journal on December 15 but could not include Portuguese coauthors without written permission. That provoked a reply. On December 11, the director general wrote that he would not agree to publication of the papers in their present form because they could harm tourism. I was crushed. With my supervisors' coaching, however, I painfully made many small changes in the papers that I should have made in the first place, trimming some place and brand names and stressing (accurately) the Portuguese government's vigorous and appropriate response to the epidemic: case investigations; tetracycline treatment of contacts; no mass vaccinations; public health education; chlorinating water; closing the Fonte do Bispo and the Vimeiro springs, spa, and bottled water plant; recalling the bottled water; monitoring bottled water quality; and accepting CDC collaboration. I sent the director general the revised papers, a detailed list of the changes, and a properly humble letter, and by May 1976, he approved publication. The papers were finally published in 1977.[3,4]

Our investigations' impact on Portugal is difficult to judge. The 1974 cholera epidemic was ending as we arrived, and thus, we could not take any credit for controlling that epidemic; however, we showed how epidemiologic investigations could systematize and quantitate the things that health officials had suspected, proving some and disproving others. Unlike 1971, when the cause of the cholera outbreak in Lisbon remained a mystery, our investigations in 1974 showed that cholera may have been imported from Angola by the military, that contamination of the Fonte do Bispo infected many people and helped amplify the number of organisms in the environment, that contaminated shellfish caused many cases in southern Portugal and could have disseminated cholera throughout Portugal, and that pollution of two springs north of Lisbon caused many cases in visitors to the springs and in people in Lisbon, Faro, and possibly throughout Portugal who drank bottled uncarbonated spring water. We hope that statistical incrimination of these vehicles helped stiffen prevention measures and thus helped prevent future epidemics.

Our investigations contributed to scientific knowledge about transmission of cholera, including the most conclusive evidence ever presented that cholera could be transmitted by shellfish contaminated before harvest, the first reports that spring water contaminated before it emerges from the ground can transmit cholera, and the first report that bottled uncarbonated mineral water can transmit cholera. Because investigators sometimes focus on known vehicles and disregard possible vehicles that have not been implicated previously, publishing this information may have saved lives by alerting health authorities to these potential vehicles in prevention and control of cholera worldwide. It also had one tangible impact: The CDC changed its recommendation for international travelers to areas where chlorinated tap water is not available or where hygiene and sanitation are poor. Until 1974, the CDC recommended that one option for such travelers was to drink bottled water. After 1974, the recommendation was changed to bottled carbonated water. Carbonated mineral water is still on the list of recommended beverages for travelers.[5] Dramatic advances— many from the CDC's Enteric Diseases Branch—in understanding vehicles for cholera transmission have occurred since our investigations.[6] Foods have proven to be more important vehicles than was thought previously and include raw and cooked seafood, cooked grains and legumes, and frozen coconut milk.

This 9-week investigation shaped the rest of my career in epidemiology. It improved my epidemiologic skills and self-confidence and gave me a record of accomplishment that helped secure my career in CDC's Enteric Diseases Branch, where I worked for the next 20 years, eventually as branch chief. Cholera and other vibrio-related diseases became my special interest. The investigation made me acutely aware of the limitations of supervision by telephone and pushed me toward letting field epidemiologists use their own judgment. It enhanced my Portuguese*, leading to subsequent work in Angola, Mozambique, Brazil, and Portugal. Most important, it taught me valuable lessons—and gave me a rich source of anecdotes—that I used in mentoring EIS officers, preventive medicine residents, and other epidemiologists:

1. Matched-pair case control studies with neighborhood controls can be a powerful tool, and people with the right temperament can be trained quickly to interview subjects and select matched controls; however, supervise them carefully, and don't send them out alone until they have demonstrated competence.

---

* I wrote to my wife: "For two months I thought people were telling me that they were constipated, and I tried not to listen, but now I learn that 'constipado' means 'congested,' as in stuffy nose."

2. Take pains to develop good hypotheses before plunging into an investigation.

3. Keep an open mind about possible vehicles of transmission—the fact that a vehicle seems to be unlikely (e.g., spring water) or has not been implicated before (e.g., bottled water) does not rule it out, and experts, scientific articles, and textbooks can be wrong.

4. Without conclusive evidence, don't assume that any potential source of infection, no matter how logical and likely (e.g., decrepit water pipes and sewers in Tavira), is actually a source.

5. Scattered cases at the end of an epidemic may not provide useful information; focus on the heart of the epidemic curve, any unusual peaks, and the beginning.

6. Although it is best to investigate soon after illnesses occur, you can get a history of exposures even months later if you ask about usual practices like customary sources of water or memorable one-time exposures like travel.

7. Local investigators will tire before you do—they have different motivations and their usual work is backing up. Thus, work as quickly and efficiently as possible, and treat local investigators as colleagues and coworkers rather than as errand runners.

8. Try to understand the local officials' point of view, and adapt to it as much as possible without distorting the science—they will be dealing with the consequences of the investigation (and any publications) long after you are gone.

9. Resisting the urge to cut corners and go home can really pay off; it is better to stay in the field until you have completed the studies and preliminary analyses and identified and filled gaps in knowledge such as the distribution of incriminated products.

10. Don't pack an unused jar of thiosulfate citrate bile salts sucrose agar powder, a culture medium for *V. cholerae*, with your precious papers on your trip home; when it breaks, your papers will have a sticky green crust forever.

My experience in Portugal hooked me on epidemiologic investigations for life, and even now in retirement, I get a rush when I can contribute to an investigation. To me, the greatest joy of epidemiologic investigation is trying to solve the mystery. Initially, the situation often appears chaotic, with people becoming ill for no apparent reason; however, there is always order beneath the chaos, with everything happening for a reason. It is our fascinating job as epidemiologists to investigate, tease out the truth, and describe what happened and why it happened so that it can be stopped now and prevented in the future. The satisfaction that comes with finding out why things happen is immense.

REFERENCES

1. Baine WB, Mazotti M, Greco D, et al. Epidemiology of cholera in Italy in 1973. *Lancet* 1974;2:1370–1381.
2. Blake PA, Martin SM, Gangarosa EJ. Simple case-control studies for determining the mode of transmission of cholera. In Wood PC, ed. *Guide to Shellfish Hygiene*. Geneva, World Health Organization Offset Publication No. 31, 1976:73–77.
3. Blake PA, Rosenberg ML, Costa JB, Ferreira PS, Guimaraes CL, Gangarosa EJ. Cholera in Portugal, 1974. I. Modes of transmission. *Am J Epidemiol* 1977;105:337–343.
4. Blake PA, Rosenberg ML, Florencia J, Costa JB, Quintino LDP, Gangarosa EJ. Cholera in Portugal, 1974. II. Transmission by bottled mineral water. *Am J Epidemiol* 1977;105:344–348.
5. Centers for Disease Control and Prevention. *Health Information for International Travel 2008*. Atlanta: U.S. Department of Health and Human Services, Public Health Service, 2007.
6. Mintz ED, Popovic T, Blake PA. Transmission of *Vibrio cholerae* O1. In Wachsmuth IK, Blake PA, Olsvik O, eds. *Vibrio cholerae and Cholera: Molecular to Global Perspectives*. Washington, DC: American Society for Microbiology, 1994:345–356.

CHAPTER 4

Legionnaires' Disease: Investigation of an Outbreak of a New Disease

Stephen B. Thacker, MD, MSc

INTRODUCTION

Late on a Monday afternoon in 1976, my first day at the Washington, DC health department, I received a telephone call from my supervisor at the Centers for Disease Control (CDC) in Atlanta, Georgia. The Friday before I had completed 3 weeks in Atlanta in an intensive training course for the Epidemic Intelligence Service (EIS) as a field epidemiologist, whose responsibility is to detect and control epidemic disease. An epidemic of what appeared to be pneumonia was occurring in Pennsylvania, and I was to be in Harrisburg early the next morning to join the team that had assembled on Monday. Although a number of cases had been reported and deaths had occurred, all I knew was that the cause of the problem was unknown and that cases were being reported from across the state.

Already, epidemiologists, laboratory scientists, and statisticians were on the team, and they were ultimately joined by specialists in toxicology, pathology, environmental health, and environmental engineering. The major concern initially was the possibility of swine influenza ("swine flu"), as the initial call from a nurse at the Veterans Administration Hospital in

Philadelphia was to the influenza program, which had been established in response to the threat of a new pandemic strain of the virus. Also, because of the concern about biologic terrorism—the nation was celebrating its bicentennial and Pope Paul VI was scheduled to visit the city in August—the state and local police were involved, and investigators from the Federal Bureau of Investigation and the military had been called in to assist.

During the training course, I learned the basic steps of an epidemic investigation.[1] I was to spend the next 3 weeks in Harrisburg and Philadelphia learning on the job how to investigate an epidemic.

THE INVESTIGATION

By the time I arrived in Harrisburg, the number of cases was already in the dozens. The majority of illnesses were among men who had attended a statewide convention of the American Legion in Philadelphia in late July that had been headquartered at the Bellevue-Stratford Hotel, an elegant old building on Broad Street. To determine a baseline and gather evidence about the epidemic, the investigation team had already begun to review death certificate data, hospital data, and visits to emergency rooms for a pneumonia-like illness (Figures 4-1, 4-2, and 4-3).

On that first day, we developed a case definition of the unknown disease, trying to balance concerns about sensitivity and specificity. A case was

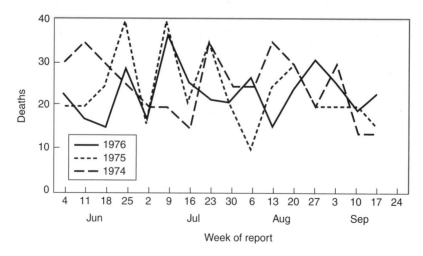

FIGURE 4-1 Pneumonia and influenza deaths, by week of report, Philadelphia, 1974–1976.

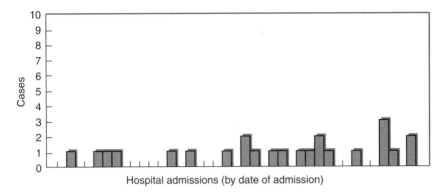

FIGURE 4-2 Illness resembling Legionnaires' disease seen in three center city Philadelphia hospitals July 1–Aug. 9, 1976.

defined as having onset during July 1 to August 18, 1976, of fever and having chest radiograph evidence of pneumonia or temperature of ≥102°F and cough *and* attendance at the American Legion convention on July 21–24, 1976, or entry into the Bellevue-Stratford Hotel since July 1, 1976.

On day 2, I was assigned to interview men and women with the disease, as well as their families, friends, and physicians. I also reviewed clinical and

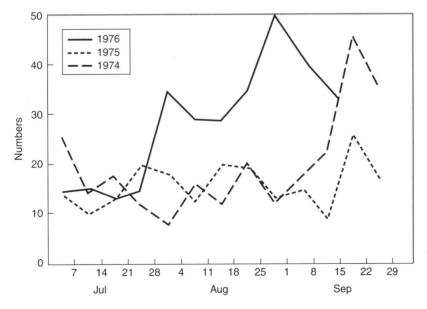

FIGURE 4-3 Emergency room visits for "Pneumonia" in 11 Philadelphia hospitals.

laboratory records as well as pathology and autopsy reports. All of the information was collected on forms developed and copied the night before. EIS officers were sent throughout the state that day to gather information on what was then approximately 50 reports of the disease, and the information was being analyzed by other team members as it came in.

That same day I was introduced to another role of an EIS officer (and anyone else in public health practice)—meeting the press. I had been assigned to room with David Fraser, MD, an EIS alumnus and chief of the CDC's Special Pathogens Branch, who I had met for the first time that day and who was leading the investigation. In the late morning, I received a message to call Dr. Fraser, and between visits to hospitals, we were able to connect. He indicated that he was under pressure to have an EIS officer meet with the media. I was relatively close by, and thus, he asked if I would be willing to meet with a half-dozen members of the media at the community hospital in Chambersburg, about an hour away from Harrisburg. Arriving at Chambersburg about 30 minutes early, I proceeded to the pathology department to review the files on a deceased patient, when I was soon approached by Lawrence Altman, MD, who identified himself as a medical reporter from the *New York Times* and an EIS alumnus. Although not an official member of the press team, he proceeded to ask questions while I spoke with the pathologist and reviewed the records.

When I arrived at the hospital director's conference room, I quickly realized that Dr. Altman's unofficial presence was not well received by the other members of the press and television media. As I reviewed what I was doing, I learned two things: The media really wanted to understand what was going on, and I already knew a substantial amount that would be of help to them without speculating on what might be going on. Afterward, wearing a mask, I proceeded to examine and interview a patient who had been critically ill but was recovering despite the distraction of the media cameras. Mr. Thomas Payne was resting comfortably on his back in a typical hospital bed when I walked in, his left hand behind his head. He was alert and comfortable and seemed less nervous than his physician and the hospital nurse. As with each visit that day, patients, their families, as well as the physicians and hospital staff were friendly and eager to be helpful, clearly looking to me as a representative of CDC and the state health department for help with a perplexing and frightening epidemic. The patient answered the long list of questions that we had developed the night before. Through this visit, I also learned how fearful people were about the disease; the media's reluctance to enter patient rooms exacerbated this fear. After the patient interview, I traveled to the university hospital in Hershey where I visited a patient in intensive care and was met by EIS alumnus Dr. Robert Aber who had recently joined the faculty in infectious disease. Then I returned to Harrisburg to debrief the team.

Beginning the following day, I was asked to maintain the line listing of all confirmed cases on a large wall chart that included epidemiologic, clinical, and laboratory information. At this time, before computers were routinely used in public health investigations, large pieces of poster board and pencil, ink, or a marker worked just as well for this purpose. Each time the team met in the morning and evening the line listing was used to summarize the information gathered to date and to provide a visual backdrop for the investigators as we planned the next investigative steps. Different hypotheses were rapidly generated and tested by the team with the data laid out in this way. Hypotheses ranged from psittacosis (parrot fever) to intentional poisoning.

The descriptive data gathered to determine the existence of the epidemic helped establish the time frame of the outbreak, which is best depicted by an epidemic curve in which all cases are entered by the date of symptom onset (Figure 4-4).[2] Because this was a state convention, cases were displayed on a map divided into American Legion districts, which depicted the geographic scope of the epidemic (Figure 4-5). The epidemic was linked to all four hotels that had housed conventioneers; however, all convention functions had occurred at the Bellevue-Stratford Hotel, and the investigation therefore led to the primary role of that hotel where delegates had spent on average more time (56.5 vs. 51.6 hours). The common site of exposure was the hotel, but no one location within the hotel or any event at the convention was recognized as a unique common exposure.

Analysis of the data collected demonstrated that delegates had higher attack rates than family members and other nondelegates who attended the convention. Men had higher attack rates than women (5.4% vs. 1.9%), and attack rates increased with patient age. It was especially concerning that this was not a mild illness. We were dealing with a pneumonia that killed approximately one of seven patients, despite the use of powerful antibiotics and supportive care. In addition, even persons who had not attended the convention were among the cases. There was a pilot who came in about noon one day, slept a few hours, and then left. There was even an older woman (at least 80 years old) who came in to use the toilet (for about 20 minutes at most) and died a couple of weeks later.

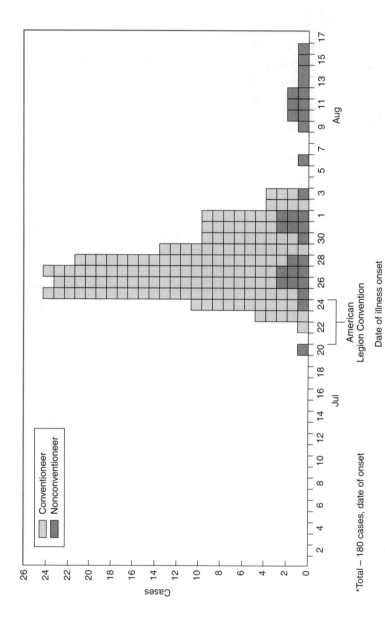

FIGURE 4-4 Legionnaires' disease,* by date of onset, Philadelphia, July 1–August 18, 1976.

From Fraser DW, Tsai TR, Orenstein W, Parkin WE, Beecham HS, Sharrer RG, et al. Legionnaires' disease: description of an epidemic of pneumonia. *N Engl J Med* 1977;297:1189–97. Copyright © 1977 Massachusetts Medical Society. All rights reserved.

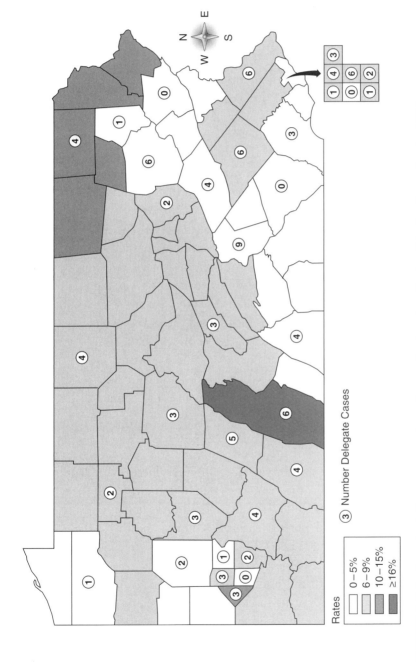

FIGURE 4-5 Legionnaires' disease cases and attack rates, by American Legion District, Pennsylvania, 1976.

Meanwhile, this outbreak had become national news, hitting television news broadcasts as well as the front pages of newspapers and the covers of *Time* and *Newsweek* magazines. Dr. Altman, who had interviewed me on day 2, published a daily *New York Times* column about the investigation. The CDC was already in the limelight because of the threat of a global influenza pandemic, and this attention only intensified when this mysterious outbreak became a political concern during this, a presidential election year. Headlines like the *New York Times'* "20 flu-like deaths in Pennsylvania. 115 ill. A mystery" captured the public's attention.

As previously noted, clearly, delegates to the convention and their families were at risk, but other cases were emerging. One at-risk population included those who had nothing to do with the convention but who had stayed at the hotel at the same time. Eventually, 20 such persons received diagnoses of the disease. Only one case in a hotel employee fit the case definition, although later serologic tests identified a limited number of others with antibodies. Possibly, this younger, healthier employee population was not at high risk. Most interesting were persons with signs and symptoms of the disease who had passed by the hotel but never even entered the facility. Our investigation team nicknamed the illness in these persons as "Broad Street pneumonia," after the street on which the hotel was located, and their data were maintained on a separate line listing. Eventually, data regarding 37 persons were placed on this list, and their illnesses were confirmed. The investigators also looked at conventions that had previously been at the hotel, seeking possible missed cases.

As we intently studied the data brought back by the EIS officers on the second and third days of the investigation, as well as data telephoned in from throughout the state by veterans, clinicians, local health departments, and the general public, the team generated hypotheses about the nature of the illness, risk factors for illness and death, sources of the exposure, modes of transmission, and potential causes. Clinical specimens were already being tested at the state and CDC laboratories for infectious agents and known chemical causes of respiratory disease. During the next weeks, specialists in infectious disease and natural and manmade biologic and chemical toxins were brought in to consult, as were specialists in pathology, environmental engineering, and even biologic and chemical weapons. A CDC engineer collected specimens from all parts of the hotel, including sleeping quarters, convention rooms, offices, the lobby air conditioner, the elevators, and the cooling tower on top of the hotel. Not all locations for sampling were based on epidemiologic data.

The immediate challenge was to design and conduct a case control study to test the multiple hypotheses that were being generated. In addition to the hotel registration records and the relevant hotel floor plans, we obtained the calendar of events for the 3-day convention. We designed a questionnaire that included basic demographic information; such behaviors as smoking, drinking, medication, and drug use; eating practices both in and outside the hotel, including local restaurants and street vendors; water drinking, including sources and amounts; time spent in different parts of the hotel, including the lobby and the elevators; and such potential exposures as pigeons.

After approximately 10 days, the focus of the investigation moved to Philadelphia. The team in Harrisburg was reduced, and some of us traveled to Philadelphia, where we stayed at the Bellevue-Stratford Hotel. As the case control study was being implemented, surveillance continued. More cases were identified. New hypotheses were proposed, and the investigation adapted to the new information. For example, to test the hypothesis that this might be a psittacosis epidemic, a woman regularly observed feeding pigeons near the hotel was interviewed. Because nickel carbonyl was a suspected cause and the metal alloys in use for scalpels and forceps contained nickel, autopsy teams were provided plastic tools.

At the end of 3 weeks, we had described an epidemic that involved more than 220 persons, including 34 deaths. Every known infectious pathogen had been sought, but none was identified. Different toxins and environmental agents had been considered, but none was identified as the causal agent. Hypotheses had been proffered, tested, and rejected. No new cases were being identified, despite active surveillance for disease. We knew a substantial amount about the epidemic, but we had not uncovered what had caused it, why it had happened when it did, why it had happened where it did, and why the Legionnaires and others exposed at the hotel were victims. In summary, the epidemic had ended without our intervention, and we had nothing to recommend specifically to prevent another occurrence. The team returned to their regular jobs but still remained actively engaged in the work both in Pennsylvania and Atlanta.

After any field investigation requested by a state, EIS officers are required to submit a written summary of their work to the state and to the

CDC director. During that fall, a detailed report of the investigation was developed, eventually totaling 71 pages; however, a discovery late in the calendar year delayed publication of the report and marked a turning point in the investigation.

The causal agent was discovered during the Christmas holidays of 1976 when Joseph McDade, PhD, who worked in the CDC's Rickettsial Disease Laboratory, was motivated to reexamine cultures after hearing criticism of the CDC's efforts in the investigation voiced at a party he attended. Hen's eggs are used to culture *Rickettsia*, and as Dr. McDade looked one more time at the egg cultures from the Philadelphia investigation, he noted a consistent contamination among the specimens. The contamination, however, was located only among the specimens from persons with disease, not from the control subjects. This Gram-negative pleomorphic rod turned out not to be a contaminant, but instead, it was the bacterium that caused the epidemic, the first human bacterial pathogen that had been discovered in decades.[3] The pathogen was confirmed as the etiologic agent of the epidemic, including the Broad Street pneumonias.[2,4] It was rapidly linked to unsolved CDC investigations in 1965[5] and 1968[6] and was later identified as the cause of other unsolved epidemics.[7,8]

Isolation of the agent led to a series of groundbreaking publications and, more importantly, provided investigators with clues to sources in the environment and airborne transmission, and ultimately uncovered the means to detect, control, and treat the disease. In fact, I was asked to review a large cardboard box full of files from 1965 and to write up the unsolved investigation of an epidemic of pneumonia at a chronic disease hospital in Washington, DC, where I was assigned as the EIS officer. It turned out this 1965 epidemic was an unsolved Legionnaires' outbreak. Legionnaires' disease has now been recognized as a much more common cause of illness, resulting in an estimated 20,000 cases of pneumonia each year. It is spread through the air and has been identified in such places as cooling towers, fresh water, and shower heads. It is also treatable with antibiotics that were available at the time of the investigation.

The approach to this groundbreaking epidemic differs little from the standard approach to any epidemic. The size and scope of the investigation, as well as the publicity surrounding it, serve to dramatize the challenging and important work undertaken every day by the practicing epidemiologist in the field. It also underscores the reality of the critical roles that members of the public health team play at every step of the investigation—from recognition of the problem to control of the epidemic and publication of the results.

PERSONAL REFLECTIONS

This investigation introduced me to the application of epidemiology to real problems in public health. My experience as an EIS officer led to a career in epidemiology and public health at the CDC (now the Centers for Disease Control and Prevention). At the CDC, I have had the opportunity to apply the tools of epidemiology to a range of public health problems, including not only infectious diseases (e.g., the initial studies of AIDS), but also toxic chemicals in the environment (e.g., dioxin exposures of soldiers and childhood lead poisoning), environmental disasters, violence and unintentional injuries, as well as chronic conditions (e.g., breast cancer and heart disease).

As the director of the CDC's epidemiology program since 1989, I have been involved in critical public health problems, including the discovery of hantavirus pulmonary syndrome in the southwestern United States, introduction of West Nile virus to the United States and its spread across the country, the emergence of the *Escherichia coli* O157:H7 bacterium as the cause of local and national epidemics, the response to the threat of Ebola virus in Central Africa, and the impending crisis of antibiotic resistance. Recently, the epidemics of severe acute respiratory syndrome (SARS), monkeypox, and avian influenza have engaged CDC epidemiologists throughout the world. The health effects of disasters, most dramatically the 2004 tsunami in Asia and Hurricanes Katrina and Rita in the United States in 2005, but also earthquakes in Central America, drought and starvation in Africa, and refugee crises related to other natural disasters and war, have involved CDC epidemiologists. Any of the leading causes of morbidity, mortality, and disability have been subject to the analytic insights of epidemiologists for both understanding the processes leading to disease and injury and for implementing effective prevention programs.

On the afternoon of September 11, 2001, a CDC team was flown from Atlanta to assist the New York City Department of Health and Mental Hygiene in responding to the tragedy of the World Trade Center terrorist attack. Included on that team were two EIS officers who were assigned to establish that night a surveillance system at ground zero to document as rapidly as possible the health consequences for both victims and workers;

their immediate actions helped target New York City's emergency response. By Friday of that week, an additional team of EIS officers were flown to the city to establish a surveillance system in 17 city hospitals to monitor the effects of the attack and to look for disease related to chemical or biologic terrorism.

On October 4, 2001, the EIS officer assigned to the Florida Department of Health was joined by the CDC staff to assist the state in investigating a case of anthrax in a 63-year-old man in Boca Raton, the first known victim of anthrax transmitted through the U.S. mail. Epidemiologists became involved in surveillance and investigation activities throughout the United States and countries around the world. All 140 EIS officers became involved, with 133 being deployed away from their assignment for weeks during the response.

Epidemiology has been called the basic science of public health. The tools of the epidemiologist help investigators extract useful information from complex data that leads to effective public health action. The work is challenging and can sometimes be risky. The rewards, however, are sizable, as one uses the best available science to work with others in addressing the major health problems that face the world's population. Although not all of my work has been as dramatic as my first investigation in Philadelphia, the gratification of seeing improvements in health stemming from the efforts of epidemiologists at the CDC and elsewhere around the world is enormous.

REFERENCES

1. Gregg MB. Conducting a field investigation. In Gregg MB, ed. *Field Epidemiology*, 2nd ed. New York, NY: Oxford University Press, 2002:62–67.
2. Fraser DWD, Tsai TR, Orenstein W, et al. Legionnaires' disease: description of an epidemic of pneumonia. *N Engl J Med* 1977;297:1189–1197.
3. McDade JE, Shepard CC, Fraser DW, et al. Legionnaires' disease: isolation of a bacterium and demonstration of its role in other respiratory disease. *N Engl J Med* 1977;297:1197–1203.
4. Chandler FW, Hicklin MD, Blackmon JA. Demonstration of the agent of Legionnaires' disease in tissue. *N Engl J Med* 1977;297:1218–1220.
5. Thacker SB, Bennett JV, Tsai TF, et al. An outbreak in 1965 of severe respiratory illness caused by the Legionnaires' disease bacterium. *J Infect Dis* 1978;138:512–519.

6. Glick TH, Gregg MB, Berman B, et al. Pontiac fever: an epidemic of unknown etiology in a health department. I. Clinical and epidemiological aspects. *Am J Epidemiol* 1978;107:149–160.
7. Terranova W, Cohen ML, Fraser DW. 1974 outbreak of Legionnaires' disease diagnosed in 1977: clinical and epidemiologic features. *Lancet* 1978;2:122–124.
8. Osterholm MT, Chin TDY, Osborne DO, et al. A 1957 outbreak of Legionnaires' disease associated with a meat packing plant. *Am J Epidemiol* 1983; 117:60–67.

CHAPTER 5

The Investigation of Toxic Shock Syndrome in Wisconsin, 1979–1980 and Beyond

Jeffrey P. Davis, MD

INTRODUCTION

In early December 1979, I had just completed my first 13 months of employment after joining the (later renamed) Wisconsin Division of Health (DOH) as the State Epidemiologist and Chief of the Section of Acute and Communicable Disease Epidemiology (ACDE). During the 5 years before beginning my tenure in the DOH, I served as an Epidemic Intelligence Service (EIS) officer assigned as a field services officer to the South Carolina Department of Health and Environmental Control and then completed the third year of my pediatrics residency and a pediatric infectious diseases fellowship at Duke University. All were formative experiences that resulted in the shaping of my career as an infectious diseases physician focused on infectious diseases epidemiology using applied methods.

In addition to wonderful staff in categorically funded programs (immunization, sexually transmitted diseases, and tuberculosis), the ACDE section included three general epidemiologists, all of whom were newly hired: Martin LaVenture, Wendy Schell, and me. Although few in number, my epi team colleagues were young, bright, and eager. I actually interviewed

Marty during my first visit to the DOH during the recruitment process for my position. Although this would be considered unusual procedure, I remember thinking that they better take my advice and hire this guy. Wendy was already in the state system as an employee at the State Laboratory of Hygiene.

The probationary period for a new employee with supervisory responsibilities was 12 months, but those 12 months flew by rapidly. Our epi team revised reporting procedures, developed a new reporting form in triplicate (copies for the local health department, DOH, and the patient's medical record), began publication of the *Wisconsin Epidemiology Bulletin*, and planned and conducted training activities. The media became interested in our investigations and recommendations as a result of the *Wisconsin Epidemiology Bulletin* distribution to 7,000 physicians, public health professionals, and media representatives.

During July and August 1979, I was directing our epi team's first large-scale investigation, which involved an outbreak of 13 cases of Legionnaires' disease in Eau Claire. After an intensive several days of initial and hypothesis generating investigation by our team that focused us on a likely source of a cooling tower on the roof of a hotel, I invited a team from the CDC to join us in an epidemic aid (Epi-Aid) investigation to help determine the extent of the outbreak and the precise mechanism of transmission of *Legionella* from the associated cooling tower. The outbreak occurrence and investigation was very visible, particularly after the CDC team arrived, and our interactions with the media were daily and generally at the same time each day, which was a valuable process. The investigation involved my first experiences with using credit card receipts as a case finding tool, isolating *Legionella pneumophila* from an environmental source (cooling tower water), and watching the application of air tracer studies to provide information regarding where the cooling tower aerosols went. In this case, it was used to demonstrate the inadvertent intake of the cooling tower exhaust down a chimney with an open damper and into a meeting room via the fireplace.[1] It was quite exciting to be involved with the successful application of these neat techniques. Our investigation team was thrilled that their epidemiologic data were supported by the laboratory findings.

In 1979, the report of a cluster of three cases of Lyme disease occurring in 1978 in individuals who cleared brush at a site in Washburn County in northwestern Wisconsin represented the first known cluster of Lyme disease to occur west of the Eastern seaboard.[2] Dick Kaslow, who at the time was working at the National Institute of Allergy and Infectious Diseases, and I initiated surveys of the distribution of *Ixodes dammini* (at that time considered to be the vector of the agent that caused Lyme disease) and another established prevalent tick (used as a control) on white tailed deer. The survey involved our epi team and additional National Institute of Allergy and Infectious Diseases, Wisconsin Department of Natural Resources, and Rocky Mountain Laboratory colleagues and numerous volunteers willing to pick ticks off of freshly killed deer at the beginning of the deer hunting season. This represented a different type of challenge: a collaborative, multiagency investigation involving detailed prospective planning. We completed the field work of our first of four surveys (1979–1982) in 1979[3] shortly after Thanksgiving and were working on shipping live ticks to Willy Burgdorfer at the Rocky Mountain Laboratory for speciation and with the intent to establish tick colonies to look for the causative agent of Lyme disease.

In the midst of this phase of our Lyme disease work, I was called by a resident in the Department of Pediatrics, University of Wisconsin Medical School, on behalf of Joan Chesney who was a colleague of mine, regarding two currently hospitalized young women from Madison with rapid onset of fever, rash, and hypotension among other findings, including acute renal failure. Joan was an infectious diseases specialist, and her husband, Russ Chesney, was a nephrologist. Both were faculty in the University of Wisconsin Department of Pediatrics and consulted on these cases from their different clinical perspectives. In essence, Joan had seen a patient with high fever, hypotension, and a rash who had acute renal failure, and Russ had seen a patient with acute renal failure who had high fever, hypotension, and a rash. While serendipitously discussing details of their cases during a dinner at home, they concluded these patients may have toxic shock syndrome (TSS), although neither had previously seen a case. After speaking with the resident, I called Joan, and she provided me with more clinical details of these two cases and told me about a third case, also in a currently hospitalized individual.

Although first reported in the 1920s, TSS is a condition initially described and named by Jim Todd of the University of Colorado and his colleagues in an article published in the *Lancet* in 1978.[4] They described a severe acute disease associated with strains of *Staphylococcus aureus* of phage group I that produced a unique epidermal toxin. His series involved seven children, 8 to 17 years old who presented between June 1975 and November

1977 with sudden onset of high fever, headache, sore throat, diarrhea, and erythroderma (a diffuse sunburn-like rash) with associated findings of acute renal failure, hepatic abnormalities, and confusion. All had refractory hypotension. One patient died, and each survivor had desquamation (peeling of the skin) of the hands and feet during convalescence.

THE OUTBREAK

Fortunately, I was familiar with TSS before publication of the article by Todd and his colleagues. I had participated in the care of an extremely ill adolescent female with TSS while I was a pediatric ID fellow in the Department of Pediatrics at Duke University. I told Joan that I felt the current three patients' clinical and laboratory findings were highly consistent with TSS. I recalled that Jim Todd's series involved sporadic cases accumulated over a prolonged period, at least 2 years. In the absence of any existing surveillance for TSS to use to estimate the expected number of cases, the Todd article was used to judge whether this was an outbreak (even if it involved only two cases at the time). I concluded that this was likely a departure from an expected number of cases because of the rarity of this condition and apparent clustering of cases in time and space. An immediate field investigation began. The next day Bill Taylor, an EIS field officer assigned to the Wisconsin DOH, and I interviewed the three patients and reviewed their medical records in an effort to begin the process of understanding host and risk factors and generating a hypothesis. We asked about a variety of work, exercise, and social activities, social venues, restaurants visited, where their groceries were purchased, whether they had traveled, and many other things. Apart from Madison-area residence, the only readily apparent common factor among these patients was being a young woman. I was struck by this. I wondered whether any of these three patients had onset of illness during menstruation. I recalled that at multiple junctures during my training I was taught of the importance of the often overlooked menstrual history, which could provide important clues regarding a variety of disease processes. Naturally, the medical records of the three patients did not contain this information, but additional interviews of the patients revealed all three had their illness onsets during a menstrual period. I immediately thought this was more than a coincidence. An aggressive case finding surveillance was established and began expeditiously.

Local surveillance was facilitated in part by Joan Chesney's contacts with hospital colleagues and a grand rounds presentation made by Joan and me. Surveillance in four Madison hospitals generated four more cases by early January 1980. All seven cases occurred since July 1979 in women. Six were menstruating at illness onset, and one premenarchal adolescent had infected figure skating-induced blisters. Of note, two had similar but milder illnesses during prior menstrual periods, suggesting that the syndrome could recur. I generated a case report form that included data on demographic features, clinical findings, clinical management and course of illness, presence and course of recurrences, and laboratory data. The form was also used to collect data on potential risk factors that included presence of skin lesions and detailed information on menstruation (onset, duration, intensity) and factors related to menstruation (catamenial and oral contraceptive product use).

Because of the striking severity and novelty of this syndrome, I prepared a mailing sent on January 31, 1980, to 3,500 internists, pediatricians, and family practice physicians licensed in Wisconsin to inform them of TSS and the currently reported case illnesses, provide management recommendations based on what we knew about these first seven case patients, establish statewide TSS surveillance with expeditious reporting to DOH, and generate appropriate specimens for culture and serologic testing to be sent to the Wisconsin State Laboratory of Hygiene (WSLH) for processing (Exhibit 5-1).[5]

Concurrently, I called Merlin Bergdoll at the University of Wisconsin Food Research Institute to discuss whether TSS could be caused by a staphylococcal enterotoxin. Merlin was the foremost authority on staphylococcal enterotoxins, and his lab was just a few miles away from our offices. At that time, there were five known staphylococcal enterotoxins (A-E), which were heat stable and primarily known for their ability to cause foodborne illnesses. Merlin thought a staphylococcal enterotoxin would be a good candidate and was most willing to collaborate and test specimens from case patients.

While expanding TSS surveillance in Wisconsin, I received a call one Sunday in January 1980 from Andy Dean, the State Epidemiologist in Minnesota. Andy learned of five cases, two cases initially and a subsequent three cases, in women hospitalized with an unusual acute illness. I said, "Let me describe it to you," which I did. The illness I described was identical to those occurring in Minnesota. Andy asked what the illness was.

Exhibit 5-1   The Initial Memorandum on TSS Mailed to Physicians in
Wisconsin on January 31, 1980

State of Wisconsin/Department of Health and Social Services
January 31, 1980

TO:	Physician in the State of Wisconsin
FROM:	Jeffrey P. Davis, MD State Epidemiologist and Chief Section of Epidemiologic Surveillance and Assessment
SUBJECT:	Toxic Shock Syndrome

The detailed information which is to follow is intended to describe a clinical entity which has recently been seen in patients in Wisconsin. The information is detailed as certain physicians in the state may not be familiar with this entity. Most physicians that will take care of such cases will manage them in a tertiary care setting. I feel that a broad description of the illness might stimulate a higher index of suspicion, facilitate any needed referrals, and enhance reporting of these cases and the communication involved with management of these patients.

Between July, 1979 and January 6, 1980 seven patients with a syndrome of toxic shock have been directly hospitalized in or transferred to Madison area hospitals. All seven patients have been women between the ages of 14 and 44, and all but one have been between the ages of 14 and 28. Each of these patients had a strong similarity in clinical onset and in clinical course, a composite clinical description follows:

Onset:	high fever (39–41 degrees C)
	vomiting (profound)
	watery diarrhea (profuse)
	headache
	myalgias that may include abdominal guarding
	sore throat
	confusion
	the onset seems to be associated with an ongoing menstrual period
Admission findings:	shock that is seemingly refractory requiring dopamine or other agents and massive fluid therapy
	acute renal failure (oliguria and azotemia with elevated creatinine)
	proteinuria
	elevated serum glutamic-oxaloacetic transaminase, serum glutamic-pyruvic transaminase, LDH, bilirubin
	prolonged protime
	hypoalbuminemia
	rhabdomyolysis (extreme elevations of serum CPK)
	leukocytosis with predominance of bands and juvenile forms (extreme shift to the left)
	thrombocytopenia
	anemia—at first seemingly hemolytic
	blood cultures are sterile

Additional manifestations:	diffuse erythematous, nonpruritic scarlatiniform rash (erythroderma) prominent on the trunk and extremities
	early fine desquamation and late peripheral desquamation
	nonpitting, subcutaneous edema
	vaginitis
	conjunctivitis, several with hemorrhages
	stomatitis, several with vesicles
	mild jaundice
	evidence if DIC in several patients
Further supportive measures:	one patient required dialysis
	three patients had evidence of the adult respiratory distress syndrome, and one required ventilatory assistance
	one patient required a D and C to control vaginal bleeding
Outcome:	All seven patients have recovered

The five patients with onsets since late November 1979 have all had staphylococci recovered from either a mucosal site (throat, NP, or vagina) or a sequestered site; further studies of toxigenicity are pending. Two of these five patients have had herpes simplex virus type I isolated from throat or oral lesion cultures; the others have had multiple site viral cultures during the acute phase of the illness which were negative. Studies of paired sera completed in two patients have been negative for antibodies to a broad series of respiratory viruses and coxsackie B viruses are pending.

A clinical entity that is identical to that just described has been reported by Todd et al in 1978 (*Lancet*; 1116–1118, November 25, 1978). Todd reported seven cases ranging from 8 to 17 years of age, all of whom had isolates of staphylococci from mucosal or sequestered sites that were noted to produce an exfoliative exotoxin (a unique epidermal toxin detected by a positive Nikolsky sign in neonatal mice). Viral cultures completed on five of these patients were negative, but the sites cultured were not stated. Each of the toxigenic strains of staphylococci were phage group I organisms. The entity was called a toxic shock syndrome-associated phage group I staphylococci. In Todd's series, five patients recovered, one patient had gangrene of the toes, and one patient died.

All seven of the patients in Wisconsin have recovered. Each of the five most recent patients has received specific antistaphylococcal antibiotic therapy as part of broad spectrum antibiotic coverage. It appears that clinical improvement has been noted after the initiation of specific antistaphylococcal therapy. This is not to say that these Wisconsin patients had toxic shock syndrome-associated with staphylococci, the diagnosis is suspected but has not been proven. Other etiologies must still be considered as potentially associated with this syndrome.

Among other diseases to consider in the differential diagnosis as bacterial sepsis; severe systemic viral infections associated with adenovirus, coxsackie B virus, herpes virus, or other viruses; Kawasaki disease (mucocutaneous lymph node syndrome); hemolytic uremic syndrome; ingestion of preformed staphylococcal enterotoxin or other exogenous toxin; and other staphylococcal syndromes. This does not represent a comprehensive list.

While the current series of Wisconsin patients are all women, the entity may not be limited to women. Males have been reported to experience this syndrome and they tend to be in the pediatric age range with evidence of focal staphylococcal disease prior to the onset of these symptoms.

(*continues*)

Exhibit 5-1   (Continued)

Recommendations:

A. Laboratory

We strongly suggest the following laboratory studies to further investigate the possibility of toxic shock syndrome and its association with staphylococci or with other etiologic agent.

1. Bacterial cultures:

   Nasopharynx and anterior nares, trachea, vagina, stool, urine, blood, and focal lesions. Blood cultures have been uniformly negative in TSS, but are needed to rule out bacterial sepsis.

   Please have your laboratory save each separate colony type of any coagulase positive or coagulase negative staphylococcus isolated from any cultured site from any patient in whom toxic shock is considered. Please call Dr. Jeffrey Davis or Dr. William Taylor at the Bureau of Prevention, 608/266-1251 to inform us of such isolates. Further arrangements will then be made with the State Laboratory of Hygiene to facilitate further studies.

2. Viral Cultures:

   These are needed to rule out the possibility of a wide range of systemic viral etiologic agents disease. Suggested sites include respiratory (throat or nasopharynx), stool, lesion cultures (most likely to be oral or genital), vagina, and urine. Please forward all material for viral isolation to the Viral Laboratory, State Laboratory of Hygiene.

3. Serum:

   Acute and convalescent phase sera are needed to diagnose viral disease and potentially screen for the presence of staphylococcal exotoxin and any potential antibody to such a toxin. Please obtain the following specimens:

   1. acute phase—as soon as possible after admission;
   2. 14 days after onset;
   3. one month after onset.

   Please obtain at least 5 cc of serum per specimen. Forward all serum specimens to the Viral Laboratory, State Laboratory of Hygiene.

Please indicate on any specimens that are sent to the State Laboratory of Hygiene that you are interested in ruling out toxic shock syndrome. Please provide the requested clinical information.

B. Management

Because the syndrome has been associated with staphylococci, institution of empiric antistaphylococcal therapy with a penicillinase-resistant penicillin or another appropriate antistaphylococcal antibiotic as part of broad spectrum coverage seems warranted as part of the patients' management. Patients in our series placed on specific antistaphylococcal regimens have demonstrated clinical improvement, but it is not clear how significant antistaphylococcal therapy is relative to other components of supportive therapy. Full attention to ruling out all clinical possibilities and maintaining full supportive management is stressed.

C. Reporting

Please call Dr. Jeffrey Davis (Wisconsin Division of Health, Bureau of Prevention) 608/266-1251 or Dr. William Taylor 608/266-1251 or 608/266-9783 as soon as you become clinically aware of any potential case of toxic shock syndrome. If you recall seeing a similar case at any point in time in the past we would greatly appreciate learning of such cases. Please feel free to call if you have any questions pertaining to any facet of this syndrome.

Further information as it becomes available will appear in the *Wisconsin Epidemiology Bulletin*.

I said that it was TSS and further described our cases, the association with menstruation, and the potential for recurrence. By the next day, these 12 cases from the two states were reported to CDC by Andy and me.

In February 1980, while planning an initial case control study, I called Jim Todd, the chief of pediatric infectious diseases at the University of Colorado Medical School, to discuss our findings. My call to him must have seemed as though it came out of left field. By then Jim knew of 35 cases from multiple states that occurred since 1975. These included 25 females with a mean age of 20 years of whom 20 had vaginitis and 10 males with a mean age of 11 years of whom 7 had focal bacterial infections. All had toxigenic strains of *S. aureus* isolated; however, one third were not associated with the unique epidermal toxin noted in his initial report and one third involved nonphage group I *S. aureus*. Jim had not studied risk factors. He could recall only one potential recurrence, and he agreed that a case control study to examine risk factors was needed.

In February 1980, Kathy Shands, an EIS officer in the Special Pathogens Branch, began the CDCs work on TSS by collaborating to generate a clinical case definition with Jim Todd and Neil Halsey of the University of Colorado, Mike Osterholm of the Minnesota DOH, and me.[6] At that time, Mike was an assistant state epidemiologist who had been investigating the Minnesota TSS cases. By April, we concurred on the case definition criteria, which became very durable in its application over time (Table 5-1).[7]

Fortunately, the response to our January 30 mailing was rapid and dramatic, particularly by physicians. After subsequent publication of my office phone number in a newspaper article about TSS by Neil Rosenberg of the *Milwaukee Journal*, a widely circulated newspaper, a large number of cases were self-reported (parenthetically, Neil developed a keen interest in TSS

Table 5-1   TSS Case Definition

Clinical Case Definition

An illness with the following clinical manifestations:

Fever: temperature greater than or equal to 38.9°C (102.0°F)

Rash: diffuse macular erythroderma

Desquamation: 1 to 2 weeks after onset of illness, particularly on the palms and soles

Hypotension: systolic blood pressure less than or equal to 90 mm Hg for adults or less than fifth percentile by age for children aged less than16 years; orthostatic drop in diastolic blood pressure greater than or equal to 15 mm Hg from lying to sitting, orthostatic syncope, or orthostatic dizziness

Multisystem involvement (three or more of the following):

> *Gastrointestinal*: vomiting or diarrhea at onset of illness
>
> *Muscular*: severe myalgia or creatine phosphokinase level at least twice the upper limit of normal
>
> *Mucous membrane*: vaginal, oropharyngeal, or conjunctival hyperemia
>
> *Renal*: blood urea nitrogen or creatinine at least twice the upper limit of normal for laboratory or urinary sediment with pyuria (greater than or equal to 5 leukocytes per high-power field) in the absence of urinary tract infection
>
> *Hepatic*: total bilirubin, serum glutamic-oxaloacetic transaminase, or serum glutamic-pyruvic transaminase at least twice the upper limit of normal for laboratory
>
> *Hematologic*: platelets less than 100,000/mm^3
>
> *Central nervous system*: disorientation or alterations in consciousness without focal neurologic signs when fever and hypotension are absent

Negative results on the following tests, if obtained:

> Blood, throat, or cerebrospinal fluid cultures (blood culture may be positive for *S. aureus*)
>
> Rise in titer to Rocky Mountain spotted fever, leptospirosis, or measles

Case classification

Probable: a case with five of the six clinical findings described previously here

Confirmed: a case with all six of the clinical findings described above, including desquamation, unless the patient dies before desquamation could occur

---

From Wharton M, Chorba TL, Vogt RL, et al. Case definitions for public health surveillance. *MMWR* 1990;39(RR-13):1–43.

and Lyme disease). We received numerous physician generated and self-reports of potential cases and laboratory specimens. Clinical and laboratory data were systematically collected using a case report form that I had generated. Line lists were created and maintained using long-hand entry—

no computers yet. Phil Wand, a bacteriologist at the WSLH, received all submitted subcultures of *S. aureus* isolates from mucous membranes of case patients to characterize, split for Dr. Bergdoll's laboratory and also stored at the WSLH. In addition, he stored paired samples of sera from case patients for future testing. It is always critical to anticipate future testing, and storing isolates and paired sera is most valuable. A very large bank of specimens evolved.

I also received numerous calls from physicians in other states who had read or heard of our mailing and wanted to discuss suspect cases and send clinical specimens to the WSLH for processing. I reported confirmed cases of TSS to Kathy at the CDC, as did other state epidemiologists. National surveillance was initially established after a description of TSS and its recent occurrence in an *MMWR* article published on May 23, 1980.[8] Fifty-five cases had been reported to the CDC, including 31 cases from Wisconsin; 95% of cases occurred in women, and 95% of 40 women with known histories had onsets during menses. The case fatality rate was 13% among all cases, but it was 3.2% among the 31 cases in Wisconsin where surveillance had been heightened for more than 4 months and 25% among 24 cases occurring in other states. This difference can be explained in part by rapid dissemination of extensive clinical and epidemiologic information to a broad group of stakeholders who included physicians, infection control practitioners, public health partners, and the media. The letter to physicians was particularly important because it had detailed description of the illnesses and known risk factors, which facilitated rapid disease recognition, including recognition of milder cases. These materials also included detailed recommendations for patient management, which facilitated rapid and appropriate clinical management that in turn enhanced outcomes and reduced mortality.

After publication of this *MMWR* article, reporting of TSS continued to be voluntary and passive, and it was further heightened by media coverage, enthusiasm regarding a newly described condition, and concern regarding its severity. Indeed, the national media response to this *MMWR* article was intense. Shortly thereafter, a group of CDC-based EIS officers, including Kathy Shands, George Schmid, Bruce Dan, and Debbie Blum supervised by Dave Fraser (who previously directed the CDC's initial investigation of Legionnaires' disease) and John Bennett, officially became the CDC TSS Task Force. During ensuing months, they would be joined by many others.

THE INITIAL WISCONSIN CASE CONTROL STUDY AND CLINICAL AND LABORATORY FINDINGS

Facilitated by the strong response to our mailing and the reporting of cases that met criteria in our case definition, I planned and we (our epi team) conducted a case control study in Wisconsin during winter and early spring 1980. Each case patient was matched to three gynecology clinic patients as controls. These controls had to be not more than 2 years of age younger or older than their respective case patients and had to be non-pregnant at the time of survey administration. All participants were Wisconsin residents. Based on information from case reports and my phone conversations with case patients, their physicians, and Joan, I created a survey instrument. This survey was used to examine potential risk factors and host factors and hypotheses, including demographic features (marital status, other), characteristics of menstruation (flow duration and intensity), catamenial products (tampons, napkins, pads) used during menstruation (including type and brand, deodorant containing or not), exertion and its extent, birth control and contraceptive methods used, and presence of herpes infection. Because all patients, except for two, had TSS associated with menstruation, the survey was focused on menstrual TSS. In late spring, we balanced the concern about the need for a sufficiently large population to assess adequately differences in the use of commonly used products with the need for important information on risk factors of a serious widespread illness. I conducted a preliminary analysis of case control data to help inform discussions of menstrual TSS occurrence. At that time, nearly all women (30 of 31 [97%]) with confirmed menstrual TSS used tampons during every menstrual period compared with a significantly smaller proportion of controls (71 of 93 [76%], $P < 0.01$). This significant difference demonstrated the initial association of tampon use with menstrual TSS occurrence.

Our study inclusive of cases with onsets through June 30, 1980, was published in the *New England Journal of Medicine*.[5] Among 38 cases meeting our case definition, 37 occurred after January 1, 1979. Thirty seven occurred in women, and 35 case illnesses had onsets during menses. We found the median time from the onset of menses to the onset of illness was 3 days (mode, 2 days; range, 0 to 9 days). Among the women with nonmenstrual TSS, one was the premenarchal girl with *S. aureus* skin lesions on her heels, and the other was a patient who had undergone menopause 5 years earlier, was bleeding from a dilation and curettage procedure performed 10 days prior to onset, and was using tampons at the onset. One patient (2.6%) died. All case patients were white. Although the minority population proportion in Wisconsin was relatively small at the time, this complete absence of minorities among the case patients was a striking finding.[5]

We found that 34 of 35 case patients (97.1%) versus 80 of 105 controls (76.2%) used tampons during every menstrual period ($P < 0.01$) (Table 5-2), findings virtually identical to those noted in the preliminary analysis. Our analysis of tampon brand data did not implicate a specific brand. We also found the practice of contraception (any method) was protective (9 of 35 cases vs. 64 or 105 controls, $P < 0.001$), and this difference remained significant when the rates were adjusted for marital status. Additionally, fewer case patients used oral contraceptives (6 of 35 vs. 38 of 105 controls, $P < 0.10$), but no single method accounted for the difference. We waxed eloquently on the meaning of this finding in our discussion that included the difference in marital status (34% of case patients were married vs. 49% of controls). We also discussed the physiology of oral contraceptives but did not understand its role.[5]

Another important finding arose when I analyzed (the old-fashioned way with calculator and pencil and paper) the clinical and laboratory data. Only 1 of 19 women who received beta-lactamase–resistant antibiotics (principally antistaphylococcal penicillins such as oxacillin, methicillin, and cloxacillin) during management of their first episode had recurrences of TSS within the ensuing 2 months compared with more than half (9 of 13) the women not receiving such antibiotics ($P = 0.0002$).[5] Similar findings were noted when the analysis involved treatment during any episode of TSS. Besides a means to prevent recurrences by encouraging the treatment of this condition with these beta-lactamase resistant antibiotics, this provided indirect evidence that staphylococci were involved in the etiology of TSS. More directly, however, 74% of 23 women tested before antibiotic treatment had *S. aureus* isolated from vaginal or cervical sites, far greater than rates of 0% to 17% cited in previously published colonization studies of healthy women.[5]

In addition to recommending treatment with beta-lactamase resistant antibiotics during the initial and recurrent episodes of TSS, we recommended that until the association of TSS was further clarified, the avoidance of tampon use for at least several menstrual cycles by women who had

Table 5-2 Results of a Case Control Study to Evaluate Potential Risk Factors for TSS Associated with Menses

Characteristic	Cases	Controls	Chi-Square*	P Value†
Number	35	105	—	—
Mean age (yr)	24.1 ± 8.6	24.8 ± 8.0	—	NS‡
Married (no.)	12	51	3.06	NS
Menses				
Flow duration (days)	5.38 ± 1.3	5.18 ± 1.4	—	NS‡
Flow intensity (no. moderate)	22	74	0.65	NS
Birth control				
Using any method	9	64	11.70	< 0.001
Using oral contraceptives	6	38	3.58	0.05 < P < 0.10
Married only: use of any method	5/12	38/51	—	0.028§
Physical exertion pattern, moderate to active**	22	66	0.00	NS
Tampon or napkin use				
Case episode period vs control pattern††	34	80	7.56	< 0.01
Deodorant tampon use	7	32	1.53	NS
Napkin usage (case episodes vs. control pattern)	6	17	0.02	NS

* The Mantel-Haenszel method for multiple controls was used unless otherwise specified.
† NS, not significant.
‡ Statistical inference for two means, unpaired core.
§ Fisher's exact test.
** "Moderate to active" denotes that a person participates in at least two vigorous exercise activities per week.
†† Number of cases using tampons during the menstrual period associated with an episode of TSS versus number of controls who always use tampons during menstrual periods.

From Davis JP, Chesney PJ, Wand PJ, LaVenture M, Investigation and Laboratory Team. Toxic-shock syndrome: epidemiologic features, recurrence, risk factors and prevention. *N Engl J Med* 1980;303:1429–1435, Copyright (c)1980 Massachusetts Medical Society. All rights reserved.

TSS was warranted. We recognized the need for a broader recommendation as well and advised that women who have not had TSS might reduce their probability of having an episode of TSS even further by minimizing their use of tampons.[5]

We also reported results of state and university laboratory testing of isolates of *S. aureus* from 15 patients with TSS (11 with cervical or vaginal isolates) that demonstrated 11 to be resistant to penicillin or ampicillin but sensitive to other antibiotics. Eleven were lysed by group I bacteriophages, including 10 lysed by phage 29, and 7 of 13 produced enterotoxins A or C, whereas 6 produced none of the known enterotoxins A–E.[5] These data indicated a unifying causative toxin had not yet been detected; however, more than half of these bacterial isolates produced enterotoxins that were already known to enhance susceptibility to lethal shock. I felt confident that Merlin and his laboratory team would soon isolate the causative toxin of TSS.

Parallel to our epidemiologic and laboratory investigations was a comprehensive examination of the clinical manifestations of TSS. Joan was the lead of this clinical investigation that involved a series of 22 cases of TSS among 22 women hospitalized in Madison during August 1977 through September 1980. This study provided an extraordinary compendium of the presence, emergence, and course of the many specific clinical features and laboratory alterations of TSS and an assessment of its clinical management.[9] During our TSS investigations, I was communicating almost daily with Joan regarding our findings, and virtually every conversation was marked with the observation of a new, previously unknown clinical or epidemiologic feature. Although we were working extraordinary hours for such a lengthy time and would expect to generate new information, we were amazed at the rapidity of the emergence of so much new information.

For example, before this outbreak, it had not been recognized that patients with TSS typically develop hypocalcemia (a low calcium level in their blood). Some of the other previously undescribed features of TSS noted in this study included hypophosphatemia, hyponatremia, hypocholesterolemia, lymphocytopenia, hypoferrinemia, vulvar cellulitis, and a disorder called telogen effluvium that is hair and nail loss occurring when the patient is convalescing.[9] These findings and associated data in the study were important to the development of the criteria in the TSS case definition. Members of our team and academic colleagues at the University of Wisconsin were also involved with a variety of associated specific studies focused on many of the clinical criteria noted in the TSS case definition.[10–12] All of the significant findings in our early studies, whether positive or negative, were valuable and lead to additional focused collaborative studies involving our epi team to understand further risk and host factors associated with TSS occurrence.

THE CDC CASE CONTROL STUDIES

In June 1980, the use of tampons as a risk factor for TSS was corroborated in a case control study (CDC-1) involving 52 cases and 52 age- and gender-matched acquaintance controls conducted by the CDC TSS Task Force and colleagues. This study did not include cases occurring in Wisconsin, Minnesota, or Utah, and it included only one case among those reported in the May *MMWR* article. All 50 case patients with onsets during menstruation used tampons compared to 86% of 50 controls.[13] Among other findings, the CDC study also showed no significant differences in tampon brand use, and 94% of 17 women with pretreatment specimens had vaginal cultures positive for *S. aureus*.

In a separate, smaller case control study conducted in Utah by Bob Latham, Mark Kehrberg, and colleagues, all 12 cases and 80% of 40 neighborhood-matched controls used tampons. A trend was demonstrated, but it was not statistically significant.[14]

Because of the common use of tampons among young women and the association of tampon use with TSS, the number of persons possibly at risk for TSS was huge. Thus, this was an extremely important public health issue. In late June, officials from each tampon manufacturer in the United States traveled to Atlanta to be advised of all case control study findings by CDC staff and me. An article presenting updated TSS surveillance data and findings of the CDC, Wisconsin, and Utah case control studies was published in the June 27, 1980, *MMWR*.[14] The article included recommendations that women who had menstrual TSS avoid tampon use for at least several menstrual cycles afterward, that beta-lactamase resistant antibiotics be administered during acute TSS episodes after appropriate specimens for culture were obtained, and that supportive therapy was important. Virtually immediately after this *MMWR* article was published, tampons became a household word, and menstruation became the topic of dinnertime conversation.

Intense investigation continued to reveal further the risk factors associated with TSS occurrence. In September 1980, Wally Schlech and many CDC colleagues conducted the second CDC case control study (CDC-2) that addressed concerns regarding study size, recall accuracy, friend controls, and dynamic changes in tampon products. CDC-2 corroborated earlier findings regarding tampon use as a menstrual TSS risk factor.[15] Cases occurred in association with multiple brands of tampons; however, among women who were exclusive users of a single tampon brand, significantly more case patients compared with age-matched acquaintance controls reported using Rely brand tampons. Rely tampons were a recently introduced and rather unconventional product that had rapidly been gaining market share. Of note, the early-phase rollout of this product in 1979 included Wisconsin. I recalled receiving free samples of Rely in the mail at my home on two occasions, which was unusual because I was single at the time.

The preliminary results of the CDC-2 were reported in the September 19 *MMWR*.[16] On September 22, Proctor and Gamble, the manufacturer of Rely, voluntarily withdrew the product from the market.

THE TRI-STATE CASE CONTROL STUDY

More pieces were soon fit into the puzzle. In August, Mike Osterholm in Minnesota, Vern Wintermeyer, the state epidemiologist in Iowa, and I, along with university and health department colleagues in each of our states, initiated a three-state collaborative comprehensive case control study of menses-associated and other potential TSS risk factors (the Tri-State TSS Study). Mike coordinated and brilliantly led this study. Mike and Bob Gibson and Jack Mandel (both faculty in the University of Minnesota system) were deft methodologists, and Bob rapidly generated complex computer-based analyses using a database incorporating data from the finely tuned 16-page study questionnaire and also proprietary tampon fluid capacity and chemical composition data for all brand styles of tampons in the marketplace through early September.[17] This was important because of the perplexing array of products within brand lines labeled as regular, super, and super plus (brand styles). The progression of such terms probably provided many women with relative knowledge about the absorbency of products within brand lines, but the consumers had no precise or even relative information regarding absorbency of products across brand lines. For example, one brand's super could be more absorbent than another brand's super plus. The proprietary data were essential to sort this out. With the assistance of legal council, Mike worked with representatives of each of the tampon manufacturers to procure these data, and to their credit, the companies willingly provided it.

Eighty women with TSS with onsets before September 19, 1980, and 160 age- and gender-matched neighborhood controls were randomly selected. Interviews were conducted in person. We found the odds ratio for developing menstrual TSS with any tampon use compared with no tampon use was 18.0 ($P < 0.001$). We were fortunate that there were some nontampon users in our study. When individual tampon brand use was compared with no tampon use, the brand-specific odds ratios were each significantly associated with TSS and ranged from 5.9 to 27. Similarly, odds ratios for individual brand style use compared with no tampon use were each significantly associated with TSS and ranged from 2.6 to 34.5.[17] In multivariate analysis, tampon fluid capacity (absorbency) and Rely brand tampon use were the only variables that significantly increased the relative risk of TSS; the risk associated with Rely was greater than that predicted by absorbency alone, suggesting that chemical composition of tampons was an important factor. We also found that significant risk factors for TSS recurrence were continued tampon use during menstrual periods after an episode of TSS and not receiving antistaphylococcal antibiotics during an initial episode of TSS. Among women with menstrual TSS, those having both of these risk factors had the greatest risk of recurrence. Those having neither factor had the least risk of recurrence, and those having either factor but not the other had an intermediate risk of recurrence.[18]

IMPACT OF THE CASE CONTROL STUDIES AND CONTROL MEASURES

Each of the studies cited used highly comparable TSS case definitions. Despite divergent methods, the association of menstrual TSS with tampon use was established in six different case control studies by late 1980: the two CDC studies[13,15] and four state-based studies (Wisconsin, Utah, Oregon, and the Tri-State Study).[5,16,17,19,20] The association with Rely use was established in four (CDC-2, Utah, Oregon, Tri-State Study).[16,17,19,20] In a review of these six TSS epidemiologic studies published in 1982, the author, Reuel Stallones, wrote this:[21]

Early cases were predominantly in menstruating women, and the use of tampons was strongly associated with the onset of illness. Because of widespread publication of this finding, the case-comparison studies had problems due to differential ascertainment and recall bias. However, the number of cases among women was so great and the relation with tampon use so marked that unreasonable assumptions are necessary if the results are to be attributed to these biases. These studies show the power of epidemiologic methods, even given the unfavorable circumstance of an uncommon condition, associated with a common practice.

In October 1980, the Food and Drug Administration published a proposed regulation stipulating that all tampon manufacturers place TSS warnings on their packages.[22] The warnings initially appeared in 1982,[23] but based on data from the Tri-State TSS Study were later enhanced to include information on tampon absorbency as a TSS risk factor, that women use tampons with the minimum absorbency needed to control menstrual flow, and ultimately a scale to indicate the absorbency of the individual units. These warnings are still protecting women.

On December 18, just over 1 year after that initial call regarding three cases in Madison, final expanded reports of the Wisconsin and first CDC case control studies were published in the *New England Journal of Medicine*.[5,13] We included an estimate of TSS rates based on 81 cases reported in Wisconsin during a full year that ended September 30, 1980. Among women of menstrual age (ranging from 12 to 49 years old), TSS incidence rates among women under age 30 years were 3.3-fold greater than among women age 30 years and older. Peak rates of nearly 15 cases per 100,000 menstruating women per year in Wisconsin were noted among women 15 to 19 years old who were regular users of tampons (Figure 5-1).[5] These rates decreased dramatically after September 1980 and during 1981 in Wisconsin and nationwide in response to the clinical management and product-related control measures and recommendations that were disseminated widely and rapidly to a nation captivated by this compelling episode in public health (Figure 5-2).[24,25]

The reported number of TSS cases that occurred in the United States during 1970 through June 15, 1983, was 2,204, among which 2,108 (95.6%) occurred in females and 90% of cases in women had onsets during menses (99% of those women were tampon users). There were over 100 reported deaths, and the case fatality rate decreased from 10% before 1980 to 5% in 1980 and 3% in 1981 and 1982.[24] In Wisconsin during

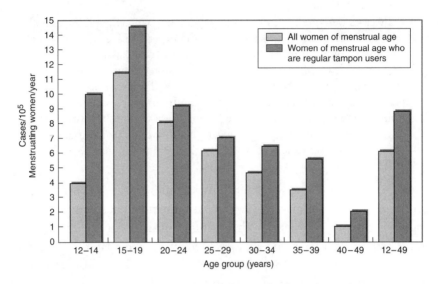

FIGURE 5-1 Minimum crude incidence of toxic-shock syndrome by age group in Wisconsin.

From Davis JP, Chesney PJ, Wand PJ, LaVenture M, Investigation and Laboratory Team. Toxic-shock syndrome: Epidemiologic features, recurrence, risk factors and prevention (Fig 2). *N Engl J Med* 1980;303:1429–35, Copyright ©1980 Massachusetts Medical Society. All rights reserved.

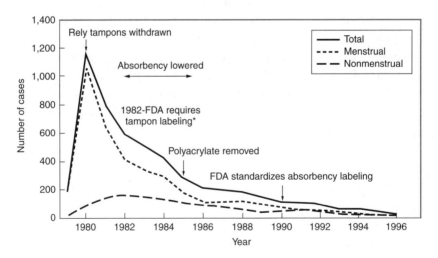

*FDA, Food and Drug Administration; includes definite and probable toxic shock syndrome cases

FIGURE 5-2 Toxic shock syndrome cases, menstrual vs. nonmenstrual, United States by year, 1979–1996. Years of important federal and voluntary measures are indicated [39].

1972 through 1982, 221 confirmed and 51 probable reported cases of TSS occurred. Among these cases, 5 (1.8%) were fatal.[23]

Within 12 months, much of the TSS unknown had been successfully revealed, and by mid 1981, reports were published of the discovery of the etiologic agent of TSS independently in two laboratories. Merlin Bergdoll at the University of Wisconsin and colleagues isolated and described a new *Staphylococcus* enterotoxin, SEF, produced by isolates from patients with TSS.[26] Similarly, Pat Schlievert at the University of Minnesota and colleagues isolated and described a new pyrogenic exotoxin, PEC.[27] These investigators and others ultimately concurred these moieties were identical, and they renamed the toxin TSST-1.[28]

THE WISCONSIN TSS TEAM: CONTINUING INVESTIGATIONS AND PERSONAL REFLECTION

After these discoveries, the seroepidemiologic features of TSS were rapidly delineated. Merlin and his staff used the purified toxin to develop an assay (radioimmunoassay) for antibody to SEF (TSST-1).[26] The assay was then used to measure the anti-SEF (anti-TSST-1) antibody in the many banked pairs of serum from case patients and sera obtained from various categories of control subjects and from the extensive WSLH general serum bank. Our Wisconsin TSS team, that now also included Jim Vergeront and Susan Stolz, along with Joan, Phil, and Merlin's laboratory colleagues and I, examined SEF-related immune responses. These included the detection and measurement of the presence of antibody in longitudinal specimens obtained from patients with TSS and in sera from controls and the detection and seroprevalence of SEF antibody markers in representative stored sera from different age cohorts ranging from early infancy to old age and in sera collected from young adults in different geographic regions of the United States.[29–31]

I have not focused on nonmenstrual TSS in this chapter, but Art Reingold and colleagues published an early, definitive article on the TSS not associated with menstruation,[30] a condition with a wide range of risk factors that did not decrease substantially in occurrence during the early 1980s.

The intense, sustained investigation of TSS, particularly during December 1979 through December 1980, was exhilarating, challenging, and humbling. It was also exhausting. The number of work hours devoted to our TSS-related studies was immense, and they accrued in parallel to my other duties as state epidemiologist including many investigations of other diseases that were reportable or newly emerging in Wisconsin. I experienced unanticipated intervals of tampon burnout, but I learned more about tampons in 1 year than I ever expected to know during a lifetime. The experience stimulated a sustained TSS-related investigative activity involving our TSS team and clinical and laboratory colleagues that, in addition to continuing to address TSST-1 related immune responses and seroepidemiologic features of TSS, also examined clinical outcomes and sequelae of TSS, epidemiologic trends and TSS surveillance methods, and other issues.[33-38] Most of all, the experience of investigating the many aspects of TSS during the initial year and the years that followed has provided me with a valued network of colleagues for which I am very grateful.

REFERENCES

1. Band J, LaVenture M, Davis JP, et al. Epidemic Legionnaire's disease: airborne transmission down a chimney. *JAMA* 1981;245:2404–2407.
2. Dryer RF, Goellner PG, Carney AS. Lyme arthritis in Wisconsin. *JAMA* 1979;241:498–499.
3. Davis JP, Schell WL, Amundson TE, et al. Lyme disease in Wisconsin: epidemiologic, clinical, serologic and entomologic findings. *Yale J Biol Med* 1984;57: 685–696.
4. Todd JK, Fishaut M, Kapral F, Welch T. Toxic-shock syndrome associated with phage-group-1 staphylococci. *Lancet* 1978;2:1116–1118.
5. Davis JP, Chesney PJ, Wand PJ, LaVenture M, Investigation and Laboratory Team. Toxic-shock syndrome: epidemiologic features, recurrence, risk factors and prevention. *N Engl J Med* 1980;303:1429–1435.
6. Osterholm MT, Gibson RW, Mandel JS, Davis JP. Tri-State Toxic Shock Syndrome Study: methodologic analysis. *Ann Intern Med* 1982;96(Pt 2):899–902.
7. Wharton M., Chorba TL, Vogt RL, et al. Case definitions for public health surveillance. *MMWR* 1990;39(RR-13):1–43.
8. Toxic-shock syndrome—United States. *MMWR* 1980;29:229–230.
9. Chesney PJ, Davis JP, Purdy WK, Wand PJ, Chesney RW. Clinical manifestations of toxic-shock syndrome. *JAMA* 1981;246:741–748.
10. Gourley GR, Chesney PJ, Davis JP, Odell GR. Acute cholestasis in patients with the toxic-shock syndrome. *Gastroenterology* 1981;81:928–931.
11. Chesney RW, Chesney PJ, Davis JP, Segar WE. Renal manifestations of the staphylococcal toxic-shock syndrome. *Am J Med* 1981;71:583–588.
12. Chesney TW, McCarron DM, Haddad JG, et al. Pathogenic mechanisms of the hypocalcemia of the staphylococcal toxic-shock syndrome. *J Lab Clin Med* 1983;101:576–585.

13. Shands KN, Schmid GP, Dan BB, et al. Toxic-shock syndrome in menstruating women: association with tampon use and *Staphylococcus aureus* and clinical features in 52 cases. *N Engl J Med* 1980;303:1436–1442.
14. Follow-up on toxic-shock syndrome—United States. *MMWR* 1980;29:297–299.
15. Schlech WF III, Shands KN, Reingold AL, et al. Risk factors for development of toxic shock syndrome: association with a tampon brand. *JAMA* 1982;7:835–839.
16. Follow-up in toxic-shock syndrome. *MMWR* 1980;29:441–445.
17. Osterholm MT, Davis JP, Gibson RW, et al. Tri-State Toxic-Shock Syndrome Study. I. Epidemiologic findings. *J Infect Dis* 1982;145:431–440.
18. Davis JP, Osterholm MT, Helms CM, et al. Tri-State Toxic-Shock Syndrome Study. II. Clinical and laboratory findings. *J Infect Dis* 1982;145:441–448.
19. Latham RH, Kehrberg MW, Jacobson JA, Smith CB. Toxic shock syndrome in Utah: a case-control and surveillance study. *Ann Intern Med* 1982;96(Pt 2):906–908.
20. Helgerson SD. Toxic shock syndrome in Oregon: epidemiologic findings. *Ann Intern Med* 1982;96(Pt 2):909–911.
21. Stallones RA. A review of epidemiologic studies of toxic shock syndrome. *Ann Intern Med* 1982;96(Pt 2):917–920.
22. Food and Drug Administration. Update on toxic shock syndrome. *FDA Drug Bull* 1980;10:17–19.
23. Food and Drug Administration. Tampon packages carry TSS information. *FDA Drug Bull* 1982;12:19–20.
24. Update: toxic-shock syndrome—United States. *MMWR* 1983;32:398–400.
25. Toxic-shock syndrome in Wisconsin. *Wisc Epidemiol Bull* 1983;5:1–2, 5.
26. Bergdoll MS, Crass BA, Reiser RF, Robbins RN, Davis JP. A new staphylococcal enterotoxin, enterotoxin F, associated with toxic-shock syndrome Staphylococcus aureus isolates. *Lancet* 1981;1:1017–1021.
27. Schlievert PM, Shands KN, Dan BB, Schmid GP, Nishimura RD. Identification and characterization of exotoxin from *Staphylococcus aureus* associated with toxic shock syndrome. *J Infect Dis* 1981;143:509–516.
28. Bergdoll MS, Schlievert PM. Toxic shock syndrome toxin. *Lancet* 1984;2:691.
29. Vergeront JM, Stolz SJ, Crass BA, Nelson DB, Davis JP, Bergdoll MS. Seroprevalence of antibody to staphylococcal enterotoxin F among Wisconsin residents: implications for toxic-shock syndrome. *J Infect Dis* 1983;148:692–698.
30. Stolz SJ, Davis JP, Vergeront JM, Crass BA, Chesney PJ, Wand PJ, Bergdoll MS. Development of serum antibody to toxic-shock toxin among individuals with toxic-shock syndrome in Wisconsin. *J Infect Dis* 1985;151:883–889.
31. Vergeront JM, Blouse SE, Crass BA, Stolz SJ, Bergdoll MS, Davis JP. Regional differences in the prevalence of serum antibody to toxic-shock toxin (anti-TST). Twenty-fourth Interscience Conference on Antimicrobial Agents and Chemotherapy, Washington DC, October 1984; Abst. 610.
32. Reingold AL, Dan BB, Shands KN, Broome CV. Toxic-shock syndrome not associated with menstruation: a review of 54 cases. *Lancet* 1982;2:1–4.

33. Davis JP, Vergeront JM, Amsterdam LE, Hayward J, Stolz-LaVerriere SJ. Long-term effects of toxic shock syndrome in women: sequelae, subsequent pregnancy, menstrual history and long-term trends in catamenial product use. *Rev Infect Dis* 1989;11(Suppl 1):550–551.

34. Vergeront JM, Evenson ML, Crass BA, et al. Recovery of staphylococcal enterotoxin F from the breast milk of a woman with toxic-shock syndrome. *J Infect Dis* 1982;146:456–459.

35. Chesney PJ, Davis JP, Chesney RW. Factors determining severity of the toxic-shock syndrome (TSS). *Pediatr Res* 1981;15:440.

36. Chesney PJ, Davis JP. Toxic shock syndrome. In Feigen RD, Cherry JD, Demmler GJ, Kaplan SL, eds. *Textbook of Pediatric Infectious Diseases*, 5th ed. Philadelphia: Saunders, 2003:836–859.

37. Davis JP, Vergeront JM. The effect of publicity on the reporting of toxic-shock syndrome. *J Infect Dis* 1982;145:449–457.

38. Hayward J, Vergeront JM, Stolz SJ, Bohn MJ, Davis JP. A hospital discharge code review of toxic-shock syndrome in Wisconsin. *Am J Epidemiol* 1986;123:876–883.

39. Hajjeh RA, Reingold A, Weil A, Shutt K, Schuchat A, Perkins BA. Toxic shock syndrome in the United States: surveillance update, 1979–1996. *Emerg Infect Dis* 1999;5:807–810.

CHAPTER 6

The Early Days of AIDS in the United States: A Personal Perspective

Harold W. Jaffe, MD

INTRODUCTION

In the spring of 1981, I was working as an Epidemic Intelligence Service (EIS) officer in the Venereal Disease Control Division at the Centers for Disease Control (CDC) in Atlanta. My stint in EIS was rather atypical in that I had first come to the CDC in 1974, fresh out of internal medicine training. I stayed for 3 years but left when I had the opportunity to do an infectious diseases fellowship. Soon after I returned to the CDC in 1980, the newly elected Reagan Administration decided to reduce the federal workforce, including CDC staff. Fortunately, the EIS was considered as a training program, exempt from the cuts, and thus, serving in EIS kept me employed!

It was a bit strange to be working on infectious diseases at a time when the public health community seemed to feel that many of the problems posed by infectious diseases had been solved, at least in the developed world. We had vaccines for most of the childhood infections and a broad range of antibiotics available to treat bacterial and even some viral diseases. I recall hearing a lecture by Dr. Robert Petersdorf, a very eminent infectious diseases physician from the University of Washington, in which he argued that the demand for infectious diseases specialists was likely to diminish.

At the same time, however, our group at the CDC was busy studying the newly emerging problem of penicillin-resistant gonorrhea and the increasing rates of syphilis in men who had sex with men (MSM). During my time as an infectious diseases fellow in Chicago, I had "moonlighted" at a sexually transmitted diseases (STD) clinic caring for MSM and had treated many of them for gonorrhea and syphilis. Unfortunately, the era of infectious diseases was not over for them. Thus, when I saw the first report of a strange illness occurring in MSM in Los Angeles, I was more than a little interested.

THE BEGINNING

The report had come to CDC's Division of Parasitic Disease from Dr. Wayne Shandera, an EIS officer assigned to the Los Angeles County Health Department. Wayne had received reports from Dr. Michael Gottlieb, an immunologist at UCLA Hospital, and from several other Los Angeles physicians who had seen young MSM with *Pneumocystis carinii* pneumonia (PCP). These cases were highly unusual because PCP typically occurred in adults with a known cause of immune suppression, such as the receipt of cancer chemotherapy or drugs to prevent rejection of a transplanted organ, but none of these men had these predisposing risk factors.

The first report of these cases, which appeared in the CDC's *Morbidity and Mortality Weekly Report* (*MMWR*) on June 5, 1981,[1] raised a series of questions. First, was this really a new disease, or had similar cases occurred in the past without being reported? Second, were cases being seen elsewhere? Third, were other unusual diseases also occurring in MSM, and fourth, why were the cases occurring in MSM? These questions led to fundamental epidemiologic steps that are essential to ask as one begins to investigate a possible outbreak. Verify whether there really is a new outbreak or an outbreak at all. Determine the extent of the problem by searching for additional cases within and outside of the area of the initial report. More thoroughly examine the problem through case investigation, and consider performing a risk factor analysis to identify whether information can be learned that could create a prevention strategy to decrease the extent of or terminate the outbreak.

To answer the first question, the CDC turned to its Parasitic Disease Drug Service, which supplied American physicians with medications to treat unusual parasitic infections. (At the time, *Pneumocystis carinii*, was considered to be a parasite; more recently, it has been reclassified as a fungal species, *P. jiroveci*) The only drug available to treat PCP in 1981 was pentamidine isethionate. A record review revealed that almost all previous pentamidine requests had been for persons with an obvious cause of immune suppression. Beginning in the second half of 1980, however, a few requests had been received for persons fitting the profile of the Los Angeles cases.[2] Thus, the disease might have begun a bit earlier than 1981, but not much earlier.

The answers to questions two and three came soon after the report from Los Angeles. MSM with PCP were also being seen in San Francisco and New York City. Some of these men were developing other severe infections typically seen only in immunosuppressed persons (called opportunistic infections, or OIs). At a meeting I attended in San Diego soon after publication of the Los Angeles report, I also heard that MSM in San Francisco were developing a very unusual skin cancer, Kaposi's sarcoma (KS), a disease typically seen in older men and organ transplant recipients. I was so worried that I would forget the strange name of the disease that I wrote it on a slip of paper and put it in my wallet so that I could discuss it when I returned to Atlanta. For lack of a better name, we began referring to this new disease as "KS/OI." Why it was occurring in MSM remained a mystery.

EARLY INVESTIGATIONS

Whatever this new disease might be, it did not fit neatly into any of CDC's organizational units, and thus, a "KS/OI Task Force" was set up under the direction of Dr. James Curran. Because there seemed to be so many aspects to KS/OI, the membership of the Task Force was very diverse and included experts in cancer epidemiology, parasitology, virology, immunology, and STDs. I was asked to join the group because of my experience in working with MSM and was happy to do so. Our initial Task Force meetings included perhaps a dozen people and were mainly brainstorming sessions about what might be going on; however, we all agreed that we needed to begin national surveillance for KS/OI and for that we needed a case definition (Exhibit 6-1). We distributed the case definition to health departments and major teaching hospitals. By the end of August 1981, over 100 cases meeting the definition had been reported. (Subsequently, the CDC began funding health departments, starting with New York City, to

---

Exhibit 6-1 Case Definition of KS/OI (1981)

- Biopsy-proven KS and/or biopsy- or culture-proven life-threatening opportunistic infections
- Previously healthy persons less than 60 years of age
- Patients excluded with conditions known to cause immunosuppression such as congenital immunodeficiency, lymphoreticular malignancy, and therapy with immunosuppressive agents

---

establish systematic hospital-based surveillance, a program that remains in place today.)

It was apparent, however, that little information sharing about cases was occurring at the local level. Physicians seeing cases at one hospital were often unaware that similar patients were being seen at other hospitals in the same city. In New York City, Dr. David Sencer, the former CDC director and now the New York City Health Commissioner, recognized the problem. To break down these communication barriers, he established monthly meetings at the health department, at which clinicians from all of the major New York City hospitals would come to discuss their cases and hear updates from health department staff.

At this point, we thought it would be important for the physicians on the Task Force to see persons with KS/OI, both to appreciate the clinical presentation of the disease and to start developing an epidemiologic profile of these patients. I was asked to go to San Francisco, and I spent several days talking to patients cared for at University of California, San Francisco. I was struck by how sick these young men were. They had lost large amounts of weight. Those with PCP were on ventilators in intensive care units, and those with KS were covered with purplish lesions (Figure 6-1). In speaking with the men who were able to talk, it became apparent that they were highly sexually active and had used a variety of recreational drugs.

When we gathered again in Atlanta to discuss what we had seen, the profiles of KS/OI patients sounded very similar, whether they were from California or New York. Thus, we again asked ourselves our fourth question, "Why MSM?" Two ideas seemed most plausible. First, we might be dealing with a new STD. Rates of other STDs had been dramatically increasing in MSM, and the men we had interviewed had been very sexually active. The second hypothesis involved an environmental exposure,

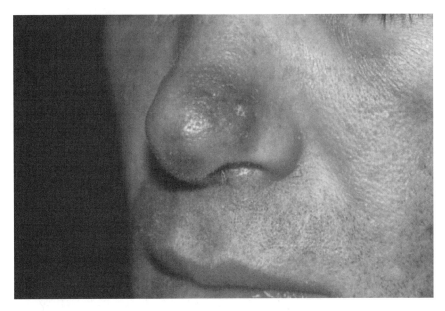

FIGURE 6-1 Kaposis' sarcoma in a patient with AIDS.
Courtesy of David Hines, MD, not from the early 1980's.

perhaps to street drugs or an exposure in gay bath houses. I hoped the second hypothesis was right because it would certainly be easier to eliminate something from the environment of MSM than to control a new STD.

Regarding the environmental hypothesis, we were particularly interested in nitrite inhalants or "poppers," whose use to enhance sex was thought to be especially common in MSM. To look at this possibility in more detail, Dr. Bill Darrow, a CDC research sociologist, and I made a visit to the Club Baths, a gay bath house in Atlanta. With the permission of the manager, we interviewed customers about their use of poppers. (We were rather obvious, as we were the only ones wearing clothes!) Although the customers had no particular reason to trust us, most were very willing to sit down and talk for a few minutes. We found out that popper use was almost universal and that poppers could be purchased in bath houses and other gay venues in bottles with names such as "Rush" or "Bolt." In fact, our visit coincided with "Popper Night," with a 50-cent discount offered on each bottle. We subsequently learned that poppers could also be bought in gay bars and bookstores in unlabeled bottles. To find out what was in these bottles, we purchased them in several cities and brought them back to Atlanta for chemical analysis. (My wife was not amused to find them stored in our home refrigerator!) We thought we might find some sort of contaminant, but the bottles contained butyl and isobutyl nitrite, chemicals not associated with immunosuppression.

By the end of the summer of 1981, the Task Force decided to do a case control study of KS/OI. The study would examine a wide range of possible causes but would focus on infectious and environmental risk factors. Because of the sensitive nature of the questions, we decided to conduct all of the interviews in person. The cases would be MSM with PCP and/or KS, but the selection of control patients was more problematic. We thought these persons should be apparently healthy MSM matched to the cases within an age range and by race and city of residence. How should we select them? After much debate within the Task Force, we decided to recruit three MSM control groups and separately analyze our case data in comparison to data from each of the control groups: persons attending public STD clinics, persons cared for by private physicians with predominately MSM practices, and friends of cases who had not been their sexual partners. It was very telling that many of the case patients could not name an MSM friend who hadn't been a sex partner.

To do the interviews, we sent teams to Los Angeles, San Francisco, and New York. Being originally from Los Angeles, I was put on the California team. Although the men we interviewed could have had many reasons to distrust us, I was very impressed by how open they were in discussing the most intimate details of their lives. I think this was likely the result of fear in the MSM community, where increasing numbers of men were sick or dying. We did the interviews in our hotel rooms, creating much puzzlement among the desk clerks who must have wondered why all these young men were asking to see us. Taking no particular precautions (we did not wear gloves), we also drew blood from these men in our rooms. In retrospect, we were very foolish, although this was an accepted practice in medical facilities at the time.

The analysis of the case control study indicated that KS/OI was most strongly associated with having a large number of male sex partners.[3] For example, case patients had a median of 61 partners per year as compared with 27 partners for the control patients from STD clinics. This was an especially striking difference given that the STD clinic patients would be expected to be highly sexually active. Although we felt the findings were most consistent with a sexually transmitted cause of KS/OI, we could not entirely exclude the environmental hypothesis because sex and drug use were highly associated in this population.

The epidemiologic proof of a sexually transmitted cause of KS/OI did not come until the spring of 1982. Dr. David Auerbach, the EIS officer who had taken over for Wayne Shandera in Los Angeles, called me to say that he had heard through contacts in the MSM community that some of the men with KS/OI had been sexual partners. He wanted to interview the men to confirm these rumors but had never done this sort of interviewing and needed help. Thus, we sent Bill Darrow to work with him. In just a few days, Darrow and Auerbach were able to confirm the sexual links between these cases. Furthermore, they found that four men with KS/OI in Southern California had sex with a French-Canadian flight attendant who himself had developed KS. This flight attendant, referred to in a published report as Patient O, could also be linked to four other KS/OI patients in New York. As the investigation expanded, a total of 40 patients living in 10 North American cities could be linked by sexual contact.[4] When reported in the popular press, Patient O was described as the "source" of the North American epidemic. Although this was a misinterpretation of the study findings, it did seem likely that a small number of men who were both highly mobile and very sexually active, like Patient O, could have quickly spread the disease among MSM.

AN EXPANDING PROBLEM

By the summer of 1982, more pieces were being added to the KS/OI puzzle. The clinical spectrum of illness began to expand to conditions beyond those initially identified. For example, reports of generalized lymph node enlargements among homosexual men suggested that this condition might be a precursor of KS/OI. Some homosexual men were also reported with unusual forms of non-Hodgkin's lymphoma.

The groups of persons developing KS/OI also expanded beyond the homosexual men initially reported. By June 1982, 13 of the 355 reported KS/OI cases were in women, more than half of whom had used intravenous (IV) drugs. Haitians residing in the United States, particularly in Miami, Florida and Brooklyn, New York, were reported with KS/OI. Almost all of the Haitians were young men; those interviewed all denied homosexual activity. Finally, three heterosexual men with hemophilia A were reported with PCP. All had received Factor VIII concentrate, a blood product used to treat their coagulation disorder.

The early winter of 1982–1983 proved to be a pivotal time in the investigations of what by then was called AIDS (acquired immune deficiency syndrome). The case total in the United States was approaching 800, with a mortality rate of about 40%. Although cases were still concentrated in New York City, San Francisco, Los Angeles, Newark, and Miami, other cities were beginning to report cases. The first key event of this period was the December 10, 1982, *MMWR* publication of a possible case of transfusion-associated AIDS.[5] Dr. Arthur Ammann, a pediatric immunologist at University of California, San Francisco, was caring for a 20-month old infant with unexplained severe immunodeficiency. Although AIDS had not been previously described in children, the features of this child's illness more closely resembled AIDS rather than other forms of pediatric immunodeficiency. The child had received multiple transfusions shortly after birth to treat erythroblastosis fetalis (a condition that results from a blood group incompatibility between mother and fetus). Investigation of the blood donors by the San Francisco Department of Public Health revealed that 1 of the 19 donors was a man who developed AIDS 9 months after donation. Although initially reported with no known risk factors, subsequent investigation by David Auerbach determined that the donor was a homosexual man.

Only a week later, the *MMWR* reported four other infants with unexplained immunodeficiency.[6] These infants, born in New York City, Newark, and San Francisco, had not received transfusions. Two of the infants had Haitian mothers, whose health status was unknown. The mothers of the other two infants reported IV drug use; one of these mothers died of AIDS, whereas the other had early signs of the disease.

Finally, in early January 1983, the CDC published a report from New York City of two women who each had developed immunodeficiency after repeated sexual contact with a man who had AIDS.[7] One of these men was an IV drug user, whereas the other was bisexual. Neither woman had any other known risk factor for the disease.

Taken together, these three reports plus the "Patient O" investigation strongly suggested an infectious cause of AIDS. Evidence from case ascertainment and analysis of descriptive epidemiologic data supported that the putative agent could be transmitted through sexual contact, either homosexual or heterosexual, from mother to child, and through blood and blood products. Furthermore, the source of transmission could be a person who had not yet developed the disease, implying that the agent could be carried asymptomatically.

In addition to the epidemiologic importance of these reports, they also had a major impact on the media's interest in AIDS and the public perception of the disease. Until this time, the mainstream media paid relatively little attention to AIDS; most of the coverage had been in the gay press. With these new reports, however, AIDS could no longer be regarded as simply "the gay plague." Suddenly, Americans realized that transfusion could put them at risk. My own wife refused to sign a hospital consent form to allow transfusions to be given to her during the birth of our first child unless either she or I agreed that they were absolutely necessary. Infants with the disease, portrayed as "innocent victims," gave special poignancy to the story. I remember seeing camera crews and reporters from all of the major television networks lining up to do interviews with CDC staff to meet the sudden demand for news about AIDS. Although I was glad that the mainstream media was finally paying attention, I wondered why it had taken them so long.

Unfortunately, while the problem was increasing, resources were not. The Task Force continued to operate without a clear organizational home within CDC. Many of our staff had been "detailed" from other programs. With no specific appropriations forthcoming from Washington, the money to support our work came from funds that had been appropriated for other purposes, particularly STD control.

The lack of interest from the administration was exemplified by an October 1982 press briefing when President Reagan's press secretary, Larry Speakes, was asked whether the President was aware of the growing AIDS epidemic. His first response was "what's AIDS?" When told that it was affecting gay men, Speakes replied, "I don't have it. Do you?"[8] The President himself made no public remarks about AIDS until 1987.

AIDS AND THE BLOOD SUPPLY

The growing concern about the safety of the blood supply gave rise to an important meeting held at the CDC in January 1983. From our perspective at the CDC, the purpose of the meeting with the U.S. Food and Drug Administration, the National Hemophilia Foundation, blood banking organizations, and groups representing MSM was to describe the occurrence of AIDS in transfusion recipients and persons with hemophilia and then discuss potential prevention measures. Prevention options included excluding blood donation from persons known to be at risk for AIDS (such as MSM) or those with laboratory findings known to correlate with AIDS risk (such as a positive hepatitis B antibody test).

As well described by Randy Shilts in his book *And the Band Played On*, the meeting quickly became a contentious debate rather than a constructive discussion.[9] Although the CDC presented a series of cases thought to be AIDS resulting from receipt of blood or blood products, the representatives of the blood banks and hemophilia treatment community said they were not convinced that the disease was AIDS and were unwilling to accept our evidence that the "AIDS agent" was contaminating the blood supply. At one point in the meeting, Dr. Donald Armstrong, Chief of Infectious Diseases at Memorial Sloan-Kettering Cancer Center in NYC, stood up to say that he could hardly believe these comments. In his mind, there was no question that these were AIDS cases and that something needed to be done, but the other participants simply ignored him.

The other participants also rejected the concept of using a "surrogate," such as the hepatitis B antibody test, to exclude potential donors. In part, this may have represented a legitimate concern about the possibility of creating a blood shortage. In my view, however, much of the discussion simply reflected denial. The blood-banking and hemophilia treatment communities were unwilling to accept the notion that blood and blood products, seen by them as lifesaving, could be transmitting a lethal infection. This decision would later cost millions of dollars in lawsuits. Similar sorts of decisions were made in France in 1985 that resulted in the 1992 imprisonment of officials judged to be responsible.[10]

Needless to say, CDC staff members were very disheartened by the outcome of this meeting. We felt that we had made a convincing case, but the case had been rejected. Fortunately, private discussions held over the next few months proved to be more productive, and in March 1983, the U.S. Public Health Service published the first comprehensive set of recommendations for the prevention of AIDS.[11] The recommendations noted that "available data suggest that the severe disorder of immune regulation underlying AIDS is caused by a transmissible agent." Although no test existed to detect this agent, those at highest risk were noted to be those with symptoms or signs suggestive of AIDS, the sexual partners of AIDS patients, sexually active MSM with multiple partners, Haitian entrants to the United States, past or present IV drugs users, patients with hemophilia, and sexual partners of persons at increased risk for AIDS. The publication then went on to recommend avoiding having sexual contact with persons known or suspected to have AIDS and noted that having multiple sexual partners increased the risk of AIDS. Furthermore, as a "temporary" measure, members of these risk groups were advised not to donate plasma or blood. These recommendations were derived from the epidemiologic data available at the time. In the absence of a screening test for the transmissible agent, this was a rational strategy for decreasing the risk of AIDS transmission though blood and blood products.

Several features of the recommendation might strike contemporary readers as puzzling. First, why not restrict all MSM from blood donation rather than only those with "multiple sexual partners" (a term not further defined)? This recommendation represented a compromise between public health officials, who wanted a wider prohibition, and gay rights advocates, who wanted the prohibition to be as narrow as possible. Because the risk of AIDS correlated with the number of sexual partners, the "multiple partners" language was seen as an acceptable compromise. Second, why were all Haitian Americans excluded from donation when relative few seemed to be at risk for the disease? Here the problem was that no particular behaviors had been shown to correlate with AIDS risk, and thus, the donation restriction could not be limited to a specific subgroup of Haitians. Undoubtedly, this decision resulted in unwarranted discrimination against Haitians living in the United States. Even in retrospect, however, I think this was the correct public health decision at the time. With the subsequent availability of tests to screen donated blood for HIV, the restriction on Haitians was eventually lifted but remains in effect for MSM and injection drug users.

Putting these controversies aside, I think the most remarkable aspect of the recommendations was that they were essentially correct, even though the cause of AIDS had not yet been discovered. It was not until May 1983 that Luc Montagnier and his associates at the Institute Pasteur in Paris identified a novel retrovirus in the lymph node of a homosexual man.[12] Another year then passed before Robert Gallo and his associates at the U.S. National Institutes of Health could prove that the virus, called HTLV-III by his laboratory, was the cause of AIDS.[13] Thus, the investigations done by the CDC Task Force and many others showed the power of the epidemiologic method to establish the likely transmission routes of a new infectious agent, as well as to develop basic prevention recommendations, before the identity of the agent was known. Furthermore, those investigations helped focus the work of the laboratory scientists who were trying to find the agent.

Unfortunately, the AIDS epidemic did not stop with the identification of the causative agent. Despite the release of the recommendations intended to help prevent further cases of AIDS in the March 1983 *MMWR*, case counts continued to rise. There were many factors that kept these recommendations from being as immediately useful as the removal of the pump handle by John Snow during the 19th century London cholera outbreak. It would be later learned that the virus had a long latency period from infection to AIDS such that these recommendations were too late for many persons who had acquired the virus weeks, months, or years earlier. Much remained and still remains to be learned about how to change human sexual behavior to prevent disease transmission. Almost a million Americans have been reported with AIDS since 1981, and almost 40 million persons are now living with HIV/AIDS worldwide.

CONCLUSIONS

I've often been asked what it was like to be one of the early AIDS investigators. To me, at least, it all began as a medical mystery, just like many other outbreak investigations. I was caught up in being a "medical detective" without much thought of the broader significance of what we were investigating. Perhaps some of my colleagues were astute enough to have seen the future, but I wasn't. As time went on, however, I gradually began to see that what we were studying was something much bigger than I had imagined. Once it was clear that the disease was sexually transmitted, we knew that the disease would not be limited to MSM. After we knew that the agent was in the blood supply, we knew many more people were at risk. The medical mystery would soon become the global pandemic.

ACKNOWLEDGMENT

An adaptation of this chapter was printed in the following: Jaffe HW. The early days of the HIV-AIDS epidemic in the USA. *Nat Immunol* 2008; 9:1201–1203.

REFERENCES

1. CDC. *Pneumocystis* pneumonia—Los Angeles. *MMWR* 1981;30:250–252.
2. Centers for Disease Control Task Force on Kaposi's Sarcoma and Opportunistic Infections. Epidemiologic aspects of the current outbreak of Kaposi's sarcoma and opportunistic infections. *N Engl J Med* 1982;306:248–252.
3. Jaffe HW, Choi K, Thomas PA, et al. National case-control study of Kaposi's sarcoma and *Pneumocystis carinii* pneumonia in homosexual men: part 1, epidemiologic results. *Ann Intern Med* 1983;99:145–151.
4. Auerbach DM, Darrow WW, Jaffe HW, Curran JW. Cluster of cases of the acquired immune deficiency syndrome: patients linked by sexual contact. *Am J Med* 1984;76:487–492.
5. CDC. Possible transfusion-associated acquired immune deficiency syndrome (AIDS)—California. *MMWR* 1982;31:652–654.
6. CDC. Unexplained immunodeficiency and opportunistic infections in infants—New York, New Jersey, California. *MMWR* 1982;31:665–667.
7. CDC. Immunodeficiency among female sexual partners of males with acquired immune deficiency syndrome (AIDS). *MMWR* 1983;31:697–698.
8. The White House. Office of the Press Secretary. Press briefing by Larry Speakes, October 15, 1982. http://findarticles.com/p/articles/mi_m0HSW/is_401/ai_n6078340.
9. Shilts R. *And the Band Played on. Politics, People, and the AIDS Epidemic.* New York: St. Martin's Press, 1987.
10. Weiberg PD, Hounshell J, Sherman LA, et al. Legal, financial, and public health consequences of HIV contamination of blood and blood products in the 1980s and 1990s. *Ann Intern Med* 2002;136:312–319.
11. CDC. Prevention of acquired immune deficiency syndrome (AIDS): report of inter-agency recommendations. *MMWR* 1983;32:101–104.
12. Barre-Sinoussi F, Cherman J-C, Rey F, et al. Isolation of a T-lymphotropic retrovirus from a patient at risk for acquired immune deficiency syndrome (AIDS). *Science* 1983;220:868–671.
13. Gallo RC, Salahuddin SZ, Popovic M, et al. Frequent detection and isolation of cytopathic retroviruses (HTLV-III) from patients with AIDS and at risk for AIDS. *Science* 1984;224:500–503.

CHAPTER 7

Verify the Diagnosis: A Pseudo-outbreak of Amebiasis in Los Angeles County

Frank Sorvillo, PhD

INTRODUCTION

Struggling through the laboratory section of Larry Ash's notorious course "Protozoal Diseases of Humans" in the spring of 1978 as part of my master's in public health curriculum at UCLA's School of Public Health, I repeatedly questioned my sanity in taking this six-unit class that had a widespread reputation of brutalizing students. Professor Ash is regarded as one of the leading parasitologists of our era. His discovery of an animal model (the Mongolian jird) for filariasis was considered a major scientific breakthrough that led to numerous significant achievements against a disease that is now considered a target for eradication. Moreover, Ash and his colleague Tom Orihel had produced two highly acclaimed texts, considered the "bibles" of diagnostic parasitology, *Atlas of Human Parasitology* and *Parasites in Human Tissues*.[1,2] They would also go on to produce a series of bench aids for the World Health Organization for use in the diagnosis of parasitic infections. These aids are considered among the most important tools in the recognition and control of parasites of global public health significance. Despite the challenge, Ash's classroom lectures had

117

made the subject of parasitology so captivating that I changed my focus from cardiovascular disease to infectious disease epidemiology. Nevertheless, hours of reviewing hundreds of stained slides, wet mount preparations, and countless baffling artifacts were both exhausting and humbling, and none of us bargained for examining our own stool specimen! The benefits of this torment were realized some time later when, working as an infectious disease epidemiologist with the Acute Communicable Disease Control unit of Los Angeles County's Health Department, I was assigned to the surveillance of parasitic diseases.

Sue Nagamine, the lead secretary for the Acute Communicable Disease Control unit, advised me that an anxious caller from a large, local health maintenance organization (HMO) "needed to speak to someone about parasites." I answered the phone and could quickly sense the obvious concern in the person's voice. It was October 1983 and an outbreak of amebiasis was unfolding in their patient population. Over 30 cases had been diagnosed, and they were anxious for the health department to investigate and find the source.

Amebiasis is caused by the protozoan parasite *Entamoeba hystolytica* and is endemic in most areas of the developing world. Globally, an estimated 50 million cases of amebiasis occur each year, causing approximately 100,000 deaths.[3] Although infection is often asymptomatic, when symptoms do occur, it typically induces diarrhea and dysentery but can cause severe and even life-threatening disease when it becomes invasive and affects tissue of the liver, lungs, or brain. The term histolytica in fact refers to the ability to "lyse tissue," which allows dissemination of the parasite beyond its gastrointestinal niche. Fulminant amebic colitis and cerebral infection, although rare, have a particularly poor prognosis.

Concern about *E. histolytica* had been heightened in the early 1980s with the recognition of very high prevalence rates (20% to 30%) in communities of men who have sex with men. One of the first reports of this phenomenon was Most's classic article entitled "Manhattan: a 'Tropical Isle'" in which he documented the frequent occurrence of pathogenic protozoa among gay men in the New York City area, a phenomenon that typically was seen only in resource-limited areas of the world.[4] Recent immigrants from endemic regions, residents of long-term care facilities, and travelers to developing countries were also known risk groups.[5-7]

The call from the HMO was taken very seriously. We knew that amebiasis could occur in outbreak form with significant accompanying mortality

Table 7-1 Reported Common Source Outbreaks of Amebiasis, United States

Location	Year	No. Cases	No. Deaths	Source
Chicago	1933	1400	98	Water
Chicago	1934	123	Unknown	Water
South Bend	1953	31	4	Water
Colorado	1978–80	36	6	Colonic irrigation device

(Table 7-1). A major waterborne epidemic of amebiasis had occurred during the 1933 World's Fair in Chicago, with over 1,400 cases and 98 deaths recorded.[8] Sewage contamination of drinking water led to the outbreak. Other waterborne outbreaks in the United States had been recognized in Chicago and South Bend Indiana.[9,10] Moreover, in 1982, just 1 year prior, Greg Istre, then an Epidemic Intelligence Officer with the Centers for Disease Control assigned to Colorado, had published in the *New England Journal of Medicine* a report of an outbreak of amebiasis linked to "colonic irrigation" exposure.[11] Thirty-six cases were reported with six deaths.

Colonic irrigation, also known euphemistically as "colonic hydrotherapy," is administered through a bizarre, almost medieval contraption that provides a series of enemas over a short period of time. Historically, some proponents of colonic irrigation have contended that many conditions, including everything from impotence to cancer, are caused by fecal impaction of the colon and that these conditions can be cured with colonic irrigation. Practitioners of this procedure include "colon therapists" and naturopaths, as well as some chiropractors. It is a procedure that, regrettably, is often sought by persons who may not have access to conventional medical care for treatment of their ailments or by individuals seeking hope for conditions that may not be curable.

Given the bohemian nature of Los Angeles and penchant for the unconventional, we were well aware of the procedure. It is not uncommon to find advertisements in various Los Angeles publications trumpeting in large boldface font that "Death Begins in the Colon!" while encouraging people to get their colons "cleansed." Our most bizarre experience with colonic irrigation occurred in the summer of 1988 when a young man in tennis shoes, jeans, and a t-shirt walked into our office carrying a huge contraption that we recognized immediately as a colonic irrigation device. He was a Los Angeles police department vice squad officer, and they had seized the "machine" as part of a raid on what he termed a "bondage and dominance parlor" in the central city area. Anyone entering the establishment had to first submit to a colonic irrigation. Because no police officer would agree to this personal invasion, they were unable to go undercover. The detective had brought the colonic irrigation device to us to see whether we had any information that might be of use for their case against the operation. Because a small amount of cloudy liquid remained in the reservoir (a glass tank capable of holding about 4 to 5 gallons of water), we took several swabs of the liquid for bacterial culture. Our bacteriology laboratory subsequently isolated *Aeromonas hydrophila* as well as several *Pseudomonas* species (which are commonly recovered from water). *A. hydrophila* can cause gastrointestinal illness, and this was the first time that a pathogen had been recovered from one of these devices. Believing that this was important information to share, we documented our findings in a letter format submitted to the *Journal of the American Medical Association*. Wanting a catchy title for this letter, one of the co-authors (Dr. Laurene Mascola, then chief of our unit) suggested that we use "The Holistic Runs." Pleased with this title, we submitted our letter and received an enthusiastic response from the *Journal of the American Medical Association* with one suggestion—that we change the title to "Bondage, Dominance, Irrigation and *Aeromonas hydrophila*: California Dreamin."[12] We had to admit that the *Journal of the American Medical Association* editors had managed to improve substantially what we had thought was a great title.

Given the occurrence of repeated waterborne outbreaks and the colonic irrigation report, clearly the epidemic potential of *E. histolytica* was recognized. Because amebiasis is a fecal–oral transmitted disease, we were concerned that the current outbreak possibly represented the initial cases in a waterborne or foodborne epidemic.

THE INVESTIGATION

Preliminary information indicated that a total of 38 cases of amebiasis had been identified over the 3-month period from August through October. Most of the patients reported acute diarrhea and had improved after treatment with antiprotozoal therapy. Gratefully, none of the cases had died. Based on historic data, the expected number of cases diagnosed at the HMO during this time period was just three (approximately one *E. histo-*

lytica infection per month). We determined that there had been no increase in specimens submitted for "ova and parasite" examination that might explain a jump in cases. Given this information, the number of cases recognized substantially exceeded typical baseline levels and therefore met the criterion of an outbreak.

As often occurs with such circumstances, we initiated several activities concurrently. Two senior epidemiologists, Mike Tormey, a marathon runner who had graduated from that bastion of parasitology, Tulane University, and Marc Strassburg, one of the elite cadre of individuals who had worked on smallpox eradication, provided help (as well as their typical dose of usually valuable criticism). Our preliminary investigation failed to implicate a possible common source of infection. Although this centralized laboratory served several healthcare facilities, there was no clustering of cases from any particular site(s). Moreover, early information indicated that the affected patients were not from recognized risk groups such as recent immigrants or men who have sex with men. At this point, information was not available on possible exposure to colonic irrigation. A review of county-wide reported amebiasis cases and a quick survey of other major laboratories and selected physician groups did not reveal an increase in cases beyond that reported by this HMO. Although this information was reassuring, we still had a sizable outbreak yet to resolve.

In his protozoal diseases laboratory section, Larry Ash had drilled into us that *E. histolytica* was a difficult parasite to diagnose. On his dreaded laboratory exams, taken under the duress of 1-minute timed stations, complete with the pressure of a loud timer annoyingly ticking off the seconds, he had always included artifacts or "fake parasites." From this torture we learned that not only could a number of common nonpathogenic protozoa be confused with *E. histolytica* but fecal leukocytes (white blood cells), notably polymorphonuclear neutrophils and macrophages, were routinely mistaken for *E. histolytica* (Table 7-2). Nevertheless, this was a highly respected laboratory that had followed approved procedures for the diagnosis of intestinal protozoa. Their methods were solid. As recommended, permanently stained smears were prepared from polyvinyl alcohol-preserved stool specimens using the Gomori-trichrome staining method. The laboratory had also done well in proficiency testing (independent testing to assure quality control).

Given this information, we were confident in the capability of this laboratory. Nevertheless, infectious disease epidemiologists are indoctrinated

---

Table 7-2   Artifacts and Organisms that
Can Be Mistaken for *E. Histolytica* Infection
and Lead to a False-Positive Diagnosis

Artifacts
    Polymorphonuclear neutrophils
    Macrophages
    Epithelial cells
Organisms
    Entamoeba coli
    Entamoeba hartmanni
    Entameoba polecki

---

that it is essential early in an outbreak investigation to verify or "confirm the diagnosis." Not expecting to find anything irregular, we nevertheless went to the HMO facility, where we found a large operation with state-of-the-art equipment. To my relief, we were greeted by a very cooperative laboratory director, a woman with many years of experience in clinical laboratories. We asked whether there had been any recent changes to staff or procedures in the parasitology section. She advised us that there had not been any significant changes of note. A single technician was responsible for reading the parasitology slides and had been employed for the previous 4 years. The established protocol was for all positive findings to be reviewed by a supervisor. The only recent modification was that a new staff member had been assigned to prepare the initial fecal smears. The laboratory director stated that, because of this change, the slides had become "less dense" and were "easier to read." This made sense because organisms can be difficult to see when smears of stool are too thick.

Based on the information provided and our observations of their operation, we had no reason to believe that there may have been a laboratory error and became more concerned that we needed to find a source of the outbreak. In spite of this, just to be thorough, I asked the laboratory director whether I could review the "parasite" logs. In 1983, most logs were large notebooks with entries that were recorded by hand. Going down the list of entries, the benefits of Larry Ash's grueling parasitology course were finally realized. Most of the *E. histolytica*–positive entries had recorded in the comments section that "many white blood cells were observed." Few

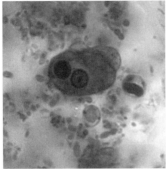

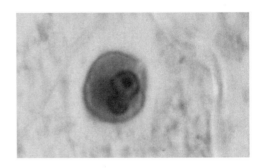

A: Entamoeba histolytica   B: Fecal leukocyte
   trophozoite

FIGURE 7-1 Comparison of *Entamoeba histolytica* (trophozoite) and fecal leukocyte from trichrome stained fecal smears under oil immersion. Courtesy of Lawrence R. Ash.

specimens from other patients had such comments. Because white blood cells are commonly mistaken as amoebae, we now suspected that our epidemic of amebiasis was perhaps not an outbreak at all but rather a pseudo-outbreak caused by false-positive lab findings. The similar appearance of *E. histolytica* and fecal leukocytes is illustrated in Figure 7-1. We asked to take 12 of the positive slides back to the Los Angeles County Public Health Laboratory's Parasitology Section, where Kay Mori, the unit supervisor, reviewed the slides. Kay had decades of experience and, in the early 1980s, was one of the first to recognize the rare protozoan parasite, *Entamoeba polecki*, in Vietnamese immigrants. Each year her lab processed thousands of stool specimens for "ova and parasite" exam. In just a few hours, Kay called to tell us that none of the 12 slides were positive for *E. histolytica* but that frequent leukocytes were observed!

Eventually, 71 slides from the 38 patients were reviewed either by the Public Health Laboratory or UCLA's Clinical Laboratory.[13] A total of 67 (94.5%) specimens from 36 patients were negative for amebiasis; just 4 slides from 2 patients could be confirmed as *E. histolytica* positive. This meant that 95% of the patients were incorrectly diagnosed. Specimens from 34 of the 36 unconfirmed cases were found to have polymorphonuclear neutrophils and/or macrophages. In the remaining two cases, nonpathogenic protozoa were observed. Thinner, "less dense" slides can make the morphology of cells, including leukocytes, more defined, and those features of white blood cells that can mimic *E. histolytica* may become more pronounced. The change in procedure by the new technician had resulted in misdiagnosis.

It is likely that some of the patients in this pseudo-outbreak mistakenly diagnosed with amebiasis may have actually had bacterial gastroenteritis. Such bacterial infections can elicit gastrointestinal inflammation, and the presence of fecal leukocytes is commonly observed in infections such as *Salmonella*, *Campylobacter*, and *Shigella*.[14] Moreover, because these infections are typically self-limited, it could explain the apparent, yet coincidental, response to antiamebic therapy. It is also possible that some patients may have had inflammatory bowel disease, a condition that may mimic amebiasis and one in which white blood cells frequently occur in stool specimens. It was amusing that although the laboratory director informed the patients' physicians of the misdiagnoses, a number of incredulous clinicians called to challenge us stating, "My patients must have had amebiasis because they improved on antiamebic therapy." We listened, politely assuring them of our findings and advising them that the observed patient improvement was simply coincidental.

The microscopic diagnosis of *E. histolytica* can be challenging and requires highly skilled technicians.[1] Krogstad and colleagues investigated seven suspected foci of amebiasis and determined that a number of laboratories had substantially overdiagnosed amebiasis with the principal error found that leukocytes in stools were reported as *E. histolytica*.[15] Two of these laboratories were in community hospitals, and one was in a teaching hospital associated with a medical school and a school of public health. These three laboratories may have mistakenly diagnosed as many as 1,200 cases of amebiasis a year for 20 years. In independent proficiency testing conducted by the Centers for Disease Control using a stool specimen that contained no parasites but had numerous leukocytes, none of 17 reference laboratories reported the presence of parasites; however, 74 of 528 other laboratories (14%) erroneously reported one or more parasites, most commonly *E. histolytica*.[13] Missing the presence of parasites (i.e., false-negative findings), including *E. histolytica*, is another common error, and together, the frequency of underdiagnosis and overdiagnosis speaks to the larger issue of having qualified and quality controlled laboratory personnel in diagnostic laboratories.

DISCUSSION AND CONCLUSION

This pseudo-outbreak of amebiasis underscores the need to verify the diagnosis as one of the initial important steps in outbreak investigations. Failure to do so can waste valuable time and resources, as well as induce unnecessary alarm. Pseudo-outbreaks are not rare. Such events, across a variety of infectious agents and circumstances, have been routinely reported in the biomedical literature and may be more common than appreciated. These apparent outbreaks can be caused by many different factors (Table 7-3). Among the more unusual of such events included a spurious outbreak of gastrointestinal *Pseudomonas aeruginosa* infection that resulted when stool culture samples were taken from feces that had already been excreted in toilets rather than captured in a clean container.[16] An apparent outbreak of pharyngeal gonorrhea was attributed to false-positive test results caused by the presence of commensal oropharyngeal *Neisseria* species.[17] Storing transport media in uncovered bottles under a sink allowed contamination by tap water and led to a pseudo-outbreak of multidrug-resistant *Pseudomonas*.[18] A contaminated ice machine was the source of transient respiratory tract colonization with *Mycobacterium fortuitum*.[19] The following briefly details factors that have been implicated as causes of pseudo-outbreaks and includes accompanying examples.

Improper Specimen Collection Techniques

The pseudo-outbreak of *P. aeruginosa*, referred to previously here, occurred among 10 patients in a hematology unit.[16] Because *P. aeruginosa* is not a recognized cause of diarrheal disease, this was an indication that something might be wrong. In investigating the apparent outbreak, it was observed that nurses obtained specimens for cultures from feces in the toilet. *P. aeruginosa* genetically identical to the "patients'" strain was recovered from toilet water. Pseudomonads are ubiquitous in water sources, including municipal water, and it would be expected to be found in toilet water.

Laboratory Error

A variety of factors can lead to false-positive laboratory findings and the occurrence of pseudo-outbreaks. Such factors include misidentification of nonpathogenic organisms or artifacts (fake parasites) as disease-causing agents as occurred in the amebiasis outbreak detailed here or the pseudo-outbreak of pharyngeal gonorrhea referred to previously.[17] The use of

Table 7-3 Factors Implicated in Pseudo-Outbreaks and Examples of Reported Incidents

Cause	Circumstance	Agent	Setting	Number of Cases	Reference Number
Improper specimen collection techniques	Sampling from feces in toilet	*Pseudomonas*	Hematology unit	10	16
Laboratory error					
Misidentification	Commensal organism misidentified	*Neisseria gonorrhoeae*	Prostitutes	Unknown	17
Incorrect test cutoff	Antibody testing	*Legionella pneumophila*	Community-wide	7	20
Inappropriate test performed	Antibody testing	Epstein-Barr virus	College students	285	21
Contaminated equipment	Inadequate disinfection of bronchoscope	*Pseudomonas, Serratia*	Private hospital	41	22
Contaminated media/reagents	Transport media stored under a sink	*Pseudomonas*	Infants	16	18
Cross-contamination from control strains	Cross-contamination at time of processing	*Mycobacterium scrofulaceum*	Veteran's hospital	3	24
Airborne contamination	Laboratory construction	*Aspergillus sydowii*	Ophthalmology ward	23	25
Transient colonization	Contaminated ice machine causing respiratory tractcolonization	*M. fortuitum*	Hospital ward for persons with HIV	47	19

Inappropriate testing material	Tuberculosis skin testing	*Mycobacterium tuberculosis*	Residential facility staff	9	27
Improper reading (e.g., skin test)	Tuberculosis skin testing	*Mycobacterium tuberculosis*	Prison	73	28
Enhanced detection	Expanded culturing by laboratories	*Escherichia coli* 0157:H7	Community-wide, New Jersey	46	29
Sporadic cases mistaken for an outbreak	Unrelated cases viewed as cluster	*Mycobacterium tuberculosis*	Poultry plant workers	4	30
Automated Identification System errors	Software update	*Enterococcus durans*	Community hospital	29	26
Use of probiotics	Stool cultures taken after probiotic administration	*Bacillus cereus*	Hospital	3	23
Misinterpretation of testing (low positive predictive value)	Usually antibody testing	Variety of agents	NA	NA	31

incorrect test cutoff values as has been reported for Legionnaires' disease,[20] poor laboratory technique, and using the wrong diagnostic test, which has been documented for infectious mononucleosis,[21] can also result in false-positive findings.

Contaminated Equipment

An apparent outbreak of both *P. aeruginosa* and *Seratia marcesans* occurred among 41 hospitalized patients who had undergone bronchoscopic procedures.[22] It was determined that contamination and inadequate disinfection of bronchoscopes were responsible for the pseudo-outbreak.

Contaminated Media or Reagents

The spurious outbreak of multidrug-resistant *Pseudomonas* mentioned previously occurred among 16 infants and was linked to contaminated transport media stored under a sink where a number of bottles were found to be open and without tops.[18] Tap water splashing from the sink was considered the likely mode of contamination.

Use of Probiotic Supplement

An apparent clustering of diarrheal illness thought to be caused by *Bacillus cereus* was linked to the use of probiotic medication.[23] Three patients were given the probiotic supplement after developing diarrhea. Genetically identical *B. cereus* was recovered from the probiotic that had been administered to the patients.

Cross-Contamination from Control Strains

Microbiology laboratories retain reference strains for use as controls to assist in confirming identification of cultured organisms and as a quality control measure to ensure that techniques are reliable. An apparent cluster of three cases of *Mycobacterium scrofulaceum* was linked to cross-contamination of patient specimens with a laboratory reference strain.[24] Because infection with this agent is rare and had not been identified by this laboratory for 10 years, an investigation was initiated. Testing of the patient isolates and reference organism indicated that they were identical.

Airborne Contamination

A pseudo-outbreak of *Aspergillus sydowii* keratitis in 23 patients in an ophthalmology ward and clinic was associated with recent construction and probable airborne contamination of culture media.[25] It was noted that many colonies formed outside of the inoculation zone of the agar plates and that *Aspergillus* was recovered from air sampling in the clinic.

Transient Colonization

As previously discussed, a contaminated ice machine led to transient *M. fortuitum* colonization of 47 HIV-infected patients on a hospital ward.[19] The patients had consumed water with ice from the contaminated machine. After thorough disinfection of the ice machine with vinegar and bleach, no additional cases were observed.

Automated Identification System Errors

The use of automated systems for identification of infectious agents, particularly in large laboratories, has been increasing. An apparent outbreak of 29 cases of *Enterococcus durans* followed an error in the updated system software.[26] Using alternative methods of identification, it was determined that these isolates were likely misidentified.

Improper Testing Material

Nine staff of a residential facility converted to skin-test positive for tuberculosis; however, it was determined that an inappropriate concentration of purified protein derivative (250 tuberculin units) was used for the skin testing. Retesting with the standard 5 tuberculin units yielded no reactions.[27] Improper reading of PPD skin tests can also result in spurious outbreaks.[28]

Enhanced Detection

A community-wide pseudo-outbreak of *E. coli* O157:H7 resulted from expanded culturing of the organism by laboratories. Often, clinical laboratories will not routinely test for pathogens that may be considered rare or less important unless specifically requested by a physician; however, when such agents begin to become more common or well-known, laboratories will increase testing with the result that these agents are more frequently identified. Such enhanced detection of sporadic cases can be mistakenly perceived as an outbreak.[29]

Sporadic Cases Mistaken for an Outbreak

The occurrence of four cases of *M. tuberculosis* in poultry workers initially appeared to be a localized outbreak[30]; however, investigation found that they were unrelated cases that were erroneously viewed as a cluster.

Low Positive Predictive Value

An underappreciated problem is that even highly specific diagnostic assays will result in false-positive findings and subsequent over diagnosis. For example, a test with 95% specificity will have a 5% level of error. That is, 5 of every 100 noncases will be false positives. In low-prevalence populations, where the large majority of individuals are negative, most of the positives will, in fact, be false positives, and the test will have a low positive predictive value; therefore, in such circumstances, imprudent interpretation of diagnostic test results can lead to the incorrect presumption that an outbreak exists. This phenomenon was encountered in the early years following the discovery of the Lyme disease agent (*Borrelia burgdorferi*) where there was a veritable explosion of testing for this infection using a new serologic test; however, given the protean (many and varied) manifestations of Lyme disease that include dermatologic, arthritic, cardiac and neurologic conditions, huge numbers of patients, many of whom were not even at risk, were now being tested. Moreover, patients with a variety of chronic conditions that were nonresponsive to therapy requested that their physicians test for Lyme disease. During this time, I spoke with many persons who actually desperately wanted to have Lyme disease. Because the infection is treatable with antibiotics, they held the hope that their chronic illness was Lyme disease, which meant that they could be cured with a course of antibiotics. During this period, we began receiving scores of reports of Lyme disease among residents of Los Angeles despite the fact that repeated surveys of local tick populations failed to find the agent. The rapid expansion and national epidemic of Lyme disease was caused, in part, by overdiagnosis through misinterpretation of serologic testing.[31]

Epidemiology has been described as "reasoning under uncertainty."[32] Most epidemiologists are either born skeptics or acquire the trait through repeated indoctrination. The saying "believe none of what you hear and half of what you see" could very well have been coined by an epidemiologist. The pseudo-outbreak of amebiasis detailed here should reinforce the admonition to keep an open mind and question everything, even apparent diagnoses from highly regarded sources. It demonstrates that verifying the diagnosis is an essential element of any outbreak investigation.

REFERENCES

1. Ash LR, Orihel TC. *Atlas of Human Parasitology*, 5th ed. Chicago: American Society for Clinical Pathology, 2007.
2. Orihel TC, Ash LR. *Parasites in Human Tissues*. Chicago: American Society for Clinical Pathology, 2007.
3. Petri WA Jr, Haque R, Lyerly D, Vines RR. Estimating the impact of amebiasis on health. *Parasitol Today* 2000;16:320–321.
4. Most H. Manhattan: "a tropical isle." *Am J Trop Med Hyg* 1968;17:333–354.
5. Arfaa F. Intestinal parasites among Indochinese refugees and Mexican immigrants resettled in Contra Costa County, California. *J Fam Pract* 1982;12:223–226.
6. Thacker SB, Simpson S, Gordon TJ, Wolfe M, Kimball AM. Parasitic disease control in a residential facility for the mentally retarded. *Am J Public Health* 1979;69:1279–1281.
7. Steffan R. Epidemiologic studies of travelers' diarrhea, severe gastrointestinal infections, and cholera. *Rev Infect Dis* 1986;8(Suppl 2):S122–S1230.
8. National Institutes of Health. *Epidemic Amebic Dysentery: The Chicago Outbreak of 1933*. National Institutes of Health Bulletin no. 166. Washington, DC: Public Health Service, 1936.
9. LeMaistre CA, Sappenfield R, Culbertson C, et al. Studies of a water-borne outbreak of amebasis, South Bend Indiana. I. Epidemiological aspects. *Am J Hyg* 1956;64:30–45.
10. Hardy AV, Specter BK. The occurrence of infestations with *E. histolytica* associated with water-borne epidemic disease. *Public Health Rep* 1935;50:323–334.
11. Istre GR, Kreiss K, Hopkins RS, et al. An outbreak of amebiasis spread by colonic irrigation at a chiropractic clinic. *N Engl J Med* 1982;307:339–342.
12. Sorvillo FJ, Kilman L, Mascola L. Bondage, dominance, irrigation and *Aeromonas hydrophila*: California dreamin. *JAMA* 1989;261:697–698.
13. Centers for Disease Control and Prevention. Epidemiologic notes and reports, pseudo-outbreak of intestinal amebiasis—California. *MMWR* 1985;34:125–126.
14. Thielman NM, Guerrant RL. Acute infectious diarrhea. *N Engl J Med* 2004; 350:38–47.
15. Krogstad DJ, Spencer HC Jr, Healy GR, Gleason NN, Sexton DJ, Herron CA. Amebiasis: epidemiologic studies in the United States, 1971–1974. *Ann Intern Med* 1978;88:89–97.
16. Verweij PE, Biji D, Melchers WJ, et al. Pseudo-outbreak of multiresistant *Pseudomonas aeruginosa* in a hematology unit. *Infect Control Hosp Epidemiol* 1997; 18:128–131.
17. Verzijl A, Berretty PJ, Erceg A, et al. A pseudo-outbreak of pharyngeal gonorrhea related to a false-positive PCR-result. *Ned Tijdschr Geneesk* 2007;151:689–691.
18. Heard S, Lawrence S, Holmes B, Costas M. A pseudo-outbreak of *Pseudomonas* on a special care baby unit. *J Hosp Infect* 1990;16:59–65.
19. Gebo KA, Srinivasan A, Perl TM, Ross T, Groth A, Merz WG. Pseudo-outbreak of *Mycobacterium fortuitum* on a human immunodeficiency virus ward: transient

respiratory tract colonization from a contaminated ice machine. *Clin Infect Dis* 2002;25:32–38.

20. Regan CM, Syed Q, Mutton K, Wiratunga K. A pseudo community outbreak of legionnaires' disease on Merseyside: implications for investigation of suspected clusters. *J Epidemiol Community Health* 2000;54:766–769.

21. Centers for Disease Control and Prevention. Pseudo-outbreak of infectious mononucleosis—Puerto Rico, 1990. *MMWR* 1991;20:552–555.

22. Silva CV, Magalhaes VD, Pereira CR, Kawagoe JY, Ikura C, Ganc AJ. Pseudo-outbreak of *Pseudomonas aeruginosa* and *Serratia marcescens* related to broncho-scopes. *Infect Control Hosp Epidemiol* 2003;24:195–197.

23. Kniehl E, Becker A, Forster DH. Pseudo-outbreak of toxigenic *Bacillus cereus* isolated from stools of three patients with diarrhoea after oral administration of a probiotic medication. *J Hosp Infect* 2003;55:33–38.

24. Oda GV, DeVries MM, Yakrus MA. Pseudo-outbreak of *Mycobacterium scrofulaceum* linked to cross-contamination with a laboratory reference strain. *Infect Control Hosp Epidemiol* 2001;22:649–651.

25. Freeman J, Rogers K, Roberts S. Pseudo-outbreak of *Aspergillus* keratitis following construction in an ophthalmology ward. *J Hosp Infect* 2007;67:104–105.

26. Singer DA, Jochimsen EM, Gielerak P, Jarvis W. Pseudo-outbreak of *Enterococcus durans* infections and colonization associated with introduction of an automated identification system software update. *J Clin Microbiol* 1996;34:2685–2687.

27. Grabau JC, Burrows DJ, Kern ML. A pseudo outbreak of purified protein derivative skin-test conversions caused by inappropriate testing materials. *Infect Control Hosp Epidemiol* 1997;18:571–574.

28. Weinbaum CM, Bodner UR, Schulte J, et al. Pseudo-outbreak of tuberculosis infection due to improper skin-test reading. *Clin Infect Dis* 1998;26:1235–1236.

29. Centers for Disease Control and Prevention. Enhanced detection of sporadic *Escherichia coli* O157:H7 infections—New Jersey, July 1994. *MMWR* 1995; 44:417–418.

30. Kim DY, Ridzon R, Giles B, Mireles T. Pseudo-outbreak of tuberculosis in poultry plant workers, Sussex County, Delaware. *J Occup Environ Med* 2002; 44:1169–1172.

31. Sorvillo FJ, Nahlen B. Lyme disease. *N Engl J Med* 1990;322:474–475.

32. Greenland S. Probability logic and probabilistic induction. *Epidemiology* 1998; 9:322–332.

CHAPTER 8

Measles Among Religiously Exempt Persons

Charles E. Jennings

During January 1985, I was working for the Illinois Department of Public Health's Immunization Section in Springfield, Illinois. My primary duty was to administer the disease surveillance/outbreak control section for the vaccine preventable diseases. Prior to this, I started my career in public health by coordinating the "Swine Flu" efforts for the central and southern areas of Illinois back in 1976. After concern about the "Swine Flu" vaccine being unsafe with resulting shut down of the "Swine Flu" program, I continued to work for the Immunization Section by conducting school-based immunization clinics as part of the Centers for Disease Control's (CDC) measles elimination efforts.

On February 13, 1985, I received a report through interstate reporting procedures of a suspected measles case in a Missouri resident who was also one of 714 students at Principia College in Southwestern Illinois.[1] This was an unusual report because measles was uncommon thanks to the success of measles vaccine in the United States, and it was a unique population that may have been exposed to measles. Principia College is a college run by Christian Scientists for Christian Scientists. That same day, while I was investigating this report, I received a call from a public school nurse in the area that had heard a rumor of a 17-year-old female that died at a hospital in Alton, Illinois with a suspected rash. Alton, Illinois is a relatively

133

small town, but it was the closest city to Principia College with medical facilities that serve a wide area of southwestern Illinois. I immediately contacted the hospital, and they confirmed that a 17-year-old female had died of severe dehydration, rash, and a remarkably high temperature of 107°F (41.7°C). I learned that measles was suspected, but no report was made to health authorities although measles is a class I–reportable illness. In Illinois, our surveillance system mandated that class I–reportable diseases must be reported to health authorities within 24 hours by telephone when there is a suspicion of disease.

After further questioning, I was told that the girl's body was returned to the family for cremation. This was troubling because such an unexplained hospital death should have been referred to the coroner. Fortunately, I contacted the Jersey County coroner and learned that tissue samples had been preserved.

During this very busy day, I received a call from "Cathy" (not her real name) who identified herself as a "nurse" from Principia College. She said that she wanted to comply with the law and to report six students currently in the college sick room with measles. She also said that she had previously reported cases to the Jersey County Health Department but had not received any feedback. I asked how she could confirm measles, and she stated she identified it from a picture in a book. She stated that all cases felt warm and had a rash similar to the picture. Before I could formulate my next questions, she proceeded to explain that as a Christian Scientist nurse she cannot take temperatures or blood pressure measurements or provide any care other than to make the person comfortable, assist with drinking and eating, and guess what something is from text books. I then asked about the 17-year-old female that had died, and she confirmed that she was a student there, including having been in the sick room; however, the family chose to remove her from Christian Science care and seek medical attention. Not liking the way this all sounded and the way the day was going, I consulted with the Jersey County Health Department and left immediately to begin an investigation.

That evening, the Jersey County Health Department Communicable Disease staff and I met to plan our strategy to begin an investigation of this suspected measles outbreak. The items that we discussed included the case definition that we would use in an investigation. The CDC case definition of measles at that time included a fever of 101°F (38.3°C) or greater if measured, a generalized rash lasting 3 or more days, and at least one of the following: cough, coryza, (inflammation of mucous membranes, i.e., running nose) conjunctivitis, or photophobia. We decided to modify the case definition for this outbreak because temperatures were not taken; however, a feeling of warmth could be reported. We also discussed how we would approach the investigation the next morning. They further discussed with me their relationship with the college in the past, the people they work with, and about the community of Elsah, Illinois, where the college is located.

Principia College is located high on the bluffs overlooking the Mississippi River on very prime real estate. The college is completely fenced and has only two gates guarded 24 hours a day with tightly controlled access. The village of Elsah, just outside the main gate, is an old rustic sort of town featuring quaint bed and breakfasts, restaurants, and arts and crafts stores. Most residents of the town are closely associated with the college and are either faculty, staff, or former students settling there. The health department said they maintain a good relationship with the college in regards to mandatory food and sanitation inspections and a few communicable diseases in the past.

The Jersey County Health Department admitted that a few rash cases had originally been reported to them by the college but had at this point failed to act on those reports. They would later be penalized during health department accreditation hearings for this lapse. Arrangements were made to meet with the college administration the next morning. Later that first night, I visited the county coroner, who was also a local funeral director, and was given lung tissue, bronchial fluid, and heart blood for shipment to the CDC laboratory. The results that came later from the CDC showed massive Gram-negative bronchial pneumonia with purulent tracheobronchitis and some areas of bronchopneumonia associated with *Staphylococcus* and *Streptococcus*. Measles is often complicated by pneumonias such as these, particularly among adolescents and adults with no prior histories of exposure to circulating measles virus or vaccine.

On February 14, 1985, representatives from the Jersey County Health Department led by Nola Kramer, RN, administrator, and me drove the 20 miles to the campus. This was my first visit to Elsah and the college, and I was very impressed with what I saw. The town of Elsah was like stepping back into time, and I was awed by the beauty of the college campus. Grand old buildings were mixed with modern architecture. They overlooked the Mississippi River and could be seen for miles in all directions. After arriving at the guarded gate, we were told precisely where we needed to go to meet the college administrators and were escorted there by college staff. We were very enthusiastically received and were introduced to the college president, the dean of students, and a representative of the office of information for the Church of Christian Scientist out of Chicago, Illinois.

After all the formalities, I explained what I suspected (measles occurring on campus), what I wanted to do (investigate), and if indeed measles was occurring that we could make efforts to control and contain the disease, including offering clinics for vaccinating students, staff, and families. The college administration stated that they were Christian Scientists and that their religion teaches them to live by the laws of the land but to strive to continue to practice their religion. I stated that I respected their wishes and beliefs but that it was my role to protect the public health of everyone both on the campus and the general public outside the gates of their campus. I requested access to the campus as needed. They arranged for me to visit their "sick room." The sick room on campus is a separate building where students, staff, and families stay when they are sick. This is also where the Christian Scientist "nurses" work from. Here I met "Cathy," who placed the earlier phone call to me. She explained again that as a Christian Scientist nurse she could only observe and view pictures of illness to determine what might be wrong.

To my amazement, there were currently 16 students who had a rash and felt warm in the sick room facility. There was no attempt at isolation of these rash illness cases, and thus, these students in the sick room were sharing common space with other ill students. Being the first part of February, it was my opinion (as I also was responsible for influenza surveillance for the state of Illinois) that influenza was also circulating on campus as well as in the community and this region of the state. The girl that had died was in the sick room at the same time as others with influenza-like symptoms. If someone who was debilitated with one disease should become infected with another disease, the outcome could be more severe than would normally occur. In fact, the 17-year-old that died was in the sick room with influenza-like illness while incubating measles.

Over the next 6 days my investigation continued. On the second day after arriving at the sick room, the building was surrounded by students singing and praying for those in the sick room. On the same day, the college agreed to close the campus, not allowing people to enter or leave with out some proof of previous vaccination. This, I thought at the time, was actually a huge step, as I had been told the day before that as Christian Scientists they do not believe in medical care or immunizations. They did, however, only tell the students that if they had a vaccination record at home they could have someone send it to them but would not agree to making these records a part of the students file. We learned later that this "quarantine" of the campus was not enforced to any extent, as sport teams, visiting families, and other groups were allowed to enter and leave the campus freely. Students also knew how to sneak their way off campus through the fence. Serious isolation and quarantine would come later as the outbreak became more serious. Suspected measles cases and those considered susceptible (persons with no history of immunity from past disease or vaccine) need to be isolated from the outbreak for up to 21 days after the onset of rash of the last known case. Measles is a highly communicable virus and is spread by respiratory droplets so that strict airborne isolation is necessary; however, their restrictions on access did not apply to families of staff attending school at Principia College's grade school and high school across the river in Missouri.

Our access to ill students was limited. Although college officials stated that we could have all of the access we needed, we were always escorted by school officials, and they were always present during any interview. One of my goals was to be able to draw blood for measles specific IgM, for confirmation that measles was occurring. When a student would agree to let me draw blood, he or she eventually would change his or her mind after talking with a school official. I even suggested obtaining throat swabs for viral isolation, as this would be less invasive to the body, but this too was denied. By the third day, school officials were visiting each student before I was allowed to talk to them.

The Christian Scientist nurses were as helpful as possible. They explained to me that if a Christian Scientist is ill, it is because their thoughts and minds are not right with God. While a student is in the sick room, a Christian Scientist reader will come and sit with them for hours reading to them from the bible and from the literature of Mary Baker Eddy,[2] the founder of the Church of Christ, Scientists. They explained that with the girl that died they would read to her and rub her neck to get her to swallow water. When the family decided to put her in the hospital, all Christian Science spiritual assistance stopped. Above the Christian Scientist nurse is the Christian Scientist practitioner (considered the "doctor" of Christian Science). An ill person can hire the practitioner to provide the spiritual care to get the persons mind right with God; however, that spiritual help ends when a person chooses medical care.

The interviews that I conducted with the ill students typically went like this. The school official would introduce me as a new friend here to meet them who would like to talk to them about their being here in the sick room. I would then attempt to do an epi-investigation; however, many factors would hamper the collection of good data. I asked, "How long have you had this rash?" The answer more often than not would be, "What rash?" I came to learn as the investigation progressed that the students would drape towels over their mirrors so that they would not see the rash, as being ill meant that their mind was not right with God. Denial of symptoms seemed to be the norm. If they didn't see it, they didn't have it.

It was also on the third day of investigation that I was told by college officials that a 19-year-old male student had died, but it turned out that he had not been included among the students I had interviewed, which further led me to believe I was not being told everything and/or not being told of all suspected cases. This student who died had been found unresponsive in the bathroom of his dorm, and CPR was attempted to revive him. I immediately asked why CPR was attempted on him when medical care is generally not allowed. I was told that this student while being read to went into the bathroom and fell and hit his head, and thus, it was considered an accident and not because of any illness. I was further told that when an accident happens (i.e., a sports injury) that first aid is appropriate. This was confusing to me because the investigation showed this young man to have met the case definition, and an autopsy showed massive Gram-negative bronchopneumonia.

As we attempted to make home visits to interview ill family members, we would see evidence of persons ill in the home (such as bowls out in the open, probably used for vomiting); however, it was believed that ill children were being moved from house to house ahead of our team. We believed this, as not all of the children could be found when visiting homes. Some families would tell us of sick children in other homes, but having to make "appointments" to visit the homes, we would find that the suspected case would be visiting friends or relatives at another location.

At this time, I requested assistance from CDC and was immediately sent Steven G. F. Wassilak, MD, an Epidemic Intelligence Service officer, to assist in this investigation further. Dr. Wassilak came with a lot of measles experience and was eager to hit the ground running. Steve immediately started analyzing the data and offered suggestions on the investigation. As the investigation continued, three acute-phase IgM measles-specific serum specimens were obtained. The first confirmation of measles came from the sister of the 19-year-old male that died. She was hospitalized with measles and was not a practicing Christian Scientist. The other two confirmed IgMs were from students whose parents agreed to having the blood drawn despite the college administration's wishes.

During our initial discussions with the college administration, they had expressed a desire not to include the news media. I agreed that no information would come from the Illinois Department of Public Health and should something get out they would be the ones to handle it; however, in situations like this, the news media is all over it. After the outbreak leaked to someone in the media, it became a full time job just trying to respond to them. My hotel was 12 miles from the campus. On one morning, I actually had two cars and one helicopter follow me to the campus. The news media set up camp outside the gate and helicopters even attempted to land on campus. I encouraged college officials to arrange for a news conference on campus, where they could control what was presented to the media. The college agreed but asked me to take the lead. This was a good opportunity to let the media know what was happening, and I was able to introduce Dr. Wassilak as an expert on measles, which probably helped the media view our work with enhanced credibility and focus on and accept the facts rather than speculation, which could have gone awry given the two deaths. After the news conference was over, the media was satisfied with updates every day, and they left us alone to do our work. The news media seemed to be most happy getting updates of the numbers of cases.

One evening I visited one of the measles cases in the hospital. It was the sister of the 19-year-old that had died. Her father, who was in town to make arrangements for his son's body, was visiting, and we had the opportunity to sit and talk for several hours.

We talked about many things, but I took the opportunity to explain measles and how vaccine can prevent illness. I explained how I needed to get the college to accept vaccine. After he and I shared a tearful 2 hours, he stated that he wished he knew the things we talked about before he lost his son. He asked me whether other parents really knew what was going on, to which I responded that I could not answer that because the college controlled the communication with the parents.

That night I received a phone call at my hotel from the dean of students asking me how quickly could I offer vaccine on campus. He also stated that a 16-year-old female, the daughter of a faculty member, had now died too (another case we knew nothing about!). Without showing just how excited I was, I said we could have a clinic set up by 8:30 a.m. the next day. I learned later that the father to whom I had explained the public health facts about measles, along with many other parents, had put pressure on the college. He had contacted us to allow us to do whatever was necessary to control the outbreak.

At about this same time, I received a call from the Illinois Department of Children and Family Services. They were concerned about a number of complaints that there may be children in this community that were ill and not receiving appropriate health care. They were consulting with me about the possibility of filing child abuse charges against parents and even the college. I approached the college administration to let them know what this state agency wanted to do. I offered that I could encourage the department to not pursue the issue if the college would allow us the opportunity to have all ill persons be examined by a physician of our choice. Dr. Wassalak was chosen to do this, as he had developed a strong relationship with the college administrators; however, the college stipulated that he examine only minor children. One of the minor children that Dr. Wassalak examined, a 12-year-old female, was the sister of the 16-year-old female who had recently died. The parents agreed to allow the ill child to be examined; however, the parents stated that they were only agreeing to the exam because of the agreement we had with the college. They made it very clear that no further medical care was to occur, no matter what Dr. Wassalak determined. While sitting in their home while the exam was being conducted, a little dog was running around the house. The mother of the girl being examined stated that the poor little dog had been sick that day and that they had just taken it to the vet. With a great deal of surprise I had to ask how they were able to seek medical care for the dog but would refuse it for their children. I was told that the dog is not able to think for itself and that it does not have the thought processes as the humans do, and thus, they need to make the decision for the dog. Humans are capable of thinking and that God has given every person the chance to keep their minds right with God or be punished with an illness.

Because this was my first major outbreak situation in my new role of surveillance/outbreak control, I was fortunate to have had great people to work with. The administrator of the Illinois Immunization Program, Mr. C. Ralph March, and the Division of Disease Control Chief, Byron Francis, MD, were great in allowing me the leeway and the authority that I needed to be able to negotiate and compromise in our effort to contain this outbreak. My immediate boss, Mr. March, and I had an agreement that I should do as I see fit to control the outbreak and that he would do the politics associated with state government. If I made an unpopular decision (politically or medically), he would work to smooth it over. This partnership was important for the eventual containment of this outbreak and demonstrated a trusting administrator–program staff relationship that allowed me to thrive in my job.

By 8:30 a.m. the morning after the college allowed a clinic on campus, staff members from the Illinois Department of Public Health and the Jersey County Health Department were set up and ready to begin vaccinations. I had suggested to college officials earlier that if we could set up a clinic we could use the jet injector device. This is a device that injects vaccines and other injectables directly into the body using hydraulic pressure that pinpoints the stream of vaccine. As there is no needle, I convinced college officials that this method would be less invasive to the body. They requested that this is what they wanted. Another incentive that I offered was that if anyone agreed to vaccination they could immediately have access off campus with no further restrictions. I realized that some who received vaccine could still be incubating disease but that this was a compromise necessary to get the clinic approved. In fact, only one person that received vaccine developed a rash within 7 days of being vaccinated.

That day vaccine was administered to 403 students, staff, and families. One hundred thirty five more were able to prove prior vaccination, and 50 students that declined vaccine were quarantined on campus for up to 21 days after onset of rash of the last case. This quarantine was strictly enforced. An additional 127 persons sought vaccine off campus.

Before it was finally controlled, this outbreak (Figure 8-1) was sustained for six generations of cases with 125 cases among the 714 students and 121 staff and resident family members (overall attack rate of 15.0%). It was shown that the index case was a student who had traveled to Alaska over the Christmas holidays returning to the college on the 9th of January and developing rash on the 11th of January.

There were 11 associated cases. Three died, two students and one 16-year-old child of a staff person residing on campus (case fatality ratio = 2.2%). The case fatality ratio for the United States at that time was (< 0.01%). The 11 associated cases were among persons who were not students, faculty, staff or family members and were reported from outside the

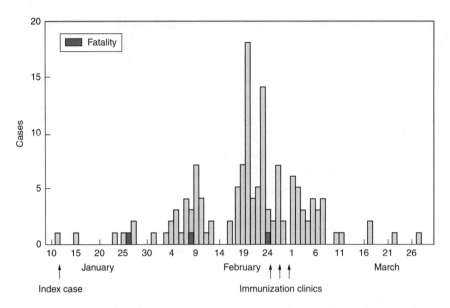

FIGURE 8-1 Measles cases in a Christian Science college in Illinois by date of rash onset, 1985.

Novotny T, Jennings C, Doran M, March CR, Measles outbreaks in religious groups exempt from immunization laws. *Public Health Reports* 1988;103:49–54. Republished by permission of the Association of Schools of Public Health, Public Health Reports.[1]

college and immediate community but had been exposed by students, faculty, or staff.

This outbreak was one of the most important to occur during my career with the Illinois Department of Public Health. I learned many valuable lessons that carried on through many outbreaks of many vaccine preventable diseases. Most of the lessons learned were called on again during April and May of 1994 when another measles outbreak occurred among the same Christian Scientist community.[3] One hundred forty one persons with measles were reported from Illinois and Missouri among the college, an elementary school, and a high school. The same family names were again involved with this outbreak that was part of the 1985 outbreak. This time I was prepared to handle the college administration. They knew just what we needed, and I knew what I needed to do. This time I went directly to the parents of the students, as I found that many times perhaps only one parent was Christian Scientist, and found that they were always very cooperative. Most of the families could present immunization records so that I could determine who may be immune. The college was also prepared to enforce strict isolation and quarantine. The college even agreed to allow students to include immunization records as a part of their school records. Following this 1994 outbreak, I do not recall any further outbreaks reported for this community.

During outbreaks, religiously exempt groups (Exhibit 8-1) generally cooperate during health emergencies. Disease-control personnel should learn to understand and develop working relationships with the various leaders of the several diversified groups of people opposed to immunizations. All persons need to be aware of reporting laws and the advantages to early reporting. This will allow disease control personnel to control the disease more rapidly while providing protection to the general public. Disease control personnel must be willing to negotiate and compromise to accomplish the tasks necessary to control and end outbreaks. Sensitivity to the beliefs of these diversified groups needs to be balanced with

---

Exhibit 8-1   Religious Groups Possibly Opposed to Immunization

- Amish
- Church of Christ in Christian Union
- Church of Christ, Scientist
- Church of the First Born
- Church of God (several types)
- Church of Human Life Sciences
- Church of the Lord Jesus Christ of the Apostolic Faith
- Church of Scientology
- Disciples of Christ
- Divine Science Federation International
- Faith Assembly
- Hare Krishna
- Hutterites
- Kripala Yaga Ashram
- Mennonites
- Netherlands Reform Church
- Rosicrucian Fellowship
- Worldwide Church of God

Source: McLaren N. *A Study of Immunization Attitudes.* Presentation to the Center for Health Promotion and Education, CDC. August 25, 1982.

enforcement of the rules and regulations that are the public health laws of the city, county, or state. It is a difficult and delicate challenge to investigate an outbreak in this setting, but with good communication skills and a good working knowledge of what is required for the control efforts, a successful outcome is ultimately possible.

REFERENCES

1. Novotny T, Jennings C, Doran M, March CR. Measles outbreaks in religious groups exempt from immunization laws. *Public Health Reports* 1988;103:49–54.
2. Eddy MB. *Science and Health with a Key to the Scriptures*. Boston: Christian Science Board of Directors. 1934, Revised 1994.
3. Outbreak of measles among Christian Scientist students—Missouri and Illinois, 1994. *MMWR* 1994;43:463–465.

CHAPTER 9

An Outbreak of Fulminant Hepatitis B in a Medical Ward in Israel

Ronald C. Hershow, MD

My path to a public health career in infectious disease epidemiology was a circuitous one. During my internal residency at Washington Hospital Center, in Washington, DC, I was fortunate to do a 2-month elective providing emergency medical care in a Khmer refugee camp in Thailand. While there, I was exposed to the challenges of providing food, shelter, and health care to 140,000 persons who had been displaced by a genocidal Cambodian civil war. This powerful introduction to international health crystallized a desire to expand beyond the primary care focus that had defined me since I had first applied to medical school. Envisioning a possible career in international health, I decided to stay on and do an infectious disease fellowship at Washington Hospital Center. I was first told about the Centers for Disease Control's (CDC) Epidemic Intelligence Service (EIS) by Terry Chorba, a friend from residency who had just begun his EIS fellowship. He enthusiastically described a Cleveland outbreak of Parvovirus B19 that he was investigating. I was hooked. While still an infectious disease fellow, I was accepted to the EIS and subsequently underwent a frenetic week of interviews in Atlanta. I was drawn to the Hepatitis Branch because of a strong mentorship team led by Steve Hadler and James Maynard, the

145

potential for involvement in international investigations, and a diverse group of diseases that exemplified different types of epidemiology. It turned out to be one of the best decisions I ever made.

During my infectious disease fellowship, I had acquired only a rudimentary knowledge of viral hepatitis and had to learn quickly. That early immersion in viral hepatitis was a wonderful period of discovery. I learned just how fascinating my "new" diseases were by delving into their natural history, diagnosis, epidemiology, and prevention. This process affirmed my selection of the Hepatitis Branch in the same way that living in a newly purchased home reveals many unanticipated pleasures. One thing that I came to appreciate was the value of the hepatitis A and hepatitis B serologic assays; in 1986, these had only been available for a few years. For an infectious disease epidemiologist, they are powerful tools, and their development led to an explosive growth in knowledge regarding the epidemiology of these diseases.

Because this chapter concerns a nosocomial outbreak of hepatitis B virus (HBV) infection, I'll begin by discussing how HBV serologic tests aid the epidemiologist. In the context of an outbreak, the hepatitis B surface antigen (HBsAg) assay is useful because approximately 30 days after the virus is acquired, the liver begins to manufacture virus that spills into the bloodstream and is detectable by this assay; however, among adults, more than 90% of the time, this period of viremia resolves within 6 months as the immune response successfully neutralizes and resolves the infection. Before resolution occurs, most adults will experience a symptomatic acute hepatitis syndrome, with onset generally beginning 60 to 120 days after HBV acquisition, although incubation can range from 45 to 180 days.

Although successful resolution of HBV infection is due to a complicated combination of cellular and humoral responses, the antibody to the HBsAg (anti-HBs) plays a key neutralizing role, and thus, detecting anti-HBs in the blood generally coincides with the resolution of hepatitis B viremia. Soon after anti-HBs titers rise, the HBsAg assay will no longer detect circulating virus; this generally occurs within months of the acquisition event; however, 2% to 6% of acutely infected adults fail to resolve acute infection and progress to chronic infection. For such individuals, the anti-HBs response never develops, and the HBsAg assay remains positive, generally for the rest of that patient's life. Thus, although a positive HBsAg response may signify acute, recently acquired infection, most often it identifies an individual who has developed ongoing, chronic HBV infection.

Fortunately for the epidemiologist, there is a serologic marker that indicates recently acquired infection. In the typical course of an evolving HBV infection, two separate types of antibody appear. One is the already mentioned anti-HBs, but even earlier, the immune system produces antibody to a core structural element within the HBV, the antibody to the hepatitis B core antigen (anti-HBc). Early on, IgM and IgG anti-HBc are elaborated, but within 6 months of the acquisition event, the IgM class anti-HBc becomes undetectable. In contrast, the IgG anti-HBc generally remains detectable for the rest of the person's life.

These four assays used in combination provide the epidemiologist with a powerful toolkit. In the context of an epidemic, the IgM anti-HBC (generally used in combination with the HBsAg) provides a way of identifying recently infected individuals. Indeed, HBV viremia may resolve so quickly and subclinical or mild disease presentations are so common that the IgM anti-HBc may be the only way to identify some patients infected during an epidemic. The IgG anti-HBC assay is important to the epidemiologist because it accurately indicates whether a person has ever acquired HBV infection and thus has utility as an epidemiologic tool that allows epidemiologists to measure the seroprevalence of HBV infection in different populations. Such sero-surveys can be used to cross-sectionally map cumulative incidence of HBV infection by country or geographic region, and the assay can be used to screen populations to assess whether given individuals need hepatitis B vaccination. Those with a positive anti-HBc will not require immunization because they have already acquired natural infection and are either naturally immune for life or, less commonly, have developed chronic infection. The anti-HBs are almost as useful to screen populations but will not be positive among those who have gone on to develop chronic infection. Those who have developed chronic infection and are persistently HBsAg positive are at heightened risk of progressing to chronic hepatitis, cirrhosis, and hepatocellular carcinoma, although the majority live out their lives as healthy carriers.

Epidemiologically, the pool of chronically infected persons are of central importance, as they are able to transmit infection to others through sexual contact, through overt parenteral exposure (as occurs when injection drug users share syringe needles), or through less apparent parenteral exposures that occur through contact with blood or blood-derived skin exudates in household settings or during skin-to-skin contact as might occur when children engage in rough play. Skin diseases or lacerations can provide portals of exit or entrance in these situations. Most pertinent to the outbreak described in this chapter is the possible role of patients or providers as sources of HBV-contaminated body fluids in healthcare-related exposures that on occasion result in nosocomial HBV acquisition.

My involvement in this outbreak began with a single phone call. As an EIS Officer, it was my job to answer the phone 2 days a week. A great majority of these calls were routine and could be handled by anyone with a thorough knowledge of "Recommendations for Prevention of Viral Hepatitis,"[1] an incredibly helpful set of recommendations that had been published in the *Morbidity and Mortality Weekly Report* in 1985. In a year of answering questions from concerned individuals, I had heard most of the standard variations. The priest who was worried about offering communion wine to a hepatitis B carrier parishioner for fear that the wine glass would be contaminated, a police cadet who was told that she couldn't be a police officer because she had tested positive for hepatitis B, and loads of people worried about the safety of immune serum globulin in view of the burgeoning AIDS epidemic. In these examples and on most calls, my job was to reassure that risk was negligible; however, on this particular day in August 1986, a call came in from Haifa, Israel that was of a different sort entirely.

The call was from the Rambam Medical Center in Haifa, Israel, and the facts were as follows. From June 7 to June 26, 1986, four patients were admitted to their medicine ward A (or "aleph" in Hebrew) with fulminant and ultimately fatal acute hepatitis B. Remarkably, all four patients had been hospitalized on the same medical ward between April 23 and May 8, 1.5 to 2 months before their terminal admission. Recognizing that this cluster of cases probably represented a hospital outbreak, a local investigation ensued that did not identify a cause of the outbreak. As part of this investigation, serologic testing was conducted in late May and early June to identify additional case patients who may not have been ill enough to have been rehospitalized. All living patients who had been on the ward in late April and early May were serologically tested. This revealed a fifth case (IgM anti-HBc positive) who was the only apparent survivor of the outbreak. On August 17, 2 months after the first cluster, a sixth patient was admitted with fulminant hepatitis B. This patient had been previously hospitalized when patients from the first cluster had been present on ward A. Concerned that an ongoing source of virulent hepatitis B had gone unidentified after the first cluster and that a second cluster was about to emerge, hospital officials decided to seek epidemic aid from the CDC. I happened to pick up the phone when they called.

Things developed very quickly from that point. International investigations were often led by senior staff, but fortunately for me, my superiors were all busy with other projects. When I had started in the EIS program, I had selected the Hepatitis Branch in part because of its involvement in international projects; however, an investigation in Israel exceeded my expectations. As a Jew, I had always felt a special connection to Israel and had been there once before. Five years previously, my wife and I had gone to Israel after 6 months volunteering at a mission hospital in Kenya. Even though we had never been there before, our stop in Israel before heading back to the United States felt like an early homecoming. On that first trip, we flew on the Israeli Airline El Al, and I was surprised when my eyes filled with tears as the chant Shalom Aleichem was piped into the airplane before landing. We were welcomed warmly by the people we met, and several even suggested that we might want to consider immigrating to Israel. Although I had always supported Israel in my political views and through donations to charitable causes, those commitments now seemed paltry and effete compared with the daily challenges of the Israelis that we met. I often reflected on that trip and thought that I would like to make some meaningful contribution to Israel; this investigation might provide a chance to do so.

Nonetheless, preparing to depart for an investigation is always hectic. Although I had already been an EIS officer for a year, I had never worked on a hospital outbreak and had to familiarize myself with the ways that the HBV might be acquired in a hospital. In addition, I had to temporarily disentangle myself from all current projects and family commitments. The call had come in just before Labor Day, and my wife's parents were coming for a visit soon. I had even rented a house on a lake in the Smoky Mountains for a late summer getaway. My family enjoyed it without me because in a few days I was on my way to Israel, with a briefcase full of articles hastily copied in the CDC library.

After I boarded the plane, my life simplified, and during the long flight, I was able to review the basic facts of the outbreak and to synthesize what I had learned by reviewing reports of other hospital-based hepatitis B outbreaks. The first cluster of cases with onset dates occurring within a circumscribed 3-week period in June was remarkable in several respects. First, the high mortality rate among cases was extremely unusual, if not unprecedented. Acute hepatitis B generally has a case fatality rate of less than 1%. Even considering that the patients involved in this outbreak were older persons, surveillance data suggested an expected mortality rate of 5%, not the 80% rate that had occurred in the first cluster. Second, assuming that hepatitis B infection was acquired during their earlier admission, the cases had short incubation periods ranging from 1.5 to 2 months, at the lower end of the 1.5- to 6-month textbook description of incubation period for hepatitis B. Third, none of the patients had been exposed to traditional hospital-related sources of hepatitis B infection. Specifically, none had received hemodialysis, blood products, or surgery during the initial hospitalization when HBV infection had likely been acquired.

In pretrip briefings with my mentors (Stephen Hadler, Miriam Alter, and Mark Kane), we identified goals for my investigation. The first centered on confirming that an outbreak had in fact occurred. Laboratory error was ruled out by testing serum specimens from case patients for the serologic marker of acute hepatitis B infection (IgM anti-hepatitis B core antigen positive) in the CDC viral hepatitis laboratory. Soon after arrival, I also confirmed that the cluster of hepatitis B cases observed on the medicine A ward exceeded expected Haifa background rates. Indeed, review of district health office surveillance data and laboratory results from the virology laboratory at the Rambam Medical Center revealed that excluding the ward A cluster, less than 10 cases of acute hepatitis B had been reported in Haifa in the first 8 months of 1986. Furthermore, cluster-associated case patients lacked plausible ways of acquiring infection outside of the hospital. They were older, debilitated patients who tended to live alone so that acquisition by illicit injection drug use or homosexual sex was considered exceedingly unlikely by care providers. Clearly, the tight cluster seen on one ward in Rambam Hospital in June exceeded expected background rates and hospital acquisition seemed virtually certain.

My second goal was to ascertain whether case patients possessed co-factors that might predispose them to fulminant disease and to explore other explanations for the high mortality rate in this outbreak. One hypothesis to explain the high case fatality rate was that case patients may have been co-infected by the hepatitis D (or delta) virus, a highly virulent companion virus that literally parasitizes the HBV that it is dependent on it for its replication and clinical expression; however, all specimens from the six case patients were negative for total delta antibody by a CDC in-house assay that was more sensitive than the commercially available assay that had already been used by the Israelis to investigate this possibility. Furthermore, other than their older, debilitated status, case patients had no specific underlying illnesses or medication exposures that were likely to affect the liver and potentiate the risk of fulminant hepatitis. Ultimately, the reason for the high case fatality in this outbreak remained obscure for many years, but I will return to that issue later.

My preeminent goals while in Israel were to ascertain the mechanism of transmission for the first cluster of five cases in June and to determine whether the sixth case in August was part of a second cluster and, if so, to discover the mechanism of transmission of that second cluster. The first of these goals was daunting because with only five case-patients it would be difficult to identify and statistically link specific hospital exposures with development of hepatitis B infection. In addition, by the time I undertook the investigation, the period of likely acquisition of hepatitis B infection (in late April and early May) was already 4 months in the past. Thus, in attempting to reconstruct hospital exposures, I was almost completely limited to medical record review. I was concerned that medical records might be inadequate to identify important exposures. Furthermore, medical records were in Hebrew, making me totally dependent on the translator who had been assigned to me. Finally, as I got to know my Israeli collaborators, it became increasingly clear that they were extremely competent. The fact that they had conducted an investigation already and failed to identify a cause did not augur well.

In pretrip briefings, my mentors at the CDC had brainstormed with me about possible mechanisms for this outbreak. These included the possibility that there was a HBV-infected staff member who could have transmitted infection to cases through contamination of open wounds or breaks in the skin of case patients. Indeed, there were outbreaks described in the medical literature caused by this mechanism, but they tended to involve transmission from hepatitis B-infected dentists or surgeons to patients during surgical procedures,[2-6] and most often involved practitioners with dermatologic problems affecting their hands (from which plasma derived exudates could contaminate wounds) or technique problems that led to sharp instrument accidents while working in confined operative spaces. In any event, the Israelis had already effectively ruled out this possibility by testing virtually all staff that had been associated with these patients in late April and early May; no hepatitis B carrier or acutely infected staff members were identified.

A second mechanism would implicate patients concurrently on the ward as a potential source of HBV infection. If there was a hepatitis B carrier patient on the unit in late April and early May, body fluids from that patient could infect surrounding patients through a few mechanisms. First, if such patients bled into the environment, patients could be contaminated directly through splashes onto nonintact skin or into the mouth or eyes. Although this seems unlikely, patients with chronic hepatitis B infection can experience catastrophic bleeding from esophageal varices, and bleeding from any site may be exacerbated by coagulation problems caused by advanced liver disease. Blood may contaminate the environment or equipment, and patients may be indirectly exposed to hepatitis B through contact with these sources.

In addition, blood from source patients can occasionally contaminate multidose injectable preparations. For example, Miriam Alter briefed me on a dialysis-related outbreak that she had investigated.[7] This particular dialysis unit was unusual in that dialysis patients were taught to carry out simple nursing functions to facilitate their care. These included going to a common preparation area where several multidose injectable preparations were kept. One of these multidose injectables was a local anesthetic (bupivicaine) that some patients asked dialysis staff to use to anesthetize their skin before the percutaneous insertion of the dialysis canula. Patients were instructed to draw up the anesthetic into a syringe and have it ready for the dialysis technician. In this outbreak, use of bupivicaine was significantly associated with being a case. There were two known HBsAg-positive carriers on this unit who used the bupivicaine. One of them had recently had a minor stroke and had some residual hand weakness and tremors. It is postulated that she jabbed her finger with the syringe needle while attempting to advance it into the rubber stopper of the bupivicaine vial. Instead of discarding the syringe, it is thought that she persisted and readvanced the contaminated needle into the vial, effectively inoculating its contents with her blood. From that point on, other patients who used that vial of local anesthetic were directly injected with hepatitis B-contaminated fluid. In fact, of 11 susceptible patients who had used bupivicaine and received dialysis after the implicated HBsAg carrier, 10 (91%) subsequently seroconverted to HBsAg positive.

Armed with these potential mechanisms, I arrived at Lod Airport and was met by Dr. Edna Ben-Porath, an accomplished virologist who had participated in the Israeli investigation of the first cluster. She drove me to my hotel in Haifa, and I admired the view from the top of Mount Carmel. To be honest, however, as nice as that hotel was, I mainly remember only the bed because from then on I was working the typical 16-hour day of an EIS officer on assignment.

At a meeting the next day, I learned about the basic structure of internal medicine inpatient care at the Rambam Medical Center. The internal medicine inpatient wards at the Rambam were denoted alphabetically, and as mentioned, this outbreak occurred on the medicine A ward. Inpatient medical wards were staffed continuously by a core group of attending internists who served as faculty for house staff who rotated through that particular medical service. During residency training, house staff members were assigned to one of these teams and remained attached to a given unit throughout their 3-year training period. Attending physicians and residents saw a panel of internal medicine outpatients, and if these patients required hospitalization, they were admitted to ward A. This system differed markedly from the one used by my residency training program. At Washington Hospital center, the medical units were staffed by different attending physicians every month, and I was assigned to month-long rotations on these inpatient units several times a year. I did have a panel of outpatients that I followed, but when these patients required admission, they were assigned sequentially to one of the inpatient units in the order that they were admitted to the medical service. As a result, I rarely cared for my own clinic patients when they were hospitalized. It is interesting to speculate whether this outbreak would even have been detected in my training hospital as patients were not automatically linked to one inpatient unit of the hospital. It was the continuity in staffing of the Medicine A ward and the medical staff's familiarity with their panel of patients that led to the easy recognition of this outbreak when the same group of patients was admitted and then readmitted months later with fulminant hepatitis B.

At that first meeting in the hospital, I was also introduced to Dr. Nahum Egoz, a medical attending on the medicine D ward who would serve as translator and would slog through medical records with me during many long evenings. Although not part of the medicine A staff, he was assigned to me in part to insure that he would remain objective and unbiased as we conducted the investigation. We got along extremely well, and I learned much about the Israeli medical system through our acquaintance. Although Nahum maintained a "full-time" position at the Rambam, a public hospital, he also maintained a private medical practice. Attending physicians at the Rambam were generally done with ward rounds by 2 p.m., which left time for this type of dual practice.

I met a number of people who I came to like and admire as the investigation proceeded. Dr. Gideon Alroy was the chief of medicine A at the Rambam. He was an inspiring, vigorous leader, all the more remarkable because he suffered from end-stage kidney disease and was dependent on peritoneal dialysis administered in his home. Early in my stay, he invited me to dinner at his home (as did Dr. Ben-Porath and many others), and I developed a friendship with his daughter, Tamar, who was an artist. In rare moments, when I had some free time, she was kind enough to show me parts of Haifa. Once she took me to see the first segment of the recently released film "Shoah," a poignant documentary that provides insights into the day to day operation of the Nazi Death Camps by interviewing not only survivors, but also persons who had worked at the death camps or who lived in communities where Jews were being systematically removed. We were riveted for 4 hours, and both of us were speechless after seeing it.

In preliminary discussions, the Israelis had briefed me on the findings of their investigation. Following the June cluster, they had astutely performed serologic testing on all patients who had resided on the medicine A ward in late April and early May for hepatitis B serologic markers. Their testing window was based on the observation that all four patients with fulminant hepatitis B in June had all been previously together on the unit on only 1 day, April 29th. Around this date, a 1-week interval was constructed. They identified 58 patients who had been on the unit from April 26 through May 2. Of these, five later developed hepatitis B in June. Eighteen died before they could be reached for serological testing. Twenty one were tested and found to be negative for all hepatitis B serological markers. Eleven were tested and had evidence of remote prior hepatitis B infection, and four were chronic hepatitis B carriers who were known by medicine A clinicians to be positive for HBsAG even before the Israelis conducted this serologic investigation. These results raised some obvious questions. Could one of the four hepatitis B carriers be the source of hepatitis B in this outbreak? In addition, the fact that 18 of the 58 (or 31%) of these patients had died within a few months of their April/May admission seemed to be excessive and raised the possibility that some of these individuals may have been unrecognized victims of the outbreak. Unlike the 5 case patients, these 18 had not been subsequently admitted to ward A, but died elsewhere.

I asked the ministry of health to provide death certificates for these 18 patients to see whether there was any suggestion that they had died a liver-related death. Nahum and I then proceeded to examine the medical records of the five case patients. All case patients were older, but they had little else in common. They had been initially admitted to medicine A with a variety of apparently unrelated illnesses and had not shared common hospital rooms while in ward A. This lessened the possibility that the outbreak was due to catastrophic bleeding from one of the hepatitis B carrier patients. Indeed, subsequent review of the medical records of the four hepatitis B carrier patients revealed no episodes of bleeding during their residence on ward A. We also noted that all five of the case patients had some form of intravenous access devices in place during their admission. This represented a potential portal of entry for HBV, but without a control group for comparison, it was difficult to say if it was unusual. Thus, we entered the case-control phase of our investigation with a vague hypothesis that having an intravenous access device in place may have played some role in the acquisition of hepatitis B.

Fortunately, we had an obvious source of control patients. The serologic testing that the Israelis had done revealed that 21 patients were negative for hepatitis B serologic markers and therefore susceptible to hepatitis B. Why had these 21 patients avoided infection, whereas 5 unfortunate ward-mates had not? Nahum and I pored over the records of these 21 patients culling out demographic information, bed placement, exposure to medications (particularly injectables), medical examinations patients had undergone, and presence of indwelling intravenous devices. There was only one significant finding; although cases and controls were equally likely to have intravenous devices in place during their hospital stay, the five case patients were more likely to have a heparin lock in place. In fact, from April 26 to May 2, all five cases had had this device at some point compared with only 5 of 21 of susceptible controls (24%) ($P = 0.004$).

I knew a few basic things about heparin locks from my internal medicine residency. A heparin lock is a small tube connected to a catheter that is maintained in a vein to allow convenient venous access. If someone needs periodic but not continuous infusions of a given medication, that medication solution can be run into the heparin lock at scheduled intervals through a needle that is inserted into a rubber port in the barrel of the heparin lock tube.

I was ignorant, however, about how heparin locks were maintained and went back to the ward the next day eager to follow up on this lead. I asked for an interview with the head nurse of the unit. I was careful to begin with some questions about other, unrelated procedures on the ward. Eventually, I asked the critical question, "Could you tell me about the insertion and maintenance of heparin locks on the unit?" The head nurse told me that heparin locks were inserted using aseptic technique, like any other indwelling intravenous catheter. The only difference between the maintenance of an intravenous line and a heparin lock was that the barrel of the heparin lock tube was flushed at regular intervals using heparin solution. This is done so that the blood in the heparin lock barrel will not clot off and eliminate access to the vein.

I probed further and asked whether the heparin flush solution came directly from the pharmacy. The nurse stated that no, in general, the heparin solution was prepared on the unit once a day, usually just after the morning change of shifts. Routinely, at 7 a.m., a nurse would draw up a defined quantity of heparin from a vial and inject it into a rubber-stoppered vial of sterile normal saline. Trying to sound offhand, I asked whether each patient had his or her own designated heparin flush solution vial or whether one vial served as the flush solution for all patients on the ward who needed heparin lock maintenance. She stated that the heparin flush solution was kept at the nurse's station and that nurses would draw up solution as they needed it. All heparin locks on the unit were generally flushed in sequence every 8 hours. I asked whether the same syringe was used to flush multiple heparin locks and received a shocked look. "No, of course not. A new, prepackaged, sterile syringe is used to draw up heparin flush solution, and the same syringe is never inserted into the heparin lock of different patients." Even a fledgling epidemiologist knew enough to be skeptical about that kind of blanket pronouncement.

With further questioning, I established a few other facts. The April 26 to May 2nd interval that we were scrutinizing coincided with Passover, an important Jewish holiday. As a result, ward A staffing was minimal, much as it would have been during the Christmas Holidays in the United States. Although record keeping did not permit the identification of specific persons who had performed the heparin lock flushes during this interval, it was clear that such persons would have been overworked during this time interval. I postulated that under these circumstances a mistake could have been made. If one of the hepatitis B carriers housed on ward A had a heparin lock in place during this interval, an overburdened staff member might have reused a syringe that had been contaminated while flushing that carrier's heparin lock. By readvancing it into the multidose heparin/saline flush solution, the solution itself would have been contaminated. Adding to the plausibility of this mechanism was the fact that additional medical record reviews revealed that of the four hepatitis B carriers on medicine A in late April and early May, only one was in the hospital on April 29, the day when all five cluster patients had been on the unit on the same day. This carrier individual had a heparin lock in place from April 23 through the morning of May 1. Although there was no way to definitively prove it, I had a highly plausible explanation for the first cluster. This explanation was biologically plausible, consistent with available data, and credible given the tendency for error when staff are rushed or overburdened. With some excitement, I called my supervisor, Steve Hadler, and he agreed that I had identified the probable cause of the outbreak but suggested one additional analysis to bolster my case.

He speculated that the kind of mistake I was hypothesizing would probably be a one-time event because it represented a gross breach of standard practice. As we now knew, the heparin/saline flush solution was changed every 24 hours. Steve therefore suggested that I examine the association between heparin lock placement on each day of the April 26 to May 2 interval (Table 9-1). Of special interest were the data from April 29th, the only day when all five cluster patients were on the unit. On this date, the

Table 9-1 Percentage of Cases and Susceptible Controls With In-Dwelling Heparin-Lock Placement on Medicine A on Consecutive Days in late April and Early May

Date	4/26	4/27	4/28	4/29	4/30	5/1	5/2
% Cases (n)	75 (4)	100 (4)	100 (4)	80 (5)	67 (3)	100 (3)	100 (3)
% Controls (n)	11 (9)	36 (11)	9 (11)	0 (9)	11 (9)	11 (9)	14 (14)
P (Fisher's exact)	.052*	.051*	.004	.005	.127*	.018	.015

*P not significant
n = number of cases or controls present on Medicine A on specific dates.

heparin lock association was nearly perfect. Specifically, four of five cases had a heparin lock on that day compared to none of nine controls.

How could I explain the one patient who did not have a heparin lock in place on the 29th? I carefully reviewed the medical record again and found that he was admitted to medicine A from the coronary care unit on the 29th on continuous intravenous therapy. From my own experience as a resident, I knew that when a patient is transferred from one unit to another the patient is jostled and transferred from bed to stretcher and that transient interruptions in intravenous fluid administration may frequently occur. It was possible that while being transported, this case patient's intravenous line clotted off. If so, a staff person on ward A may have flushed the line with the contaminated heparin normal saline solution soon after the patient arrived on ward A. This would be done to salvage the line and avoid the need to reinsert an intravenous line at a different site. Statistically, significant associations are demonstrated on other calendar days in the April 26 through May 2 interval, but no other date included all five case patients. Furthermore, it did not surprise me that other days would show an association; a patient who requires a heparin lock on any given day is likely to continue to require it on ensuing days.

Although I remained busy during the following days, it mainly amounted to tying up loose ends. Death certificates from those 18 medicine A patients who had died after their April/May admission did not reveal any hint of a liver-related cause of death. Furthermore, the hepatitis B serologic testing performed on patients who had been co-residents of the patients who died of fulminant hepatitis in the June cluster on ward A revealed no other patients with evidence of acute hepatitis B. Thus, the sixth case that had occurred in August was an isolated event, not part of a second cluster, and in fact, he did not have a heparin lock in place. He did, however, undergo a bone marrow biopsy during his stay, had a permanent cystostomy in place, and had an indwelling intravenous line for much of his stay. Three of the dying June cluster patients were present on the ward during his admission. All of these patients had marked coagulopathies, and one was noted to have ongoing blood oozing from his intravenous line insertion site. We hypothesized that the sixth case may have acquired hepatitis B through cross-contamination with blood derived from the June cluster hepatitis patients. This blood may have been present in the environment or have been transported to the patient on the hands of staff members and gained entry through breaks in the skin of case 6 provided by indwelling lines and invasive procedures.

After completing the basic investigation, it was time to brief the staff of the Rambam Hospital on my findings and to make recommendations. In that presentation, I reviewed my findings carefully, not only summarizing my positive findings but refuting other potential mechanisms. Further strengthening the case for a common-source, multidose exposure was the tight temporal clustering of the cases and the short incubation periods. The short incubation period favored a high inoculum exposure like that which might result from the direct injection of a contaminated injectable, rather than that which would result if small amounts of infected materials were splashed or rubbed onto an intravenous site.

After completing my presentation, I was taken aback when the chief of staff raised his hand and said that I had left out one important possible explanation for the outbreak—intentional sabotage. He was concerned that a disgruntled or criminal employee had obtained hepatitis B contaminated fluid and intentionally injected it into these patients. I thought about this and asked why a saboteur would inoculate only those with a heparin lock when intravenous lines would provide equivalent ease of access to the blood stream of patients. Without hesitation, he stated that heparin locks have a flat rubberized port, whereas intravenous systems have a rounded rubberized section for introducing needles. With the latter, it is easier to poke yourself, which might have deterred a saboteur. I advanced other arguments against the sabotage theory, pointing to the fact that use of potassium chloride or poisons would be a more typical approach, but these were countered by the assertion that they would have raised greater suspicion of foul play. In the end, I inserted the following sentence into my final report: "The deliberate injection of HBsAG-positive material through the heparin lock cannot be definitively ruled out but accidental inoculation seems far more plausible and has occurred in other outbreaks."[7,8]

It was time to say goodbye. I had acquitted myself well during the investigation and had made a good impression. Before I departed, I was offered a position at the Rambam Hospital and the challenge of developing an infectious disease service there. I seriously considered this offer and even inquired about potential positions for my wife, Judy, who was also a physician. They assured me that something would be arranged. I did not want to leave the EIS program at that point, however, and by the time my tenure in that program ended, the idea had faded in light of family obligations and practical concerns. I said goodbye with sadness, however.

At the end of my stay in Israel, I was told that the outbreak investigation was to be kept strictly confidential. Israeli media had not been informed of the outbreak on medicine A. Families of the cases would have to be told first and then the decision about publication would be reassessed. I was disappointed in part because it meant that the work might not be published, which affected me personally, but also because the wider world could not benefit from the findings of our investigation.

At the airport, when I was getting ready to board my airplane to return to the United States, I was interviewed by security. They asked me what I had been doing in Israel. I was not prepared for this. As a representative of the U.S. government working for the CDC, I did not want to lie to Israeli security. With some trepidation, I told them that I had been working on a scientific investigation in Haifa with colleagues at the Rambam Hospital. The security agent must have sensed my unease and continued to probe for increasingly specific details of my investigation. Eventually, I divulged that I had been working on an outbreak at the Rambam Hospital. The security official left me alone for a few minutes, and when she came back, I was told I could leave. A few weeks after my return to the United States, I found out that the story had been "leaked" to the Israeli media. I've always wondered if I was that leak. In any event, the outbreak investigation was eventually published.[9]

One last issue remained to be illuminated. There was as yet no explanation for the high mortality rate in this outbreak. At the time I did the investigation, the CDC did not have the capacity to clone and sequence viral DNA from HBV strains that had infected these individuals; however, serum from these individuals was carefully stored in Israel, and 5 years later, Edna Ben-Porath and colleagues at Harvard Medical School were able to do so. Specifically, the presence of HBV was identified by polymerase chain reaction amplification of viral DNA in serum from the hepatitis B carrier patient identified as the likely source of the infecting strain by our investigation, the five patients with fulminant hepatitis B, and five controls with acute, self-limited hepatitis B. The amplified viral HBV DNA samples were then cloned and sequenced. Sequence analysis of viral DNA established that the same HBV mutant with two mutations in the precore region was present in the source patient and the five patients with fulminant hepatic failure, but not in control patients. They concluded that naturally occurring viral mutations in the HBV genome may predispose the infected host to more severe liver injury.[10] This report was gratifying not only because it helped to explain the high case fatality rate in the outbreak, but because it confirmed that we had correctly identified the hepatitis B carrier patient who was the common source for this tragic outbreak.

After this outbreak, I returned to the hepatitis branch and finished up my EIS career. I still consider those 2 years the most exciting professional experience that I've ever had. Toward the end of my tenure in the EIS program, I was offered a few jobs at the CDC that I would have considered the fulfillment of a dream when I first started. There was one position that involved measles control in Africa that was particularly exciting; however, during my EIS years, my son Charlie was born. The measles job would have required at least 4 months of international travel a year, and I chose instead to assume an academic position at University of Illinois at Chicago (UIC). My daughter, Rebecca, was born soon after we arrived in Chicago. The UIC position allowed me to return to the clinical practice of infectious diseases and to garner a joint appointment at UIC's School of Public Health. My background in viral hepatitis proved invaluable. Shortly after my arrival at UIC, the cause of non-A, non-B hepatitis was identified, and the study of hepatitis C virus natural history and epidemiology has been a major focus of my research ever since. Also, because hepatitis B and C share epidemiologic similarities with HIV infection, my training in viral hepatitis proved to be excellent preparation for work that increasingly focused on HIV infection. Shortly after arriving at UIC, I was fortunate to become a co-investigator on the Women and Infants Transmission study. The study of HIV infection as it affects women and substance users has been another important research area for me.

Nonetheless, there have been times that I have wondered about the roads I didn't take. Both of my children have graduated from high school now, and as I finish this chapter, I can hear the call of the muezzin from a nearby Mosque. I am in Jakarta, Indonesia launching the first international investigation I have undertaken since I left Israel 22 year ago. I am doing a pilot investigation to identify effective ways to promote successful antiretroviral therapy among injection drug users in Jakarta and Bali. Who knows? Maybe it's time to start planning a sabbatical in Israel.

REFERENCES

1. Centers for Disease Control. Recommendations for prevention of viral hepatitis. *MMWR* 1985;34:313–324, 329–335.
2. Prentice MB, Flower AJ, Morgan GM, et al. Infection with hepatitis B virus after open heart surgery. *BMJ* 1999;304:761–764.
3. Polakoff S. Acute hepatitis B in patients in Britain related to previous operations and dental treatment. *BMJ* 1986;293:33–36.
4. Rimland D, Parkin WE, Miller GB, Schrack WD. Hepatitis B outbreak traced to an oral surgeon. *N Engl J Med* 1977;296:953–958.
5. The Incident Investigations Team and Others. Transmission of hepatitis B to patients from four infected surgeons without hepatitis B e Antigen. *N Engl J Med* 1997;336:178–184.
6. Reitsma AM, Closen ML, Cunningham M, et al. Infected physicians and invasive procedures: safe practice management. *Clin Infect Dis* 2005;40:1665–1672.
7. Alter MJ, Ahtone J, Maynard JE. Hepatitis B virus transmission associated with a multiple-dose vial in a hemodialysis unit. *Ann Intern Med* 1983;99:330–333.
8. CDC. Outbreaks of hepatitis B virus infection among hemodialysis patients: California, Nebraska, and Texas, 1994. *MMWR* 1996;45:285–289.
9. Oren I, Hershow RC, Ben-Porath E, et al. A common source outbreak of fulminant hepatitis B in a medical ward. *Ann Intern Med* 1989;110:691–698.
10. Liang TJ, Hasegawa K, Rimon N, Wands JR, Ben-Porath E. A hepatitis B virus mutant associated with an epidemic of fulminant hepatitis. *N Engl J Med* 1991; 324:1705–1709.

CHAPTER 10

What Went Wrong?
An Ancient Recipe
Associated with Botulism
in Modern Egypt
J. Todd Weber, MD

INTRODUCTION

Terrorism, War, Religious Observance and a Holiday

On Wednesday, December 21, 1988, Pan Am Flight 103—a Boeing 747-121 named Clipper Maid of the Seas—was destroyed by a bomb. The ruins fell in and around the town of Lockerbie, Scotland. Experts showed that plastic explosive had been detonated in the airplane's cargo hold. The death toll was 270 people from 21 countries. The first leg of Pan Am Flight 103 began as PA 103A from Frankfurt International Airport, West Germany to London Heathrow Airport. An unaccompanied bag had been routed onto Pan Am 103 on an Air Malta flight to Frankfurt and then by flight PA 103A to Heathrow. This unaccompanied bag contained the bomb. The investigation of the bombing went on through 1990, and findings of various groups recommended and led to increased airport security.[1]

The Gulf War began on August 2, 1990, with the invasion of Kuwait by Iraq. Saddam Hussein was known to be developing biological weapons. After defeat by an allied coalition of 34 countries, the war ended on March

163

3, 1991, when Iraq accepted a ceasefire. Approximately 400 coalition forces died during the war, including 10 from Egypt. The United States estimates that at least 20,000 Iraqis were killed.[2]

In 1991, the month-long Islamic holiday of Ramadan began on March 17 and ended on April 14–15. Ramadan occurs in the ninth month of the Islamic calendar, a lunar calendar, changing dates on the Gregorian calendar each year. In the month of Ramadan, Muslims fast during the day, eating at night and avoiding salty foods. (Because the rules of Ramadan prohibit drinking during the day, foods that make you thirsty are undesirable). There are exceptions to the requirement of fasting, including for those who are menstruating, pregnant, postpartum, traveling, ill, or in battle—an important point because the Gulf War had only recently ended and coalition troops were still present in the region.

In 1991, the Egyptian Holiday *Sham-el-Nessim* fell on April 8, coincidental with Ramadan. *Sham-el-Nessim* is an annual springtime holiday; it is nonsectarian and is celebrated by Islamic and Coptic Egyptian citizens. It is a public holiday occurring annually on Monday, the day after the Coptic Easter Sunday. Its origin reportedly dates back millennia. The rough translation of *Sham-el-Nessim* is "sniffing the breezes." Typically, families spend the day together outside and share foods traditional to the holiday.

THE OUTBREAK

On the evening of April 9, 1991, the second day of the Centers for Disease Control and Prevention (CDC) Epidemic Intelligence Service (EIS) annual conference in Atlanta, Georgia, I was on call for the Enteric Diseases Branch of the Division of Bacterial and Mycotic Diseases at CDC. I joined the EIS after training as an internist at New York University in the Bellevue Hospital Center and Tisch Hospital. I received a call at home from an Ohio state health department officer. He needed botulinal antitoxin and knew that the CDC was the only place he could get it. He had received a call from a doctor in his state who was Egyptian and had relatives in Cairo. She told him there were three adults with botulism intoxication in a hospital in Cairo, all on ventilators, and wanted to know how to obtain antitoxin. After consultation with others in the branch, I recommended that this physician contact companies in Europe that produce antitoxin, as shipment from there would be faster.

In the next 24 hours, the CDC received other calls reporting more cases and some deaths. The physician for the U.S. Embassy in Cairo called. He said there were hundreds of Cairo citizens crowding the gates of the embassy and pleading for antitoxin. It was front-page news in the Egyptian newspapers, and the Minister of Health was being called into Parliament to explain what had happened and what was being done. This was the first time botulism had ever been reported in Egypt, and it sounded much larger than a typical botulism outbreak. Antitoxin was ultimately obtained from several European companies and the United States Armed Services. Ban Mishu, the preventive medicine resident in the branch, and I were invited to Cairo to investigate the outbreak. Along with luggage, laptops, printers, and laboratory equipment, we carried with us antitoxin from CDC's supply. The U.S. Agency for International Development paid for it at the request of their office in Cairo.

The Enteric Diseases Branch (now the Enteric Diseases Epidemiology Branch, Division of Foodborne, Bacterial, and Mycotic Diseases, National Center for Zoonotic, Vector-Borne, and Enteric Diseases, CDC) is available 24 hours a day to provide clinical advice to state health departments and clinicians. The laboratory provides testing for state health departments. The CDC controls most of the supply of antitoxin for the United States and through state health departments supplies it to doctors taking care of suspected cases. (The Alaska Division of Public Health and the California Department of Health Services also maintain supplies of antitoxin for reasons of population size, geography, and incidence of cases.) The CDC maintains control of the supply for two reasons. First, the CDC maintains active surveillance through requests that are received for antitoxin and for laboratory testing. Second, preventive measures may be taken on the basis of the report of a single case of botulism (Exhibit 10-1). This single case may be a sentinel for a larger outbreak, requiring an investigation to prevent further cases from occurring. Such an investigation is usually carried out by the state or local health department. The U.S. Food and Drug Administration is notified of each possible case so that suspect foods may be seized and have their production investigated. Numerous countries have requested the assistance that the CDC provides to states, but the distance to most countries makes timely delivery of antitoxin with an uninterrupted cold chain problematic. Without preservation of the cold chain, the antitoxin, scarce and expensive, can be rendered ineffective. The people in Egypt were not discouraged by this policy, and relatives contacted

---

Exhibit 10-1   Key Facts About Botulism

Three Main Forms

Foodborne botulism occurs when a person ingests toxin which then leads to illness or death within a few hours to days. Outbreaks of foodborne botulism have potential to be a public health emergency because the contaminated food may be eaten by other people.

Infant botulism occurs when the spores of C. botulinum are consumed by infants with subsequent growth of the organism in the gut and toxin is released.

Wound botulism is a rare disease that occurs when C. botulinum infects wounds and produces toxin.

Anaerobic conditions promote germination of C. botulinum spores and botulinum toxin production.

Among the seven types of botulism toxin designated by the letters A through G, only types A, B, E, and F cause illness in humans.

Classic Symptoms*

    Double vision

    Blurred vision

    Drooping eyelids

    Slurred speech

    Difficulty swallowing

    Dry mouth

    Muscle weakness

Untreated, botulism may progress to cause paralysis of the arms, legs, trunk, and respiratory muscles, leading to death.

---

* Infants with botulism appear lethargic, feed poorly, are constipated, and have a weak cry and poor muscle tone.

Derived from Botulism. Division of Foodborne, Bacterial, and Mycotic Diseases, Centers for Disease Control and Prevention. Retrieved October 21, 2008, from http://www.cdc.gov/nczved/dfbmd/disease_listing/botulism_gi.html.

state health departments and the CDC until the investigation began and the antitoxin was made available from several sources.

American surveillance picked up an Egyptian outbreak. Because there was no botulism expertise in Egypt, the CDC and the U.S. Naval Medical Research Unit 3 (located in Cairo) were asked to assist the Ministry of Health in an investigation in order to prove an association with a vehicle, to assist with management of cases, and to recommend preventive measures. The investigation was supported with resources and logistics by the

U.S. Agency for International Development in Egypt. The first stage of the investigation involved finding cases. Suspected cases were reported to the Egyptian Ministry of Health, and all of these were limited to Cairo. The outbreak was well publicized throughout the country, and we spoke with health officials in several other cities to ask whether they were aware of any cases in their districts. They reported none.

THE INVESTIGATION[3]

The Ministry of Health instructed all hospital administrators in Cairo to report cases of suspected botulism based on diagnosis by a physician and then compiled a list of reported patients. We were unable to examine hospital records systematically to determine the completeness of hospital reporting. Investigators examined only those hospital records of patients with botulism-like illness who were interviewed. Patients, family members, and attending physicians were questioned regarding age, gender, religion, date and time of onset of illness, symptoms, date of hospitalization, admission to an intensive care unit, the use of mechanical ventilation, and the type and dose of botulinal antitoxin received. Patients were asked to list all foods eaten during the 72 hours before onset of illness. We defined a case of suspected botulism as illness in a hospitalized patient whose physician suspected botulism and who had at least one of the following symptoms: dyspnea, blurred vision, or ptosis (drooping eyelids).

Ninety-one patients with suspected botulism were reported to the Ministry of Health. Of these 18 (20%) died from the illness. Before discharge from the hospital, 45 of the 73 surviving patients (61%) were interviewed between 14 and 19 April. The age of the patients interviewed ranged from 8 to 85 years, and there was a slight male preponderance (60%).

The onset of illness for 98% of patients interviewed was within 24 hours of April 8th, which was the Egyptian holiday *Sham-el-Nessim*. We made the assumption that the food responsible for the outbreak was served during the traditional meal of *Sham-el-Nessim*, and thus, the mean incubation period was 12.8 hours. This is on the shorter end of the spectrum for botulism, but if our assumption was correct, then it implied there could have been a very high dose of toxin.

Religion was noted for 33 of the patients we interviewed. Remarkably, the vast majority (26 [79%]) were Coptic Christians. Six (18%) were

Muslims, and one (3%) was Protestant. This is in stark contrast to the population of Egypt. The *2006 World Factbook* estimates that 7.6 million or 10% of Egyptians are Christian (9% Coptic and 1% other denominations).

After completing interviews with hospitalized patients, we conducted a case-control investigation to prove an association with a vehicle. Five families, found through the hospital case investigation, were chosen, and arrangements were made to interview as many family members as possible who had attended a *Sham-el-Nessim* feast. The case definition required illness in a person during the week following *Sham-el-Nessim* with at least three of these symptoms: blurred vision, dysphagia, dry mouth, dyspnea and constipation. Controls were other family members who shared the *Sham-el-Nessim* feast and did not meet the case definition. Because a detailed list of foods served could not be generated for each family, open-ended questions were asked about foods eaten during the day of the feast. Some family members had died, and the person who appeared most knowledgeable about what they had eaten was interviewed in their stead. There were 16 cases and 26 controls. Their mean ages and male to female ratios differed.

Five hospitalized patients and their family members were interviewed between 23 and 26 April 1991. The 42 people surveyed ranged in age from 5 to 60 years (median, 25); 20 (48%) were male. Thirty-seven (88%) were Coptic Christians, and 5 (12%) were Muslims. Sixteen (38%) reported symptoms of botulism meeting the case definition. The most frequently reported symptom was dry mouth (81%). Other frequently reported symptoms included blurred vision (69%), dysphagia (69%), weakness (69%), dyspnea (69%), and nausea (59%). Five family case-patients died (31%), all within 1 week after onset of illness.

All 16 of the family case-patients reported eating *faseikh* on *Sham-el-Nessim* compared with 10 (38%) of the 26 controls (odds ratio undefined, $P < 0.001$, lower 95% confidence limit of odds ratio = 6.6). Olive oil and lemon were also associated with illness. Olive oil, lemon, and onions are often put on *faseikh*, however, just before serving. When we asked cases and controls about how much they ate, everyone spontaneously described it in hands, a full hand, half a hand, a finger's worth, and so on. We did our best to represent these in fractions of hands. The mean amount of *faseikh* eaten by cases was 0.70 hands and 0.14 hands for controls ($P < 0.01$).

All five of the families in the case-control investigation purchased *faseikh* from the same store, which was in Shobra, the largest Coptic Christian neighborhood in Cairo. All of the families purchased the *faseikh* between April 7 and 9.

Assuming now that contaminated *faseikh* was responsible for the outbreak, the reason for the Coptic Christian majority among the cases becomes clear because *Sham-el-Nessim* fell during the month of the Islamic holiday Ramadan. *Faseikh* would be avoided by observant Muslims during this time not only because of rules regarding daytime fasting, but because of the very salty nature of *faseikh*, it is a highly undesirable food for the thirst that it might provoke during the day. Coptic Christians are under no such constraint and ate the *faseikh*, causing this group to make up 79% of the hospitalized patients and 88% of the family study case patients, vastly larger than their proportion of the general population. The sole Muslim case in the family case-control investigation was menstruating during *Sham-el-Nessim*. Thus, she was exempt from daytime fasting and ate a bit of *faseikh* as a snack on the day of *Sham-el-Nessim*.[4]

Of the 16 cases found in this investigation, 6 (34%) were not reported to the Ministry of Health. Of the patients who were not reported, three experienced only mild symptoms, and a fourth died at home; these four were never hospitalized and demonstrate the limitations of relying only on hospitals for data on cases that have died. Two other patients died in the hospital but were not reported through ad hoc surveillance. All of these unreported cases were found in families with at least one hospitalized patient. There may well have been families in which all cases died or whose illnesses were mild enough to avoid being hospitalized.

Estimating the actual size of the outbreak is difficult, however, because completeness of hospital reporting was not assessed directly, no population based-survey was conducted, and no records of sale of *faseikh* were available from the implicated shop.

We were told anecdotes that suggest there may have been unreported deaths and cases. In one Coptic Christian neighborhood, we came across a coffin maker. Without saying why we were asking, we asked how business was. He promptly replied that even though his sales were up about three coffins a day because of the increased deaths, he was proud to say that he had not raised his prices. The increased sale accounted for about 40 deaths. We were also told by several residents of the same Christian neighborhood that local shops had run out of mourning clothes because there had been so many families with deaths.

FASEIKH PREPARATION

As Americans have turkey as the traditional dish on Thanksgiving, *faseikh* is the traditional dish served during the fast of *Sham-el-Nessim*. Reportedly, it has been made since the time of the Pharaohs. *Faseikh* is an uneviscerated, salted fish. It is made from grey mullet (*Mugil Cephalus*). The fish are gathered from the Red Sea, several salt water lakes, and fish farms in the Nile delta region near the Mediterranean. Of note, grey mullet are found near the shore. To eat, a grey mullet points its head and mouth down toward the mud and sucks and swallows a mouthful of mud and tiny organisms. It can also filter food particles through its gills, expelling mud and debris and swallowing what it finds edible.[5] If *C. botulinum* spores are present within the unfiltered muck, that the gut or gills of the mullet would be contaminated with them when taken out of the water is conceivable. Although *faseikh* is sold throughout the year, it is especially popular on *Sham-el-Nessim*. It is very soft when it's ready to eat. When it's served, people take a portion and spread it on bread.

To understand better how *faseikh* is made, we spoke with several producers and discussed methods known to the Egyptian Ministry of Health inspectors. Fresh fish are collected and arrive in Cairo within several hours. *Faseikh* shop owners indicated that they refuse fish that arrive on ice as this indicates the fish is not fresh. This is the opposite of what I expected to hear because in the United States chilling fish is the norm to preserve its freshness. Shop owners indicated that they prepare *faseikh* themselves in their own shops or another facility. The fish is placed in large plastic or wooden draining trays that are covered with cotton cloth. We were told that the trays are placed in a dark, cool area for putrefaction, never outdoors or in the sun. One shop owner cautioned that placing the fish in the sun gives the fish a "bitter" taste. The fish are left for several hours to one day until they are optimally "swollen" and soft. If there is *C. botulinum* in the fishes' gut at the time, this creates an environment for it to grow and produce toxin, and this has been shown in the laboratory with other fish spiked with spores. Thus, unfortunately, what is good for *faseikh* is good for the organism that causes botulism. It is no surprise that the Arabic word "*faseikh*," roughly translated into English means "putrid." The final product smells pretty foul, and I do not recommend keeping it in your hotel refrigerator, as I did.

The fish are then placed in wooden barrels with coarse salt placed between layers. Salt is placed as the lowest and uppermost layers. Approximately 1 kilogram of salt is used for each kilogram of fish. Each barrel holds approximately 20 to 30 kilograms of fish plus salt. No other ingredients, such as oil, spices, or lemon juice, are added.

How quickly the salt penetrates into the bowel of the fish is unclear, and if there is *C. botulinum* there, it may still have time to grow before the salt concentration rises too high. If there is an anaerobic environment created by the barrel or if the shop owner who sold the contaminated fish did something to create one is also unclear, which might have been done by putting on an airtight cover.

The uncovered barrel remains in a dark, cool room for 1 week to 1 year. After several weeks, liquid is drawn from the fish by the salt and accumulated in the barrel; large, flat weights are place on the top layer to prevent upward flotation of the fish.

The Ministry of Health food inspectors described a different *faseikh* preparation method that included placing fish in the sun for 1 day for putrefaction and then placing them in barrels sealed with airtight lids.

We wanted to interview the shop owner, but his shop was closed. Shortly after the outbreak, we were told that the Cairo police arrested him and that he remained in jail. The authorities explained that he was in jail for his own safety because a mob might have attacked him. We were told that he denied ever making *faseikh* in his life, and thus, an interview would probably have been unhelpful.

Human botulism is typically caused by one of the serotypes named A, B, and E. It came as no surprise that this was type E because this type is associated with fish and other marine animals. The majority of Americans' experience with it comes from Alaska. There, type E botulism is associated with fermented fish heads, fish eggs, whale meat, and seal flipper that are prepared by Alaska natives using traditional methods.

During the 20 years before the Egypt outbreak, however, the recipes in Alaska changed for convenience. For example, the traditional method for preparing fermented fish heads involves putting 50 or so salmon heads in a clay pit. This changed to using plastic bags at ambient temperature. These changes undoubtedly create more anaerobic conditions as well as a temperature favorable for growth of *C. botulinum* and toxin production.

Three outbreaks of botulism resulted from kapchunka in the United States between 1981 and 1987, causing 3 deaths and 11 illnesses. Kapchunka, an ethnic food usually produced from whitefish, is also known as "rybetz," "ribeyza," or "rostov." Kapchunka is an uneviscerated, salt-cured, air-dried, whole fish that may or may not be smoked. It is consumed without further preparation, such as cooking. The fish are salt cured under minimum refrigeration conditions for a minimum of 25 days and then air dried at ambient temperature for 3 to 7 days. Kapchunka may be smoked before packing and are commonly stored under refrigeration.

The problems with these products are compounded by the difficulty in attaining sufficient levels of salt in all portions of an uneviscerated fish to inhibit the growth of the *C. botulinum*. Consequently, any fish product (greater than 5 inches long) that is salt cured and then dried, smoked, pickled, or fermented is considered by the U.S. Food and Drug Administration to be a potentially life-threatening health hazard. These products are considered hazardous by U.S. Food and Drug Administration whether stored at ambient temperature, refrigerated, or frozen, or whether packaged in air, vacuum, or modified atmosphere. Toxin may be present in these products even when there are no outward signs of microbiological spoilage or other clear indications to alert the consumer.[6]

Thus, perhaps the jailed *faseikh* producer violated the traditional methods of *faseikh* making. Perhaps, because he expected a large sale for *Sham-el-Nessim*, he put the fish in the sun to speed putrefaction. Perhaps he put in less salt, as a cost-cutting measure. Unfortunately, we just don't know what he did.

LABORATORY FINDINGS

We attempted to obtain serum and stool specimens from all hospitalized patients. The Ministry of Health Central Laboratory obtained partially eaten *faseikh* specimens from affected patients. Whole, uneaten specimens of implicated *faseikh* were obtained from a hospitalized patient. When we completed interviewing this patient, he casually asked whether we wanted some of the fish. Rather surprised, we answered yes, and he got out of bed and removed a plastic bag containing a fish from the locker in his room.

The CDC botulism laboratory received specimens from 32 patients but in such small quantity that direct toxin determination by mouse bioassay was not possible. Twenty-five percent of the specimens had positive cultures for *C. botulinum*, type E. These were from stool and postmortem stomach contents.

Faseikh was tested by the CDC and the Egyptian Ministry of Health central laboratory. The fish were reportedly from the single shop, samples of which were obtained from the patient's hospital locker and the Cairo police. These were all positive. Two specimens were titrated and had 16,000 and 64,000 mouse lethal doses per gram, respectively. One lethal human dose equals 7,000 mouse lethal doses. In other words, there was enough toxin in each gram of edible fish to kill between 2 and 10 people. Fresh mullet caught in the region can weigh approximately 1 kilogram.[7]

We traveled around Cairo and purchased samples nonsystematically from other shops, and none of these was positive for toxin or bacteria.

ANTITOXIN SOURCES AND USE

For ethical reasons, no controlled trial to document the efficacy of botulinal antitoxin has been conducted in humans; however, reports suggest that patients with type A and type E botulism who have received trivalent equine antitoxin early in the course of illness fare better than those who have not.

In response to this outbreak, trivalent botulinal antitoxins had been obtained from commercial sources within and outside Egypt by private physicians and patients' family members. The types of antitoxin used were recorded in patient records as dBIG (F(ab')2 "despeciated" heptavalent botulism immune globulin), French/Pasteur, French/Canadian, German, or a combination thereof.

Subsequent to written entreaty by the Egyptian Ministry of Health, 100 vials of dBIG were provided to the Egyptian government for compassionate use under a U.S. Department of Defense investigational protocol.[8] Available records indicated that no fewer than 54 patients in this group (59%) received botulinal antitoxin of at least one type during their hospital stay. Antitoxin regardless of type was not administered, and data were not collected in a systematic fashion that would allow valid analysis of comparative effectiveness. dBIG appeared to be as safe as commercially available antitoxins under these field conditions.

CONCLUSIONS

This outbreak was associated with *faseikh*, a traditional food, supposedly prepared safely for thousands of years; however, we don't know how this particular batch was made, and therefore, we could not assess the likelihood for recurrence.

This outbreak might have affected even more people had there not been the coincidence of the Muslim and Gregorian calendars that put *Sham-el-Nessim* during the holiday of Ramadan; therefore, Muslims were largely spared because of their holiday requirement of fasting and food preferences. This largely restricted the victims to the Coptic Christian community.

After the investigation was concluded, we recommended that the public be warned that *faseikh* can cause botulism. Given the enormous publicity this outbreak received, however, I am confident most people in Egypt were already aware of this. We also recommended a review of the *faseikh* preparation methods and laboratory studies to reproduce *faseikh* preparation methods using "spiked" fish, fish with a known quantity of spores in them. Only through these kinds of experiments can a safe method for preparation be proved, if it exists.

In 2003, the *Al-Ahram Weekly* (online) reported that 12 people died of *faseikh* poisoning and that authorities impounded approximately 38 tons of spoiled fish and arrested nine Cairo shop-keepers for selling "bad fish." The article suggests that safe *faseikh* can be identified by visual and olfactory inspection (which the U.S. Food and Drug Administration, above, states is not reliable because botulinal toxin is colorless and odorless). Nationwide, centers for the treatment of poisoning announced a 48-hour emergency, and "vaccines" (perhaps antitoxin) to treat botulism were distributed.[9]

In 2006, 171 cases of botulism were reported to the CDC. Of these, 19 were foodborne; 107 were infant botulism, and 45 were cases of wound botulism.

Because an outbreak from *faseikh* had never happened in Egypt before, because the Gulf War had only recently ended, and because Saddam Hussein had threatened biological warfare, it was suggested that this was the result of a terrorist act. We found no evidence to support this, however.

On my return to Atlanta from Cairo, I changed planes in Frankfurt. I was pulled out of the line to enter the plane by airport officials, although I do not remember having identified myself to anyone up to that point. They requested that I accompany them to the tarmac. There I saw my baggage, including the typical large, red Coleman coolers that CDC uses to transport specimens and laboratory equipment. I was asked to identify all of the cables, electronic equipment, and battery-containing items that were in the coolers. They had a list of suspicious items that I assume were detected through X-ray of the containers. These were systematically identified and shown by me within the specified coolers with several men dressed in white shirts and ties holding clipboards reviewing my activity at a distance. The officials then asked for a remaining cooler to be opened. I did this, and the officials poked their heads in and then practically leaped back in response to the smell of *faseikh*. I was ordered to close it up and to return to the check-in line.

REFERENCES

1. Pan Am Flight 103. Retrieved August 28, 2008, from http://en.wikipedia.org/wiki/Pan_Am_Flight_103.
2. Keaney T, Cohen EA. *Gulf War Air Power Survey*. Washington, DC: United States Department of the Air Force, 1993.
3. Weber JT, Hibbs RG Jr, Darwish A, et al. A massive outbreak of type E botulism associated with traditional salted fish in Cairo. *J Infect Dis* 1993;167:451–454.
4. Weber JT, Hatheway CL, Blake PA, Tauxe RV. Clarification of dietary risk factors and religion in a botulism outbreak. *J Infect Dis* 1993;168:258.
5. Artful Angler. Retrieved October 20, 2008, from http://www.artfulangler.co.uk/fishprofiles/fish_profiles_sea_Mullet.htm.
6. Compliance Policy Guidance for FDA Staff Updated: 2005-11-29 Sec. 540.650 Uneviscerated Fish Products that are Salt-cured, Dried, or Smoked (CPG 7108.17). http://www.fda.gov/ora/compliance_ref/cpg/cpgfod/cpg540-650.htm.
7. El-Gharabawy MM, Assem SS. Spawning induction in the Mediterranean grey mullet. *Afr J Biotechnol* 2006;5:1836–1845. Available online at http://www.academicjournals.org/AJB.
8. Hibbs RG, Weber JT, Corwin A, et al. Experience with the use of an investigational F(ab')2 heptavalent botulism immune globulin of equine origin during an outbreak of type E botulism in Egypt. *Clin Infect Dis* 1996;23:337–340.
9. Fish over reason, Al-Ahram Weekly Online May 1–7, 2003:636. Retrieved October 20, 2008, from http://weekly.ahram.org.eg/2003/636/eg8.htm.
10. Department of Health and Human Services, Centers for Disease Control and Prevention, Botulism. Retrieved October 20, 2008, from http://www.cdc.gov/nczved/dfbmd/disease_listing/botulism_gi.html#9.

CHAPTER 11

Controlling an Outbreak of Shigellosis with a Community-Wide Intervention in Lexington, Kentucky

Janet Mohle-Boetani, MD, MPH

INTRODUCTION

"There's a large outbreak of shigellosis in Kentucky, and we wondered if you could help out." This was the request to me from Dr. Patricia Griffin of the Enterics Branch in the first week of June 1991. Dr. Griffin was in the middle part of her career as a supervisor in the Enterics Branch for the Centers for Disease Control (CDC). She was known by the EIS officers as a supervisor who paid attention to details in an outbreak investigation. She was also very friendly, and I had often talked with her about interesting outbreaks when I ran into her in the elevator in the CDC building.

I had just about completed my first year of EIS in the Bacterial Meningitis and Special Pathogens Branch and had watched enviously as my colleagues in the Enterics Branch, just down the hall from me, were sent to investigate cholera in South America and botulism in Egypt (Todd Weber). Before joining the EIS, I went to Stanford Medical School, where I developed an interest in epidemiology from our pathology classes and worked

177

on epidemiologic studies of ovarian cancer and breast cancer. In my internal medicine residency at Stanford, I developed an interest in infectious diseases; I thought that the EIS program would be an ideal place to both further explore infectious diseases and expand my skills in epidemiology. In Atlanta, I had worked on engaging and complex projects including a cost-effectiveness analysis of preventive measures for neonatal group B streptococcal disease, but I had yet to be involved with a large epidemic, or even a sizable outbreak. Although Lexington, Kentucky didn't seem to be the most exotic location to be sent on an outbreak investigation and shigellosis could not have been a more common disease, the opportunity to work on a large outbreak outside of Atlanta was very appealing to me. I enthusiastically accepted the offer.

After a day spent reading all that I could about shigellosis and its control and packing my bags for an estimated 2-week trip, I boarded a plane for Lexington. I remember immediately being struck by the vast grasslands surrounding the airport. There were horse pastures seemingly everywhere; the health department was in close proximity to a fair ground where horses competed in weekly shows. I arrived at the health department at 9 a.m., and the office was bustling with activity. After being introduced to the Commissioner of Health, Dr. John Poundstone, and a crew of public health nurses, I set to work looking into the statistics that had been gathered on the outbreak.

There were 138 culture-confirmed *Shigella sonnei* infections with onsets from January through May; most of these cases were in persons who attended or worked at child care facilities or elementary schools. The public health nurses had been attempting to control the outbreak using standard public health procedures. Cases were defined as laboratory evidence of infection with *Shigella sonnei*. Cases were reported through standard laboratory surveillance. Each case triggered a public health investigation that included a home visit, collection of stools for *Shigella* culture from close contacts, and instruction in handwashing before meals, after toileting, and after diaper changes.

Shigella is a Gram-negative organism that is spread through the fecal–oral route or person to person and causes fever, diarrhea, and stomach cramps about 1 to 2 days after ingestion. The diarrhea is often bloody, and symptoms usually resolve within 1 week. The organism is carried (by persons who are infected but do not have symptoms) and causes disease in only humans (not in other animals). Because the infectious dose is very low and most infected people are only mildly ill and thus remain in contact with other people, outbreaks are common.

Shigella organisms were discovered more than 100 years ago by Shiga, a Japanese scientist. There are three major species of *Shigella*. *Shigella soneii* causes two thirds of infections in the United States, and the other third of infections are primarily caused by *Shigella flexnerii*. *Shigella dysenteriae type 1* cause toxic diarrheal epidemics in the developing world.

Public health professionals (primarily public health nurses) also visited all schools and child care centers that were attended by children with culture-confirmed shigellosis. All classmates of culture-confirmed cases were tested for shigellosis. Children in preschool or daycare were excluded while symptomatic (with diarrhea) day care center staff, teachers, and elementary school children were excluded from school or work until they had three consecutive stool cultures negative for *Shigella*.

In March, the health department mailed a notification to the directors of all licensed child care facilities (preschools, day care centers, and family day care homes). The notification included information about the outbreak and advised them to require handwashing on arrival to the facility, after diaper changes, after toileting, and before eating or preparing food.

Despite these meticulous and well-documented investigations, exclusion policies, and notifications, the outbreak persisted and spread throughout the community through the end of May. There was understandable frustration in not being able to control the outbreak, despite following standard public health practices. There was also concern that the outbreak would be exacerbated by summer activities. Because *Shigella* infections are spread person to person and through food handling, shigellosis typically increases in the summer because of increased congregations of people in areas without hygienic facilities (e.g., at camps) or sharing home prepared food items (e.g., weekend picnics). For these reasons, assistance in controlling the outbreak was sought first from the state health department and then from the CDC.

INITIAL INVESTIGATION AND RECOMMENDATIONS

In the afternoon of my first day, one of the public health nurses took me to a few of the child care facilities that had outbreaks of shigellosis. Despite recent training and written notifications by the public health nurses regarding the need to wash hands, we observed barriers to handwashing in most of the centers we visited. For example, the sinks were too high for children to reach, and no step stools were readily available for the children to get access to the sink after going to the toilet. Also, sinks were not easily accessible to the areas chosen for diaper changing.

After reviewing the data and conducting observations at child care facilities for a few more days, my supervisor in Atlanta, Dr. Griffin, and I developed recommendations for the Lexington Health Department. We recommended promotion of handwashing community wide, surveillance for diarrhea, and rapid diagnosis and treatment of shigellosis. We emphasized handwashing promotion over collection of stool specimens.

I worked diligently on the weekend and called Dr. Griffin at her home to check in on the wording of some of the recommendations. In the middle of one of these very intense conversations, she exclaimed "Wow, he did it!" I asked, "What?" "My son just pooped in his potty chair—his first time!" I found this particularly comical given that we had just been talking about how to phrase our recommendation to wash hands after helping children use the toilet.

An additional recommendation that Dr. Griffin and I developed was that the health department should stop collecting stool specimens from asymptomatic convalescing school children, teachers, and day care staff. We felt that these groups, even though recently infected, would be very unlikely to transmit *Shigella* if they had formed stools and could be relied on to wash their hands after going to the toilet. We also recommended against the practice of testing asymptomatic contacts of persons with shigellosis. We reasoned that the decreased burden of specimen collection, ensuring exclusions from work or school, and following up on multiple stool culture results would permit the public health professionals to focus on handwashing in key locations where people congregated and would permit a proactive rather than reactive approach.

Because we could not be certain that preschool aged children could be expected to wash their hands reliably, we recommended that asymptomatic convalescing preschool aged children be excluded from group child care until two stool cultures were negative for *Shigella*. This recommendation was a policy change from the practice of excluding children from child care facilities only during the time that they had diarrhea. Although we anticipated an increased workload in following these children, we expected that there would be a substantial decrease in workload in following cultures from asymptomatic contacts and from asymptomatic, convalescing, school-aged children and adults.

INITIAL RESPONSE

The Lexington County Health Department responded vigorously to our recommendations. On June 10th, the day after we provided our recommendations, the Commissioner of Health created a Shigella Task Force consisting of health department staff from the clinic, the laboratory, the field service section, the school health section and the environmental health division. The commissioner called a meeting with key leaders in each of these areas and presented our recommendations. I believe the commissioner created the task force to empower the leaders to take responsibility for controlling the outbreak. I credit the commissioner's leadership skills as responsible for the effectiveness of the committee. The leaders decided to implement a community-wide handwashing campaign with monitoring of handwashing at sites controlled by community services considered to be at high risk of transmission. The task force initiated onsite handwashing promotion at day care centers, summer schools, summer camps, and free lunch sites. The handwashing promotion included problem solving at each site to ensure that appropriate handwashing could be accomplished everyday.

In the 3 to 4 days after the creation of the task force, I accompanied public health professionals on several of their site visits to child care facilities, elementary schools, summer camps, and free lunch sites. At each of these sites, I observed the direct advice and problem solving of the public health professionals and recorded and photographed key areas of concern regarding handwashing. For example, we observed and recorded children lining up for free lunches without handwashing and a paucity of handwashing facilities available at summer camps. At child care centers, we observed sinks that were too high for the children to reach to wash their hands. At schools, we observed that no soap was available in some of the bathrooms; this was a safety issue because children would squirt soap on the floor and then slip on the soap. I planned to return to each of these sites in a few weeks to observe changes in the accessibility of soap and water and handwashing practices.

Watching the community join together to implement rapidly community-wide handwashing was one of the most rewarding experiences of my tenure at the CDC. After creating the task force, assistance in handwashing promotion was sought from the community at large. To engage the community, Dr. Poundstone held a press conference and sought cooperation from the media, the Parks and Recreation Office, the Community Services Agency, and the school board. A local television station aired a video several evenings each week that emphasized the prevention of shigellosis through handwashing and taught proper handwashing technique. The Community Services Agency and the Parks and Recreation provided liquid soap and water to all free lunch sites and summer camps. The school board ensured that all summer students viewed a video on shigellosis and handwashing and that all students would be monitored in handwashing on arrival to school, after using the toilet, and before eating lunch or snacks. I believe that it was Dr. Poundstone's leadership and a strong local public health infrastructure that permitted the rapid implementation of these community-wide preventive actions within a week of my arrival to Lexington.

An additional change that was implemented was enhanced surveillance for diarrhea. Child care facilities and elementary summer schools were directed to keep track of illnesses from school or day care and to advise those with diarrhea to seek rapid diagnosis and treatment at the health department clinic. The health department set up a special diarrhea clinic so that persons with diarrhea would not need to wait for an appointment to get tested and treated. All patients were instructed in handwashing in the clinic.

After observing the implementation of the handwashing campaign, I needed to leave Lexington to attend the international conference on AIDS in Florence, Italy. This was a conference that I funded on my own, to present a paper from work I had done during my internal medicine residency. Coincidentally, some of the work that I collaborated on regarding bacillary angiomatosis while I was an EIS officer was also being presented (this is an unusual systemic disease occurring primarily in immunocompromised persons due to infection with the bacteria *Bartonella quintana* or *Bartonella henselae*). As can be imagined, I had a very enjoyable week, both at the conference and traveling in Italy with my boyfriend (now husband) Mark. Mark lived in California while I was in Atlanta, and we very much appreciated any time that we could spend together.

THE SECOND PHASE

The week away was also ideally timed from an investigation standpoint. My departure from Lexington permitted the health department and greater community to implement the handwashing campaign unencumbered by meetings with me. I returned to Lexington just before the 4th of July, and I remember spending a great day with the family of one of the public health nurses; we swam in her backyard swimming pool and ate lots of watermelon. The personal relationships developed in the context of an intense outbreak investigation are a major unspoken reward of field investigations. The public health staff members that I met in Lexington were warm, gracious, and appreciative. Their dedication to public health and collaborative spirit were a large part of the inspiration leading to my decision to pursue a career in public health instead of academic medicine.

After my return to Lexington from Europe, my goals were to (1) observe the implementation of handwashing in a diversity of sites in the community and (2) conduct a study to attempt to determine risk factors for outbreaks of shigellosis in child care facilities. Although many child care facilities had outbreaks, there were several that had no cases or only one case; we wanted to determine whether there were predictors for the spread of shigellosis in child care facilities that could be modified to prevent outbreaks in the future.

My first goal was met through going back to the same sites I had originally visited in the week just before the handwashing campaign. I was elated to see dramatic changes at all of the sites that I visited. For example, at a summer camp where there had been limited access to handwashing facilities, handwashing stations were set up close to the latrines. In the outside picnic area where the children had lunch, two outside sinks were designated as handwashing sinks, and I observed the Parks and Recreation staff requiring children to line up and wash their hands before receiving their lunch. At the camp site, they even incorporated handwashing into one of their routine cheers ("Give me an H, give me an A, give me an N. . . . What's that spell?").

At a free lunch site in the middle of a housing project, soap dispensers were installed in the two outside sinks, and I observed the community service workers monitoring children in washing their hands before providing them with their lunches. At child care centers, I noted the addition of step stools to sinks to ensure that young children could reach the sinks and that nurses had worked with facilities to create diaper changing areas that were close to handwashing facilities (this was particularly challenging at times). I observed elementary schools lining children up to wash their hands before lunch. I documented all of these changes with "after-intervention" photographs. The collection of before and after photos was used to create an instructional video directed to local health departments on controlling a community-wide shigellosis outbreak.

To accomplish the second goal, I worked together with an epidemiologist from the state public health department, Margaret Stapleton, MSPH. My supervisor in Atlanta had also changed. Dr. Griffin was on a summer vacation, and Dr. Paul Blake, the Enterics Branch chief, was filling in. I found it refreshing to have a new supervisor for this phase of the investigation. By this point, I had learned a lot from Dr. Griffin about controlling the outbreak and providing recommendations to a local agency. In this next stage of the investigation, I hoped to do a field analytic study that would provide practical recommendations; I was not disappointed.

On another memorable weekend call, Dr. Blake and I developed a plan for a case-control study. In the information collected by the health department, I had noted that some child care centers had large outbreaks, whereas others had no cases. We wondered whether those centers with no cases were different than those that had large outbreaks. We reasoned that if we could determine factors associated with large outbreaks we could use them in recommendations to prevent outbreaks in the future. We decided to conduct a case-control study in which the "case" was a center with at least three cases of shigellosis among children and a "control" was a center with no cases of shigellosis. Although this method differs from the standard case-control study in which cases are defined as illness in individual people, we felt that the method should work in comparing centers with and without outbreaks.

The health department supplied me with a list of all licensed child care centers and family day care homes in the county as well as basic characteristics of those facilities and the number of culture-confirmed cases of shigellosis identified among children attending each facility. I found that all centers with at least three cases enrolled diapered children and children whose child care fees were paid through a federally funded program (indicating a low socioeconomic level). Because both having children in diapers and low socioeconomic status are known risk factors for outbreaks of shigellosis, we felt we needed to control for these factors. Given the small size of the study (only six "case centers"), we felt the most efficient method of controlling for socioeconomic status was to restrict the control centers to those with diapered children, at least five children who had fees paid by the federally funded program, and no cases of shigellosis. Thirteen centers met the criteria for control centers.

Ms. Stapleton and I collected the information for the case-control study through onsite interviews. First we created a questionnaire addressing policies and procedures and observations. Ms. Stapleton interviewed the directors about practices and policies while I asked the same questions of a staff member who cared for diapered children. We also collected the number of children by age group and the number of toilets used by each age group. Comparing notes with Margaret after our respective interviews was another memorable part of this field investigation. The discordance between the director and staff interviews was notable.

We found an association between having a food preparer (a staff who mixed formula or a cook) who changed diapers and having at least three cases of shigellosis in the facility (100% of case centers vs. 46% of control centers, $P = 0.04$). We found a greater median toddler-to-toilet ratio (the number of 3 year olds per flushable toilet) in the case centers than in the control centers (the ratio was 20 in case centers and 13 in the control centers, $P < 0.05$). We also found an association between the provision of transportation from home to the center and shigellosis (83% of case centers provided transportation vs. 15% of the control centers).

Differences in the response of directors and staff to hygiene questions were identified. Although 42% of staff reported that a cook changed diapers, only 11% of directors reported these combined duties. Directors were also more likely than staff to report that they had policies to prevent diarrhea (89% vs. 32%).

Thus, the case-control study did reveal features of centers amenable to changes that could help to prevent diarrheal outbreaks. Food should be prepared by persons who do not change diapers, if possible. The high toddler to toilet ratio found in the case centers could be a reflection of inadequate sinks to permit accessible handwashing. We felt that the finding of transportation associated with the case centers might be a reflection of a tendency to mix different age groups of children, permitting the introduction and spread of communicable diseases such as shigellosis. The discordant answers to questions by staff and directors highlights both (1) the importance of querying staff, in addition to directors, when doing investigations in facilities, and (2) that staff in child care centers may need additional training in infection control.

The second part of my investigation was also rewarding because I was able to observe a rapid decline in the reported cases of shigellosis. The epidemic curve showed an abrupt decrease in cases in the week after community-wide interventions were initiated in mid June (Figure 11-1).[1] Although in June there were 42 cases, in July there were only 10 and subsequently cases were reported at a very low rate, 2 to 14 per month. With the outbreak under control, I spent the last weekend at a horse show and visiting the Appalachian mountains (as suggested by Margaret), where I acquired a woolen blanket, hand woven by students in Berea College that I use to this day.

January 1991 – the Lexington-Fayette County Health Department receives three reports of *Shigella sonnei* infections from the University of Kentucky microbiology laboratory

January 1 through July 15, 1991 – 186 culture-confirmed *S. sonnei* infections reported to the health department

Investigation identifies that 47% of the initial 111 *S. sonnei* infections of all ages were attributed to child day care attendance

June 1991 – the health department creates a Shigella task force
• Creation of diarrhea clinic to facilitate proper diagnosis and treatment
• Intensification of infection-control training
• Intensification of surveillance for shigellosis
• Encouragement of community-based participation in prevention efforts
• Monitoring of hand washing at day care centers, elementary schools, summer camps, and free-lunch sites

Three weeks after intensive interventions initiated, a substantial decline of culture-confirmed cases is observed

FIGURE 11-1 Timeline of shigellosis outbreak in Lexington-Fayette County, Kentucky, 1991.

Data from Kolanz M, Sandifer J, Poundstone J, Stapleton M, Finger R. Shigellosis in child day care centers—Lexington-Fayette County, Kentucky. *MMWR* 1992;41:440–442.

CONCLUSION

During this investigation, I learned several lessons. First, some standard public health practices such as stool collection among contacts can divert precious public health resources from health promotion and prevention. Second, community-wide interventions are possible with strong leadership and an effectively functioning health department that is able to collaborate productively with the community at large. Third, the case-control study approach can be used with the facility as the unit (for a case or control) to determine facility characteristics that are associated with disease. Fourth, I learned the rewards of direct field investigation and developed a deep respect for local public health professionals. Finally, I learned that you don't need to be in an exotic location or work on an exotic disease to have a rewarding experience investigating an outbreak. Working on this shigellosis outbreak in Lexington, Kentucky was definitely one of the most gratifying experiences of my EIS career and was a turning point in my decision to work in public health at the local level.

REFERENCES

1. Mohle-Boetani, JC, Stapleton M, Finger R, et al. Community wide shigellosis: control of an outbreak and risk factors in child day-care centers. *Am J Public Health* 1995;85:812–816.

CHAPTER 12

Pork Tapeworm in an Orthodox Jewish Community: Arriving at a Biologically Plausible Hypothesis

Peter M. Schantz, VMD, PhD, and Mary E. Bartlett, BA

INTRODUCTION

I had known about neurocysticercosis in veterinary school and experienced it first hand in my first year postveterinary school when I spent a year (1965–1966) as an Academic Fellow at the Department of Parasitology at the Faculty of Medicine, National University of Mexico, Mexico City. It was of special interest to me because it was a cestode (tapeworm) associated with animals.

Neurocysticercosis was usually diagnosed at autopsy at that time, as computerized tomography (CT) and other powerful diagnostic imaging technology were not yet available. I knew that people died from it—seen by pathologists—killed by fatal seizures or by obstruction of flow of cerebrospinal fluid, obstructive hydrocephalus. A tiny minority of people died from the disease—many were asymptomatic.

The adult worm in the human intestine is flat (like all tapeworms), and *Taenia solium* is commonly referred to as the pork tapeworm because of a unique relationship between humans and pigs that allows this particular parasite to thrive. Humans are the only (definitive) host that can harbor the adult tapeworm. When a man or woman eats the meat of an infected pig that is harboring cysticerci (the larval stage tapeworm), the worm develops inside the intestines and attaches itself to the bowel wall. Proglottids (egg-producing factories) are then detached from the tapeworm and released individually or in small "chains" in the feces. The tiny eggs contain tinier larvae, or embryos. If the worm could consciously strategize, it would want its eggs to make their way to another pig so that the larvae can encyst in this human food source and keep the cycle going for its perpetual survival. The likelihood of successful transmission of the tapeworm is favored by the common practice of pigs to eat human feces (coprophagy). The tapeworm has been successful at this for thousands of years (at least). More is presented on the life cycle later here; however, it is pretty obvious from this life cycle that persons who eat pork are at potential risk for this disease.

As an anthropology undergraduate major, I had long been fascinated by other cultures and practices. Veterinary medicine too was a passion, and public heath was a means of merging these two interests. Dr. James H. Steele, then Chief Veterinary Officer in the U.S. Public Health Service, spoke to my class in public health at the University of Pennsylvania School of Veterinary Medicine on the role of and opportunities for veterinarians in public health; Jim has been and remains an important mentor to this day.

After postgraduate studies in epidemiology with Professor Calvin Schwabe at the University of California, Davis, I worked in South America with the Pan American Zoonoses Center (PAHO/WHO) in Buenos Aires, Argentina, where I was epidemiologist and head of the zoonosis laboratory. Before the outbreak described here, I had experienced several memorable field investigations at Centers for Disease Control (CDC) as an Epidemic Intelligence Service (EIS) Officer during 1974 to 1976. I investigated clusters of cases of echinococcosis in the Navajo, Santo Domingo, and Zuni tribes in New Mexico and Arizona. I had been recruited to CDC by Myron Schultz, MD, DVM (then Director of the Division of Parasitic Diseases).

The CDC was challenged to develop a serodiagnostic assay for neuro-cysticercosis in response to increasing numbers of clinical calls from physicians all over the country who were newly diagnosing the disease. Because of my prior experience with the disease in Mexico, I assisted in handling the clinical calls at the Division of Parasitic Diseases. At that time (the 1970s), new diagnostics were being developed that would detect cystic lesions in the brain (e.g., computerized tomography), which uniquely permitted detection and characterization of intracerebral pathology; however, the intracerebral cysts resembled some other possible pathologic conditions and a specific immunoassay for *Taenia solium* cysticercosis was needed to help confirm the nature and viability of the intracerebral lesions.

My veterinary colleague, Professor John Eckert, Director of the Institute of Parasitic Diseases at the University of Zurich, Switzerland, arranged for his graduate student, Bruno Gottstein, to come to the CDC to acquire experience working in our parasitology program. Under the supervision of Victor Tsang, PhD, Bruno developed an immunoblot assay for serologic diagnosis of *Taenia solium* cysticercosis with high specificity and improved sensitivity. Because cysticercosis is a larval tapeworm cyst disease that localizes in tissues of the brain and muscles, it was difficult to diagnose. The development of an immunoblot assay was an important advance as prior serodiagnostics were nonspecific and had poorly defined sensitivity.

THE INVESTIGATION

Physicians in the United States were not usually familiar with neurocysticercosis because the tapeworm (*Taenia solium*) was not transmitted locally in its life cycle, although cases were seen occasionally in immigrants from Mexico and some other Latin American countries.[1] The development and growing availability of CT scans in the 1980s provided a unique diagnostic technology for detection and characterization of a wide variety of pathological conditions within the central nervous system and other organs. Magnetic resonance imaging further improved technology for brain scanning. After CT and magnetic resonance imaging became widely available for scanning of the brain, together with the immunoblot test, diagnosis of this problem in the United States became more frequent. Most U.S. physicians were not familiar with this disease, and thus, they frequently consulted CDC for assistance with serologic diagnosis and clinical management decisions when they suspected it. I was the person who most often took those calls because it had become one of my areas of specialization. With rare exceptions, the patients who were subjects of these queries were immigrants from Mexico or other countries where *T. solium* was endemic.

Thus, in 1990, when we started getting calls from physicians in New York City about persons who were not the typical case seen in immigrants, but rather in persons who were born in New York City (and in fact had never traveled outside the United States), I knew we had to look more closely at the situation. Unlike some outbreaks, this one was not explosive. The number of cases was small. There were four persons who were evaluated with recurring seizures.[2] When they received brain imaging, lesions were present that were radiologically consistent with cysticerci; however, what was especially puzzling was the population that this infection was being diagnosed in. These were Orthodox Jewish persons who were 6 to 39 years old. One had been born in Morocco and lived in the United States since 1976, and another had traveled to and spent 1 week in an area where cysticercosis is known to be endemic; however, that travel was 8 years before the onset of his symptoms. It is a religious practice that Orthodox Jews do not eat pork. Thus, this question arose: "How do Orthodox Jewish people get infected with a pork tapeworm?" At this point, we needed to establish a biologically plausible hypothesis to explain what we were observing.

Knowledge of the life cycle of this tapeworm played a fundamental role in considering what questions to ask and which answers to dismiss or consider important. Persons who eat cyst-infected pork can become infected with *Taenia solium*, and the tapeworm establishes in their intestines; however, persons who ingest the tapeworm eggs (passed in the stool of persons infected with the tapeworm) become infected with the cystic larval stages of the tapeworm (Figure 12-1). Embryonic larvae (oncospheres) emerge from the tapeworm's eggs, penetrate the intestines, and migrate through the blood stream of the egg ingester and encyst widely in the body. They may encyst in the brain and produce neurologic symptoms, including those observed in the four index cases, such as seizures or aphasia (difficulty using or understanding words). Other neurological changes could occur depending on where in the brain the cyst(s) is located.

The unresolved question when facing this group of cases was how did these Orthodox Jews ingest pork tapeworm eggs if they do not eat pork and typically spend much of their time with other Orthodox Jews?

Questioning of their physicians and interviewing family members revealed that a common practice in the community was to hire persons

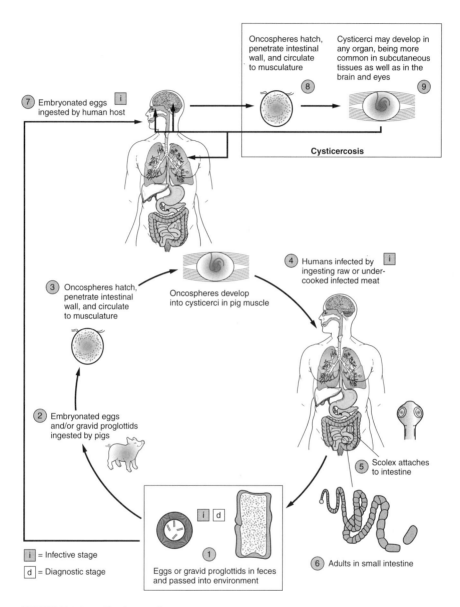

FIGURE 12-1 Cysticercosis.

From Centers for Disease Control and Prevention. Cysticercosis. Available at: http://www.dpd.cdc.gov/dpdx/HTML/Cysticercosis.htm. Last accessed October 29, 2008.

from Mexico as household laborers (domestics) with primary responsibility for food preparation and childcare. Although good hygiene, including rigorous hand washing, would minimize the possibility of exposure of other persons to the tapeworm eggs passed in the stools of infected house maids, such fastidious hygiene was apparently not uniformly practiced in this setting. It can be assumed that the tapeworm-infected domestic servants were having eggs deposited in their perianal area and, at least occasionally, contaminating their hands, which could then have engaged in preparing a salad or other food item for the family that employed them. They also could have had direct hand contact with family members (i.e., childcare) that allowed transfer of the eggs. This tapeworm can live for many months if not many years so the opportunity for someone with taenia infection to infect others may be prolonged. We discovered that there was a clandestine service that organized and facilitated transport of these household laborers from Mexico City to Los Angeles, then to New York City, and probably to other destinations. We didn't pursue the details of the labor practices and childcare, as it would have put us in a situation in which the immigrant workers might become reluctant to talk to us. This might threaten the relationship with the local community that employed them and our ability to discern the sources of infection.

For these Mexican women, this clandestine employment was a path out of poverty. They were young, unmarried, and "right off the farm," and you can probably guess what livestock species was present on that farm. In poor areas of rural Mexico, there is often a lack of disposal of human feces in a completely safe and sanitary manner, which gives roaming pigs access and opportunity to ingest tapeworm eggs shed in feces by infected humans.[1] We didn't pursue their stories, all of the details of their coming to live and work in New York City, but clearly they were coming from communities where pork tapeworm infection was not rare and pork was a common staple food.

I engaged my colleague in the Division of Parasitic Diseases, EIS Officer Anne Moore, PhD, MD, to follow-up the outbreak with a serosurvey of the extended families and other members of the involved community.[3] Serologic testing for cysticercosis antibodies was performed to detect people who had been exposed and infected with *T. solium* larva but had not necessarily developed symptoms of the disease. We drew blood on a volunteer basis anonymously. We had good cooperation in no small part because it was a very well-organized community of middle-class families in the New

York City boroughs of Brooklyn and Queens. They had an efficient communications network through the temples, and after they were advised of what was happening—that is, people were having seizures—they cooperated because they recognized it to be in their best interest to do so.

Using the enzyme-linked immunoelectrotransfer blot, 17 immediate family members of the cases were tested. Seven persons among 11 tested from families of 2 of the patients were seropositive. Among these 11 family members who went on to also have magnetic resonance imaging, lesions were identified in two of the seropositive family members (both children). They were 6 and 2 years old, respectively. Coincidentally, the day before she was scheduled to have a screening brain magnetic resonance imaging the 6-year-old had a prolonged seizure.

In the past 5 years, each of the four families had employed an average of three housekeepers from Mexico. One of these families had employed at least 10 women; however, it was not possible to identify the particular individuals who were the most likely sources of the infections because most of these women were not available for testing. In the case of the family of a 16-year-old female patient (in which none of her three immediate family members were seropositive), serum was drawn from one of the housekeepers, and it tested positive for antibodies in the CDC enzyme-linked immunosorbent assay for cysticercosis. Examining her stool revealed *Taenia* sp. eggs. When told of her results, both she and the other housekeeper refused any further interviewing or examination and left the home.[2]

COMMENTS ON THE UNIQUENESS OF THIS OUTBREAK

Taenia solium, the "pork" tapeworm, is not transmitted in its natural life cycle in the United States because swine husbandry practices rarely permit pigs to have access to human feces, a requirement for perpetuation of the life cycle of the tapeworm. Nevertheless, the disease is seen commonly in immigrants, mainly from Mexico and some other countries where the infection is endemic, who acquired their infections in their native homeland but may experience first onset of clinical disease after immigration to the United States. It is the nature of the disease that the larval tapeworm cysts (cysticerci) may exist within the brain for months or years without producing any symptoms of illness. Clinical cases of cysticercosis, larval stage *T. solium* disease, are commonly seen in hospitals and emergency clinics, usually in immigrant patients who were previously unaware of having the infection. These same individuals are also at risk of carrying the "pork tapeworm" (*T. solium*) in their intestines, which they had acquired in their home country through ingestion of uncooked pork containing the cysticerci. This intestinal-stage tapeworm infection is usually without symptoms, although the carriers may be aware of passing tapeworm segments ("proglottids") in the stools. Tapeworm carriers are important to the life cycle and maintenance of the infection if their feces are available to swine, which are the key intermediate hosts for the tapeworm. Coprophagy is a behavior characteristic of swine and allows the transmission of this infection in its human–pig life cycle. Tapeworm carriers are also the source of cysticercosis in humans when humans accidentally ingest food contaminated with feces containing the eggs of the adult tapeworm. The source of the cysticercosis may be the tapeworm carrier himself or herself as a result of direct or indirect fecal contamination.

The cause of the seizures experienced in this community was not apparent until several of the patients had been placed under specialist care with the assistance of the local New York City Health Department and the CDC. No one at the local community hospitals had prior experience with this infection and its potential dangers. Surgeons who conducted brain biopsies sent the lesions to pathologists who recognized them as cysticerci (larval stages) of *T. solium*. After the cause and source of the infections were understood, it allowed the investigations to go forward and resulted in development of educational and preventive measures that promptly prevented further transmission.

REFERENCES

1. Despommier DD. Tapeworm infection: the long and the short of it. *N Engl J Med* 1992;327:727–728.
2. Schantz PM, Moore AC, Munoz JL, et al. Neurocysticercosis in an Orthodox Jewish community in New York City. *N Engl J Med* 1992;327:692–695.
3. Moore A, Lutwick LL, Schantz PM, et al. Seroprevalence of cysticercosis in an Orthodox Jewish community. *Am J Trop Med Hyg* 1995;53:439–442.

CHAPTER 13

The Massive Waterborne Outbreak of *Cryptosporidium* Infections, Milwaukee, Wisconsin, 1993

Jeffrey P. Davis, MD

INTRODUCTION: APRIL 5, 1993

On Monday morning, April 5, Dr. Gerald Sedmak, a virologist with the City of Milwaukee Health Department (MHD), received calls from individual citizens complaining of gastrointestinal illnesses. Gerry told other MHD staff about these complaints, and in turn, these staff members began an effort to see whether there was an unusual number of individuals with similar gastrointestinal illness—indeed, there were. Kathy Blair, a registered nurse and epidemiologist with the MHD, received calls from the South Milwaukee Health Department, other local agencies, and private citizens regarding widespread occupational and school absenteeism related to diarrheal illness. Gerry, Kathy, and their colleagues could not have known at that time that these were the initial reports of what would unfold as a historically large and unprecedented waterborne outbreak in the United States. Many pharmacies on the south side of Milwaukee had or were nearly sold out of antimotility medications (medication to slow down or stop diarrhea). Additionally, many health care providers were ill and unable to work. Concomitantly, Dr. Steve Gradus, director of the MHD Bureau of Laboratories, and his colleague, Dr. Ajaib Singh, conducted telephone surveys of hospital emergency rooms and laboratories. They learned of an extreme number of weekend visits for diarrhea-related illnesses to emergency departments and increased numbers of requisitions for bacterial culture of stool specimens. The St. Luke's Hospital microbiology laboratory exhausted its supply of media used to isolate enteric bacterial pathogens. Based on this information, MHD officials suspected that the outbreak was predominantly affecting the southern part of Milwaukee and included other municipalities in southern Milwaukee County. Initial newspaper and other media reports circulating on April 5 focused on the unusual number of diarrhea illnesses, the unknown etiology of the illness, and the shortage of antidiarrhea medications. Media interest intensified rapidly.

Kathy called Jim Kazmierczak, DVM, an epidemiologist and colleague in the Bureau of Public Health (BPH), Wisconsin Division of Health (DOH; now named the Wisconsin Division of Public Health), notified him of these events, and inquired whether DOH staff were aware of an unusual occurrence of similar illnesses elsewhere in the state. Up to then we had not been told of similar illnesses elsewhere.

During my initial conversations with Kathy and Jim that morning, we discussed the potential of any one of several etiologic agents to be associated with these events and the need for good laboratory data and illness characterization. Although the agent was not yet known, my initial impression was the illness must be considered to be waterborne until proven otherwise because of the magnitude and widespread occurrence of diarrhea illness. Concomitantly, Drs. Gradus and Singh discovered that most hospital microbiology laboratory staff members were not conducting virus culture of stool specimens and that tests for ova and parasites were infrequently ordered. Accordingly, infection control practitioners were selected to facilitate collection of stool specimens for virus culture at the MHD from the next 10 patients presenting at their facilities with diarrhea illnesses.

Later, we discussed the MHD plan to widely distribute stool kits for virus testing to clinics to test individuals with acute diarrhea illnesses and the results to date of testing for bacterial enteric pathogens at St. Luke's Hospital. We sensed that this was a really big outbreak when we learned that from this one hospital on one weekend about 200 stool specimens were obtained for bacterial culture, and we were confronted with a really big clue when we learned that, despite this high volume of testing, all cultures were negative to date for bacterial enteric pathogens. I suggested testing stool specimens already known to be negative for bacterial enteric pathogens and still remaining at the St. Luke's laboratory for parasitic and protozoan infections at the MHD laboratory. The MHD laboratory was one of two public health laboratories in Wisconsin. The emerging scope and breadth of this outbreak diminished the likelihood that this was a viral illness, and it was important to consider protozoan infections, as they could be associated with large community outbreaks.

Steve arranged for this testing and also requested that microbiology laboratory supervisors begin aggressively testing of diarrhea stool specimens for protozoan infections, with specific emphasis on testing for *Cryptosporidium*. Steve also planned to review water treatment records that would be available from the City of Milwaukee Water Works (hereafter referred to as MWW), the municipal water utility. Jim Wagner, of the MWW, provided Steve with the water testing data.

Because of the apparent magnitude of the outbreak and implications for residents in multiple jurisdictions, I offered the onsite assistance of DOH staff to join the MHD in the investigation. We would need Tuesday, April 6 to structure a team and plan our activities in Milwaukee and would drive to Milwaukee from Madison early on Wednesday, April 7. The offer of assistance was accepted.

APRIL 6, 1993

On April 6, I spoke with Steve to discuss the findings of his review of the MWW water treatment records. He described some initial resistance to review the records and defense of the quality of Milwaukee's water by the MWW administrators, but he was able to review some recent water treatment records. Generally, during recent weeks, there were increases in coliform counts that were consistent with substantial rainfall at water intake points; however, chlorine levels were high, and *E. coli* counts were within Department of Natural Resources (DNR) recommendations after treatment. Steve also noted spikes in treated water turbidity (one of many measures of water quality) occurred in late March primarily at the South plant, one of the two municipal water treatment facilities operated by the MWW. Turbidity is a technical measure of particles suspended in water. Turbidity can be measured in raw, untreated water and in finished, treated water.

Steve was impressed with peaks in turbidity values of treated water on successive days.

While we were discussing these unusual turbidity test results, Steve recalled the Carrollton, Georgia, outbreak of waterborne *Cryptosporidium* infections involving an estimated 13,000 diarrhea illnesses—a lot of illness by any measure.[1] The Carrollton outbreak was associated with a filtered water supply; however, the peak filtered water turbidity was less than 1 nephelometric turbidity unit (NTU). That was surprisingly low. The NTU values in Milwaukee were considerably greater. Based on Steve's preliminary information, the potential that *Cryptosporidium* was the etiologic agent in the Milwaukee outbreak seemed increasingly likely. I requested Steve to arrange a meeting early on April 7 with the MWW directors and an opportunity for our staff to review the water treatment records. This would be our first meeting in Milwaukee after arriving on site.

Typically, notifiable enteric diseases are reported when an etiologic agent is laboratory confirmed, although in Wisconsin outbreaks were to be reported upon suspicion regardless of whether the etiology is known. Also, relatively few individuals with true notifiable infections ever get tested, and diarrhea without laboratory data is not reported by physicians. Thus, several strategic surveillance activities were planned. I contacted Dr. Dennis Juranek, the chief of the Parasitic Diseases Division in the National Center for Infectious Diseases, the Centers for Disease Control and Prevention (CDC). Dennis had extensive experience with waterborne diseases and had directed the CDC's investigation of the Carollton outbreak.[1] We discussed the Carrollton outbreak, and Dennis suggested examining illness occurrence in nursing home populations, which were geographically fixed and not likely to obtain their drinking water from other sources or sites.

Later that day Steve set up acid fast smears from three stool specimens known to be bacterial culture negative. The test would determine whether the patients were infected with *Cryptosporidium*. The specimen staining procedure required an overnight interval before the results would be known.

APRIL 7, 1993

While driving to Milwaukee early on April 7 with Mary Proctor, PhD, MPH, and chief of the BPH Communicable Diseases Epidemiology Section, I discussed our prospective and retrospective surveillance needs. We decided it would be valuable to establish immediately a surveillance focus in two settings. Mary would establish and maintain surveillance for diarrhea illness in nursing homes and emergency departments throughout Milwaukee County and its four contiguous counties.

Bill Mac Kenzie, MD, was the CDC Epidemic Intelligence Service (EIS) officer assigned to the DOH who I supervised. Bill, Jim Kazmierczak, Mary and I from the DOH, Steve and Kathy of the MHD, and Wisconsin DNR staff met with MWW officials, and we were briefed on their water treatment methods and distribution system. The DNR had purview over regulation of drinking water utilities.

Drinking water for the City of Milwaukee (1993 population estimate of 630,000) and many of the other 18 municipalities in Milwaukee County was supplied by two MWW treatment plants, one in the northern part of the city (Linnwood Avenue Purification Plant, North Plant) and one in the southern part of the city (Howard Avenue Purification Plant, South Plant). Each plant had a submerged water intake grid in Lake Michigan about 1.25 (North) and 1.44 (South) miles offshore, respectively, where water entered an enormous tunnel and flowed by gravity through additional tunnels until it reached stations to pump water to the respective plants. The North Plant was located just offshore, but the South plant was located 3.5 miles inland from the Lake Michigan south shore (Figure 13-1).

The North Plant was a strikingly beautiful structure situated on a prominence projecting into Lake Michigan that was initially opened in the 1930s, and it could be viewed from the hills overlooking Lake Michigan. I grew up in a village along the north shore in Milwaukee County, passed by the treatment plant many times, and truly appreciated the majesty of this municipal water treatment facility. The same could not be said for the South Plant, built during the 1960s. Nonetheless, both plants housed modern, large treatment facilities.

Treatment capacities of each plant were sufficiently large to supply the entire water district fully. Treated water needs in Milwaukee are great because of its large population and industrial base, which included industries such as brewing that required large volumes of pure water. Should an outage occur in one plant, the distribution infrastructures from each plant were interconnected so that either plant really could supply the water needs for the City of Milwaukee and its retail water customers elsewhere in Milwaukee County. With both plants in simultaneous operation, the South Plant predominantly supplies water to the southern portion of the district,

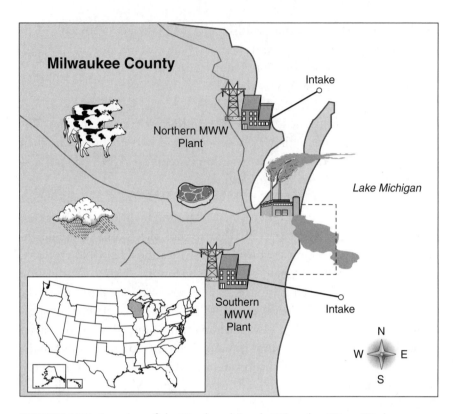

FIGURE 13-1 Location of the North and South Milwaukee Water Works water treatment plants, the water intakes for these plants, the three rivers that flow through Milwaukee County and the breakfront located in the Lake Michigan harbor.

and the North Plant predominantly supplies the northern portion. Central Milwaukee was typically supplied by both plants.

At the time of outbreak occurrence, water treatment in both plants followed the same sequence: the intake of raw water, the addition of chlorine as a disinfectant and polyaluminum chloride (PAC) as a coagulant to the raw water followed by rapid mixing, mechanical flocculation to remove solid and particulate material, sedimentation of the flocculent, and rapid filtration. The South Plant had 8 filters, and the North Plant had 16, each of which was enormous. After filtration, the water was pooled in a massive clear well at each plant (35 million gallons at the South Plant) from which it was distributed to customers (Figure 13-2). Parts of the water distribution infrastructure were very old, including large pipes, and MWW staff members were concerned that lead and copper could be leached if the pH

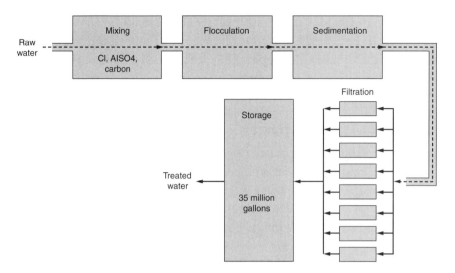

FIGURE 13-2 Schematic of the water treatment process at the South Milwaukee Water Works water treatment in March and April, 1993.

of the water was too low. To address this concern, the MWW changed coagulants in late 1992 from the venerable and time tested alum to PAC.

Testing treated water for a variety of water quality indices was required by the DNR and the federal Environmental Protection Agency (EPA) and was done three times each day at each plant before water was released from the clear wells. Tests of water quality included bacteriologic (*E. coli* testing and coliform counts), chemical (residual chlorine, residual fluoride, alkalinity, and pH), and physical (color, threshold odor, raw water temperature, and turbidity) tests. The treated water was then distributed from the clear wells. Treated water leaving the plant was referred to as plant effluent. I don't believe I have ever asked anyone whether they would like a nice tall glass of cold plant effluent.

During March and April 1993, the turbidity of water treated at the South Plant and distributed to customers increased with spikes to historically high values. Early in March there were no significant increases in finished water turbidity despite turbidity spikes in raw water; however, on March 23, the turbidity of South Plant treated water exceeded 0.4 NTU. This had not occurred in more than 10 years. Furthermore, the peak daily turbidity on March 28 and March 30 reached 1.7 NTU, even though the dosages of PAC were adjusted. When turbidity rises, the concern is that something dirty is getting into the system. The goal is to get it to precipitate out or be filtered out before it gets into someone's nice tall glass of effluent. Chemists at the South Plant aggressively tried to control the turbidity by changing the dosage of coagulant, but PAC was not the coagulant they were used to using, particularly under such extenuating circumstances. Plant staff resumed use of alum instead of PAC on April 2, but a spike in finished water turbidity to 1.5 NTU occurred on April 5.[2,3]

There were substantial differences in daily comparisons of South plant and North Plant finished water turbidity (Figure 13-3); the North Plant treated water turbidity did not exceed 0.45 NTU. MWW administrators, although mindful that treated water turbidity at the South Plant was unusually high, noted the turbidity results and other water quality measures were in compliance with state and federal regulatory standards. Turbidity related compliance was based on average results over one month. Bill Mac Kenzie and Steve Gradus thought MWW administrators viewed turbidity as less important than other measures of water quality, and more as a measure of clarity. Notably, continually during February through April

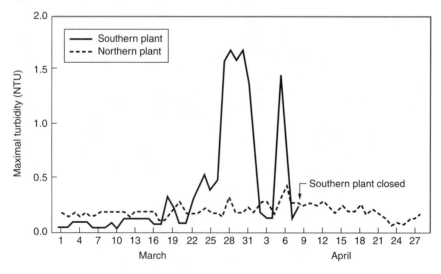

FIGURE 13-3 Maximal Turbidity of Treated Water in the Northern and Southern Water-Treatment Plants of the Milwaukee Water Works from March 1 through April 28, 1993. NTU denotes nephelometric turbidity units.

From Mac Kenzie WR, Hoxie NJ, Proctor ME, Gradus MS, Blair KA, Peterson DE, Kazmierczak JJ, Addiss DG, Fox KR, Rose JB, Davis JP. A massive outbreak in Milwaukee of Cryptosporidium infection transmitted through the public water supply. *N Engl J Med* 1994;331:161–67.

1993, samples of treated water for water quality testing obtained from both plants were negative for coliforms. Coliforms are a group of related bacteria whose presence in water may indicate contamination by disease causing microorganisms. Thus, it became strikingly apparent that the likely focus of the outbreak was the water treated in and distributed from the South Plant. Using water quality indices, there were clear differences in finished water quality between the North and South Plants during the same time interval. Nonetheless, this did not exonerate treated water from the North Plant.

Later, on April 7, raw and treated water quality records for an interval that exceeded 10 years were available from the MWW. I examined the turbidity data and plotted the monthly peaks in finished water turbidity from each plant for the past 10 years. Indeed, the initial spike in South Plant finished water turbidity of greater than 0.4 NTU represented the first time in more than 10 years that the finished water from this plant exceeded 0.4 NTU. Thus, the three major spikes occurring during March 28 through April 5 were truly historic peaks in turbidity.

After several internal planning meetings early in the afternoon, MHD Commissioner Paul Nannis and I met with the press regarding our initial impressions. I discussed the strong likelihood that this was a waterborne outbreak and that the prime focus of our investigation was the South Plant, but we would also pursue additional hypotheses. I noted that testing of stool specimens for bacterial enteric pathogens was all negative; however, results of testing these negative samples for a variety of other pathogens were pending.

While I met the press, Jim Kazmierczak and Bill Mac Kenzie were meeting with MHD staff when they received a call from Steve Gradus who reported MHD Bureau of Laboratories staff found *Cryptosporidium* oocysts in the three stool samples known to be bacterial enteric pathogen negative that he had set up the day before. In addition, staff from the St. Luke's Hospital laboratory notified Steve that they had detected *Cryptosporidium* oocysts in stools from 4 patients. These stools were obtained from 7 healthy adults who resided in the Southern half of Milwaukee. Steve also received a report of a case of *Cryptosporidium* infection in an older resident of West Allis in southwest Milwaukee County. That laboratory diagnosis was made by an astute microbiologist at West Allis Memorial Hospital who tested the stool specimen for *Cryptosporidium* oocysts even though the test was not specifically ordered. Steve, Bill, and Jim recognized the significance of these laboratory findings. Given our findings and recalling those from the Carollton outbreak that affected an estimated 13,000 people,[1] these laboratory results from only eight adult individuals were very significant.

After the press session, Paul and I were to meet with Milwaukee Mayor John Norquist to discuss our findings and investigation plans. While walking to the mayor's office, I was met by Bill and Jim and was informed of the eight laboratory-confirmed cases of *Cryptosporidium* infection. They believed *Cryptosporidium* was a highly plausible etiology for this outbreak, and I concurred. Bill raised the issue that a widespread boil water advisory involving all users of City of Milwaukee municipal water would be needed to prevent additional cases.

The meeting with the mayor involved a substantial number of MDH, MWW, DNR, mayor's administration officials and our DOH team. The water treatment and quality data and state and federal water related regulations were discussed in detail with the mayor. Based on preliminary findings and illness characteristics, an outbreak of this nature that was so widespread would be considered as waterborne unless proven otherwise. We discussed the likelihood that this large waterborne outbreak was caused by *Cryptosporidium* infection based on laboratory data that we had just become aware of. We informed the mayor of our investigation plans to consider all possible sources of these infections.

The discussion ultimately focused on what could and should be done to control the outbreak. A variety of approaches were discussed, including disinfection and a boil-water advisory. *Cryptosporidium* was a highly chlorine-resistant protozoan, thus disinfection would not be effective. To be clear, chlorine will kill *Cryptosporidium*; however, the concentration needed would be great, and treating water with a concentration of chlorine that can quickly kill *Cryptosporidium* would make the water unsafe to drink or bathe in for too long of an interval and at great expense given the magnitude of the water supply. The pros and cons of a boil-water advisory were considered. Although *Cryptosporidium* oocysts were heat sensitive and inactivated with boiling, the downside involved the need to boil all water treated in MWW plants to be used for eating and drinking, the personal injury risks associated with boiling water and with consuming recently boiled water, and the bump in energy use that would be associated with a prolonged advisory. The educational needs to conduct this activity effectively would be enormous. Plus, all of these considerations were based on limited and newly available information. Ultimately, the mayor focused his attention on a soft drink can that I brought to the meeting and asked me, "Would you drink a glass of water here, right now?" I replied, "No." Mayor Norquist then stated, "That's it. We need to go public with what our suspicions are."[4] Clearly, if I would not drink the water, he would not let Milwaukee residents and visitors drink it unless it was safe to do so.

With no pun intended, this was a watershed moment. The mayor would invoke a boil water order, and his staff notified the media of a press conference that evening. Precision was needed to provide clear instructions to all users of the water. The implications of this massive boil water advisory were enormous. Municipal staff members would need to answer many questions. That evening during the press conference, the mayor told all city residents and all users of MWW water to boil their drinking water for 5 minutes and discard all ice.

Because of the need to obtain critical water samples to document any presence of *Cryptosporidium* in water from each of the implicated treatment plants, systematic sample collections were planned for April 8, and the South Plant would be closed for an undetermined interval beginning on April 9. From April 8 throughout this undetermined interval, all drinking water in Milwaukee would be supplied by the North Plant.

This was an enormous news story with national and international implications. The local media gave this virtually unprecedented coverage. The two major (and competing) Milwaukee newspapers collaborated in publishing a special issue in Spanish. Plans for daily media updates were announced. A half-page ad for an over-the-counter antimotility medication appeared, but now that a boil water order was invoked, what would be needed to lift it? It was my responsibility to answer that question, but there were so many questions to answer and avenues to explore to describe fully the scope and all aspects of this outbreak, to generate and test hypotheses regarding how it occurred and why it was so large, and to determine whether measures were to be effective in controlling it.

THE OUTBREAK AND THE OUTBREAK INVESTIGATION

This is what was known about Cryptosporidium before April, 1993:

We needed to learn quickly what was known about *Cryptosporidium*, particularly regarding its associations with waterborne disease outbreaks.

At the time of this outbreak, relatively few public health officials had much knowledge of this protozoan parasite and its associated illnesses, nor was it well known as a pathogen by those charged with keeping local supplies of drinking water safe.

Although initially detected in animals in 1907 and for years thought not to affect humans, *Cryptosporidium* was first reported as a human pathogen in separate case reports of enterocolitis in immune competent[5–7] and compromised[8,9] patients. *Cryptosporidium* became a prominent pathogen when it was recognized in 1981–1982 as an AIDS-defining illness and opportunistic infection. The initial report in 1984 of a waterborne disease outbreak of cryptosporidiosis was associated with an artesian well in San Antonio, Texas. During 1986 to 1992, waterborne *Cryptosporidium* infections were associated with surface water exposure in New Mexico (1986), posttreatment contamination of drinking water in Aryshire, UK (1988), and filtered water supplies in Carollton, Georgia (surface, 1987), Swindon and Oxfordshire, UK (1989), the Isle of Thanet, UK (1991), and most recently in Jackson County, Oregon.[10–14] The outbreak that was most similar to ours was the one in Carollton.

Early Logistics

It was rapidly apparent this outbreak investigation would require work well beyond even the larger outbreaks I had focused on during my tenure as a state epidemiologist. Each of the outbreak's many facets would need a person in charge. Information by necessity would flow in one direction, but nominally, and those providing data needed to understand this; however, information would be continually shared with those who needed to know. Thus, organization and appropriate use of human resources were critical elements of this investigation. As the state epidemiologist and the state's lead of this multijurisdictional outbreak investigation, my time was focused on generating hypotheses, overseeing the generation of outbreak related data and information, communicating important findings, whether positive or negative, and assuring that all aspects of the investigation were proceeding in a timely, efficient way. My time would not be well spent working out the logistics of having enough staff available to conduct certain aspects of the investigation, although it was important for me to request and obtain the resources when needed. Ivan Imm, BPH Director, and John Chapin, DOH Deputy Administrator, were masterful in generating the personnel and supply resources needed and would remain on site for nearly 2 weeks to run interference. We had a large room in the Milwaukee Municipal Building for our investigation with dedicated phones, computer resources, and even a new fax machine needed on short notice for our surveillance activities that was purchased by the State Health Officer, Ann Haney. Several additional venues were established for activities requiring phone banks and dedicated teams could be rapidly deployed for survey purposes. Ultimately, nine teams each of which focused on separate investigation components and all of which involved public health personnel were created during the early phase of the outbreak investigation and were staffed by various combinations of City of Milwaukee and DOH personnel (Exhibit 13-1).

Early on we needed an experienced investigator to join our investigation and focus on special laboratory and surveillance projects. I had worked with David Addiss, MD, since 1985 when he began his 2-year term as an EIS officer assigned to our health department, and I was his field supervisor. We collaborated on many investigations since then. Dave was working as a medical epidemiologist in the Parasitic Diseases Division at the CDC and was extremely familiar with systems in Wisconsin. I invited Dave to join our investigation in Milwaukee, and fortunately, this was possible.

Review of MWW Data

Raw Water Source

The Milwaukee watershed includes three rivers that flow through Milwaukee County: the Milwaukee, Menomonee, and Kinnikinnick Rivers. Environmental sources of *Cryptosporidium* oocysts that could impact on these rivers and associated watersheds could have been agricultural, industrial (meat packing), and wildlife related. The three rivers converge a short distance before emptying into Lake Michigan within a harbor area protected by a large breakfront (see Figure 13-1). There are three major gaps in the breakfront, including a large central gap allowing boat access and egress, and smaller north and south fair weather gaps. The ambient current in the harbor and within the breakfront was southerly. The flow of water from within the breakfront through the south fair weather gap created a plume that was typically directly toward the raw water intake grid for the South Plant, which was located 7,600 feet offshore at the bottom of Lake Michigan under 50 feet of water.

Exhibit 13-1 Investigation of the Massive Waterborne Outbreak of *Cryptosporidium* Infections: Epidemiologic and Laboratory Studies Initiated and Health Education and Logistic Functions (Selected)

Studies to define the outbreak

- Laboratory confirmed case surveillance: determine outbreak trends, characterize the illness in healthy populations and in immunocompromised and other special populations, and establish case definition, collection, and storage of serologic and other specimens for future studies
- Emergency room log database and case surveillance
- Nursing home database and surveillance
- Random digit dialing (RDD) surveys:
  - RDD 1: description of clinical disease, risk factors for acquiring *Cryptosporidium* infection in the community, early estimate of magnitude
  - RDD 2: description of trends, age and zip code-specific attack rates, epidemic curve, estimates of outbreak magnitude, use of clinical services, hospitalization, economic impact, secondary transmission
  - RDD 3 and 4: survey to assess morbidity before and after reopening the South Plant
- Single day (short duration) of exposure database and surveillance: determine when problems with water treatment began, specific days that water was contaminated, incubation period calculations, quantify occurrence of secondary transmission
- Immunocompromised, AIDS/HIV assess multiple risk factors, natural history, prevention measures—large ill and well cohorts
- Surveillance in child care and daycare settings
- Satellite outbreak investigations in communities outside of greater Milwaukee areas

Environmental Studies

- MWW: plant protocols and engineering reviews, water quality data reviews
- River and estuaries data: cooperative study to monitor the Milwaukee River watershed and subwatershed, the sewage treatment plant influent and effluent, beach sites and MSS treatment plant influents and effluents. Five samplings at 21 sites through Spring 1994
- Efficacy of point of use filters in an outbreak setting
- Meteorological data analysis
- Laboratory testing of stored ice for *Cryptosporidium* and additional environmental testing

City of Milwaukee government activities (selected)

- Press-related coordination and releases, risk communication, phone banks coordination, fact sheets development, and translations and other health education related functions
- Quality assurance and inspections
- All agencies availability (24/7) and interagency coordination and committees
- Infection control and coordination with all health related facilities

The central sewage treatment plant operated by the Milwaukee Metropolitan Sewage District is located at the point where the river, created by the confluence of the three rivers, empties into Lake Michigan, and the effluent from the sewage treatment plant empties into the harbor within the confines of the breakfront.

Laboratory-Based Active Surveillance and Testing[2,15]

Steve transmitted information on *Cryptosporidium* detection to the directors of 14 clinical microbiology laboratories throughout the five county greater Milwaukee area and established laboratory-based surveillance with data to be reported to him. Compared with the usual parasitic testing of stool specimens, an additional flocculation step and special staining of the pellet with Kinyoun acid fast stain was needed to detect *Cryptosporidium* oocysts, and although it was the gold standard for testing at the time, the test was insensitive. This test was used in 13 of the laboratories. Because of the nature of the test, relatively few tests of stool for *Cryptosporidium* were requested before the occurrence of this outbreak, and these were primarily for testing patients with AIDS who had diarrhea, particularly chronic diarrhea.

Preoutbreak (prepublicity) baseline *Cryptosporidium*-related data were generated by retrospectively examining results of testing during March 1 through April 6 and were then compared with results of prospective testing during April 8 through April 16. During March 1–April 6, among 42 stool specimens submitted for *Cryptosporidium* testing, 12 (29%) were positive. This compares to 331 of 1009 specimens (33%) tested during April 8 to April 16. Of note, other pathogens accounted for only a very small proportion of the *Cryptosporidium* test-negative illnesses, and the percentage of specimens *Cryptosporidium* test positive (39%) during the Carollton outbreak was similar. The similarity in the proportion of test positive principally among immune compromised individuals with persistent diarrhea prior to the outbreak (29%) and among principally previously healthy persons of all ages in a wide range of demographic settings (33%) was striking and perplexing.

One question to be answered prospectively was the efficacy of *Cryptosporidium*-related laboratory tests that were or would be in development. To address this, Dave Addiss and a microbiologist from the CDC worked with Steve and other MHD laboratory staff members to obtain and archive stool and serum specimens for current and future testing.

Clinical Characteristics of Illness and Generation of a Case Definition[2]

The magnitude of this outbreak provided an opportunity to examine the clinical spectrum of illness among many individuals with laboratory-confirmed or clinically defined infections. Early in our investigation, we examined clinical signs and symptoms of illness and illness onset data among those with laboratory-confirmed *Cryptosporidium* infection to generate a reliable clinical case definition. We observed a virtual 100% occurrence of watery diarrhea among these individuals. Onset data suggested this outbreak emerged after March 1, 1993. We determined the illness onset interval of March 1 to April 9 would be inclusive of outbreak-related exposure until the South Plant was closed.

Although we recognized many thousands of cases likely occurred through May 15, the MHD received reports of 739 individuals with laboratory-confirmed *Cryptosporidium* infections; a more workable sample of 312 of these patients was selected, and extensive interviews were completed on 285, which was nearly a 40% sample and highly adequate for our purposes. This would be our study cohort with laboratory-confirmed infection. To understand the occurrence of illness in the community, we conducted the first of our four random digit dialed phoned surveys during April 9 to 12 to help describe clinical and other features of outbreak-related infections and generate a cohort of members with clinically defined illness to compare to the cohort with laboratory-confirmed illnesses. This first random digit dialed phoned survey (RDD 1) was administered by the DOH Sexually Transmitted Disease program staff who had substantial interviewing skills and by public health nurses, including an energetic group of retired public health nurses in southeastern Wisconsin who were a great resource and donated much time. The retired nurses, all of whom had long public health careers, literally stepped forward and asked us if they could be of service. Among 482 adult Milwaukee city residents, 42% had illness meeting the clinical case definition of cryptosporidiosis, and 6% of those individuals were hospitalized for their illnesses. We recognized the laboratory-confirmed illness cohort were ill enough to seek medical care and have their physicians order appropriate stool exams; indeed, 17% were immune compromised, and 46% were hospitalized.

We found the cohorts to be similar in mean age, gender distribution, dates of illness onset, and in occurrence of abdominal cramps, fatigue, and muscle aches (Table 13-1). As anticipated, because the case group was com-

Table 13-1 Clinical Characteristics of Case Patients with Laboratory-Confirmed Cryptosporidium Infection and Survey Respondents with Clinical Infection

Characteristic	Laboratory-Confirmed Infection (n = 285)	Clinical Infection* (n = 201)	P value†
Symptoms—number of patients of respondents (%)			
Diarrhea	285 (100)	201 (100)	NA
Watery diarrhea	265 (93)	201 (100)	NA
Abdominal cramps	238 (84)	168 (84)	0.9
Fatigue	247 (87)	145 (72)	< 0.001
Loss of Appetite	230 (81)	147 (73)	0.03
Nausea	199 (70)	119 (59)	0.01
Fever	162 (57)	72 (36)	< 0.001
Chills	65 (64)‡	91 (45)	0.04
Sweats	55 (54)‡	83 (41)	0.04
Muscle of joint aches	152 (53)	100 (50)	0.6
Headache	53 (52)‡	122 (61)	0.2
Vomiting	136 (48)	37 (18)	< 0.001
Cough	68 (24)	56 (28)	0.3
Sore throat	48 (17)	35 (17)	0.7
Mean duration of diarrhea (days)	12	4.5	0.001§
Mean maximum number of stools/day	19	7.7	0.001§
Mean maximum temperature (°C)	38.3	38.1	0.09§
Mean duration of vomiting (days)	2.9	2.0	0.07§
Mean maximum number of vomiting episodes/day	3.9	2.6	0.36§

* The criterion for clinical infection was the reported presence of watery diarrhea.

† Unless otherwise noted, Yates' correction has been applied to P values. NA denoted not applicable.

‡ Data are from 101 case patients interviewed during phase 1 of the study.

§ By Kruskal-Wallis test.

From Mac Kenzie WR, Hoxie NJ, Proctor ME, et al. A massive outbreak in Milwaukee of *Cryptosporidium* infection transmitted through the public water supply (Table 1). *N Engl J Med* 1994;331:161–167.

prised of patients ill enough to have consulted physicians and then be tested, those with laboratory-confirmed illness had diarrhea of longer duration (9 vs. 3 days), more frequent stools (median maximum of 12 vs. 5 stools daily), and higher rates of vomiting (48% vs. 18%) and fever (57% vs. 36%). Nonetheless, those with clinically defined illness were also quite ill.

Nursing Home Surveillance[2,3,15]

To determine whether and for how long gastrointestinal illness was associated with drinking water supplied by the South Plant, Mary Proctor established the aforementioned retrospective and prospective surveillance system for diarrhea illness among residents of representative samples of northern Milwaukee and southern Milwaukee nursing homes. Nursing home residents are relatively nonmobile (fixed populations) among whom information on diarrhea is collected routinely by nursing home staff. With their limited possibilities of exposures outside of their nursing homes, they represented an ideal human population to study. We defined diarrhea as three or more loose stools in a 24-hour period. Among residents of the nine nursing homes in northern Milwaukee, the prevalence of diarrhea remained less than 2% during March and April. In stark contrast, the prevalence of diarrhea among residents of six of the seven southern Milwaukee nursing homes increased to 16% during the first week of April and remained high until 2 weeks after the boil water advisory was issued (Figure 13-4c). Mary was particularly excited when she noted that the one nursing home in southern Milwaukee that did not observe an increase had a private well, and the prevalence of diarrhea among residents at that home remained less than 2% . . . serendipity at its finest. Furthermore, of stool samples prospectively collected from 69 southern Milwaukee nursing home residents with diarrhea (during April), 51% were positive for *Cryptosporidium* compared with none among samples from 12 northern Milwaukee nursing home residents with diarrhea. Clearly, if there were any doubts about the early association of illness with the South Plant, these data dispelled them.

Emergency Department Surveillance

While classically emergency department surveillance is useful during outbreak investigations, this was of greatest value to us only during the early phase of our investigation to facilitate case finding, clinical characterization, and case definition generation. To monitor the course and impact of the outbreak, other more focused surveillance activities proved to be superior.

Estimation of Magnitude of the Outbreak[2]

Because the outbreak magnitude was so large that it precluded any reasonable estimate through standard illness reporting means, we planned to generate this estimate by conducting the second of our RDDs (RDD 2). Bill Mac Kenzie, working closely with Neil Hoxie of the DOH, was the lead on this critical component of our outbreak investigation. With objectives of estimating the magnitude of the outbreak and its temporal and geographic impact, a questionnaire was created for use by telephone surveyors, and sample selection was conducted using computer-generated, random telephone numbers for the greater Milwaukee area. The survey was written by the University of Wisconsin Survey Research Institute (SRI) based on a set of key data needed by the DOH. DOH and SRI staff generated the final instrument. SRI staff members were finely honed to conduct these types of surveys and conducted all of the calls and completed all forms and data entry. DOH staff members were responsible for cleaning the data and conducting all analyses. Based on RDD 1 data, watery diarrhea with onset between March 1 and April 28 was used as a reliable definition of cryptosporidiosis. The survey included questions about watery diarrhea occurrence and frequency, other signs and symptoms, illness duration, health care visits, hospital stays, mortality, and demographic features. The survey sample included households in Milwaukee County and the four counties contiguous to Milwaukee County; the five-county greater Milwaukee area population was an estimated 1.61 million people. During April 28 through May 2, among the 840 households contacted, 613 (73%) participated representing 1662 household members from Milwaukee and the four surrounding counties. Household-related information was provided by interviewing the most knowledgeable adult member. The sample distribution was similar to the five county population distribution based on 1990 census data.

The clinical definition of cryptosporidiosis was watery diarrhea, but the time frame of onset was March 1 through April 28 to assess the impact of the boil water order and other recommended control measures. Among the 1662 household member sample, 436 (26%) had illness meeting the definition of clinical cryptosporidiosis. These data were excellent for generating

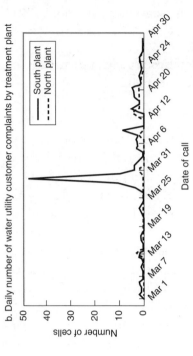

a. Daily maximum water treatment plant effluent turbidity by treatment plant

- South plant
- North plant

NTU

Date of turbidity reading

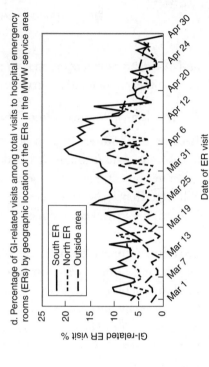

b. Daily number of water utility customer complaints by treatment plant

- South plant
- North plant

Number of cells

Date of call

c. Daily nursing home (NH) diarrhea prevalence rates per 100 residents by geographic location of nursing home in Milwaukee Water Works (MWW) service area

- South NH
- North NH

Prevalence of diarrhea

Date of symptom onset

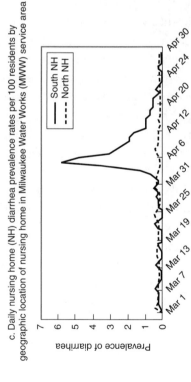

d. Percentage of GI-related visits among total visits to hospital emergency rooms (ERs) by geographic location of the ERs in the MWW service area

- South ER
- North ER
- Outside area

GI-related ER visit %

Date of ER visit

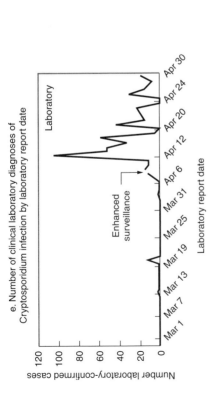

f. Daily number of cases of water diarrhea clinically defined during a random digit dialing survey

Number of clinically-defined cases

Date of symptom onset

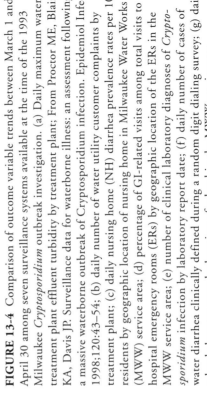

e. Number of clinical laboratory diagnoses of Cryptosporidium infection by laboratory report date

Number laboratory-confirmed cases

Enhanced surveillance

Laboratory report date

g. Daily school absentee rates by location of school in the MWW service area

Absentee rate (%)

South school
North school
Outside
Midzone

Date of absence

FIGURE 13-4 Comparison of outcome variable trends between March 1 and April 30 among seven surveillance systems available at the time of the 1993 Milwaukee *Cryptosporidium* outbreak investigation. (a) Daily maximum water treatment plant effluent turbidity by treatment plant; From Proctor ME, Blair KA, Davis JP. Surveillance data for waterborne illness: an assessment following a massive waterborne outbreak of Cryptosporidium infection. Epidemiol Infect 1998;120:43–54; (b) daily number of water utility customer complaints by treatment plant; (c) daily nursing home (NH) diarrhea prevalence rates per 100 residents by geographic location of nursing home in Milwaukee Water Works (MWW) service area; (d) percentage of GI-related visits among total visits to hospital emergency rooms (ERs) by geographic location of the ERs in the MWW service area; (e) number of clinical laboratory diagnoses of *Crypto-sporidium* infection by laboratory report date; (f) daily number of cases of water diarrhea clinically defined during a random digit dialing survey; (g) daily school absentee rates by location of school in the MWW service area.

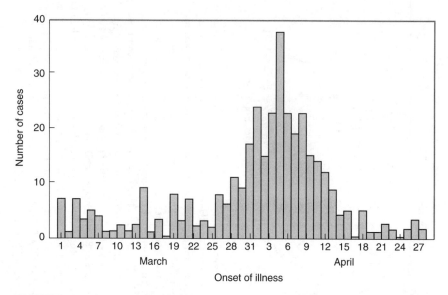

FIGURE 13-5 Reported Date of the Onset of Watery Diarrhea during the Period from March 1 through April 28, 1993, in 436 Cases of Infection Identified by a Random-Digit Telephone Survey of the Greater Milwaukee Area.

Reprinted with permission from Mac Kenzie WR, Hoxie NJ, Proctor ME, Gradus MS, Blair KA, Peterson DE, Kazmierczak JJ, Addiss DG, Fox KR, Rose JB, Davis JP. A massive outbreak in Milwaukee of Cryptosporidium infection transmitted through the public water supply. *N Engl J Med* 1994;331:161–167.

an epidemic curve to examine outbreak trends (Figure 13-5). The occurrence of watery diarrhea began with a small increase in morbidity beginning about March 18 followed by a larger increase in the five-county area beginning about March 24, a peak during April 1–April 7 with a distinct mode on April 4 followed by a rather sudden decrease in morbidity on April 13. This observed decrease in morbidity provided strong evidence that the boil water order was effective.

Among participants residing within the MWW service area in Milwaukee County, the attack rate of watery diarrhea was greatest (52%) among residents in southern Milwaukee, lowest (26%) among residents of northern Milwaukee, and intermediate (35%) in the mid-zone region in which water could be supplied by either the South or North Plants. The attack rate among participants residing outside the MWW service area was 15%; however, among residents who lived outside the MWW service area but worked within southern Milwaukee, the attack rate was 39%.

To digress momentarily, it is logical to wonder why there was such a big difference in attack rates among residents in southern Milwaukee households (52%) and residents of the southern Milwaukee nursing homes (16%) who are typically thought of as being more vulnerable. We observed attack rates in this outbreak to be age dependent, and the older population had the lowest attack rates. This is likely associated with prior immunity. There were similar outbreaks during the 1930s, each involving tens of thousands of people prior to the construction of the north plant, and I suspect that individuals who lived in Milwaukee at that time were more likely to be immune.

By projecting the overall attack rate (26%) onto the five-county population (1.61 million), we estimated that during March 1 through April 28, the number of persons with watery diarrhea who resided in this area was 419,000. Subsequently, in another RDD survey (RDD 3), a background rate of watery diarrhea among residents in this area was estimated to be 0.5% per month. Application of these background data resulted in a final estimate of 403,000 residents of the five county area with watery diarrhea attributed to this truly massive outbreak. The RDD 2 data were used to estimate health care seeking and occupational impacts. Among the 436 household participants with watery diarrhea, 50 (11%) saw health care providers (estimated 44,000 persons seen as outpatients) for their illnesses, and 5 (1%) were hospitalized (estimated 4,400 persons hospitalized). Furthermore, for each case individual, the mean days of reported lost productivity (work or school) was 1.8 days, which projected to an estimated 725,000 days lost productivity attributed to this outbreak.[2,16]

These were astounding numbers. The outbreak was the largest waterborne outbreak documented in the United States, and perhaps in the developed world! Using these data as the estimates of morbidity, several years later after appropriate hospital-, workplace-, insurance-, and government-related records were reviewed, estimates of the fiscal impact of this outbreak were generated.[16]

Cases in Visitors to Milwaukee[17]

While most BPH communicable disease epidemiologists were involved in the onsite investigation, one, Wendy Schell, remained in Madison. In addition to memoranda circulated widely to physicians, public health officials, and infection control practitioners throughout Wisconsin, on the day after the announcement of the boil water advisory, I generated a memo. This memo included information regarding the occurrence of the large waterborne outbreak, descriptive epidemiologic data, and data pertaining to the *Cryptosporidium* etiology and the boil water advisory. Wendy distributed this memo nationwide to all state and territorial epidemiologists with instructions for the reporting of cases. These memoranda were used to establish regional and national surveillance for confirmed and suspected cases of *Cryptosporidium* infection among individuals residing outside of the five-county greater Milwaukee area. This surveillance activity was very fruitful. Numerous reports of cases were received from state and local departments, and after regional and national press coverage of the outbreak and related events, the DOH received numerous self-reports of illness from individuals who resided outside the five-county region but visited Milwaukee and subsequently became ill.

As questions and hypotheses mounted, we recognized that residents of the greater Milwaukee area had too many opportunities to become infected to be helpful in addressing some of them; however, interviewing individuals with short term visits to Milwaukee would be key to determining the incubation period, how long *Cryptosporidium* was present in the water supply, and the extent of secondary transmission in households.[17]

During April 12 through May 20, out of region participants with suspected or confirmed *Cryptosporidium* infections were interviewed by phone using a standardized questionnaire focusing on demographic features, illness characteristics, length and site of stay, and water consumption; 130 of those interviewed had laboratory or clinically confirmed cryptosporidiosis, and 94 case individuals had brief (<48 hours) visits to the MWW service area. We had a unique opportunity to measure the interval during which *Cryptosporidium* was present in the water by noting the dates of the brief visits of these 94 case individuals. Among those with these brief visits, particularly the 63 with visits of 24 hours or less, we determined the incubation period by examining the intervals between dates of illness onset and dates of arrival to Milwaukee. The median incubation period was 7 days (range, 1–14 days). Among those with brief exposures, the earliest date of exposure was March 24, and the last date of exposure (with one exception) was April 5. The peak days of exposure were March 27 and 28, and based on arrival date information, *Cryptosporidium* was present in the municipal water supply continuously and daily during March 24 through April 5. Because of the brief durations of exposure, including several strikingly brief airport layovers, we could quantify consumption of tap water and beverages containing tap water while in the

MWW service area. The median amount consumed was 16 ounces, and 23% of brief exposure participants drank 8 ounces or less.[17]

Important clinical observations among this cohort included the low (5%) risk of secondary transmission within households where the index case patient was an adult; however, cryptosporidiosis during this outbreak appeared more severe when compared with cases described in previous case series reports. The recurrence of watery diarrhea after apparent recovery from clinical illness was a frequent event among short-term visitors to Milwaukee with laboratory-confirmed infections (39%) as well as in Milwaukee County residents with clinical infections (21%) and contributed a significant proportion of cases of postoutbreak diarrhea in the community.[17] The significance of this observation among the short-term visitors was that it excluded re-infection with *Cryptosporidium* as a cause of recurrence.

Response to Questions from Business

The boil water order affected many businesses in Milwaukee County. Because of the importance of beer (as an industry and as a beverage to be depended on more often than usual in the days to come), one early concern involved the cold-filtered brewing process used by a major Milwaukee brewing company; however, this company pasteurized its water before it was used in the brewing process, and its filters were sufficiently small to remove *Cryptosporidium* oocysts effectively. Before and during the outbreak, this brewing company donated a very large volume of pasteurized, purified water for individuals who were immune compromised and needed a reliable source of pure drinking water.

Many questions came from food processors and the health care industry. The only food-related industries with prevailing concerns were those that prepared food that was not to be heated to an adequate temperature to kill *Cryptosporidium* oocysts. Regional and nationwide recalls (all voluntary) of many of these types of products, such as prepared salads and dips, were needed and we depended on the Food and Drug Administration and U.S. Department of Agriculture to help with these actions.

Studies of Special Populations

Impact on Children and in Childcare Settings[18,19]

We were very cognizant of the importance of the observation of widespread school absenteeism in the recognition of this outbreak. Although much effort was focused on understanding the occurrence of illness in fixed populations, we needed to understand the impact of *Cryptosporidium* infection on children, particularly because of hygienic issues that may contribute to transmission in households, day care facilities and other settings, but also to determine the extent of asymptomatic infection and persistent shedding of *Cryptosporidium* in this population. To address these issues, two very specific Epidemic Aid investigations were generated with Dave Addiss serving as the CDC supervisor; Ralph Cordell focused on the impact of *Cryptosporidium* infections in child day care settings,[18] and Helen Cicirello focused on broader impacts among children.[19]

Ralph coordinated the screening of 129 diapered attendees of 11 day care centers in metropolitan Milwaukee and found 35 (27%) with *Cryptosporidium* oocysts in their stool, 10 of whom did not have diarrhea during the outbreak. Thus, at least in this very young population, asymptomatic or minimally symptomatic *Cryptosporidium* infection appeared to be somewhat frequent.[18] There was no systematic assessment of asymptomatic shedding of *Cryptosporidium* among those without diarrhea.

Helen coordinated a study of the clinical, laboratory, and epidemiologic features of outbreak-associated cryptosporidiosis among children who sought medical care at the Wisconsin Children's Hospital during the outbreak. As with other diarrhea illnesses for which multiple stool examinations increases the opportunity to make a diagnosis, those children who had laboratory-confirmed *Cryptosporidium* infections had stools specimens submitted more frequently and later in their illnesses than those with stool exams that were negative.[19]

HIV Infection[20]

In outbreak settings, it was not known whether *Cryptosporidium*-related diarrhea illness attack rates were greater in HIV-infected persons than in the general population. There was great concern among the public health community and the HIV/AIDS advocacy community regarding the impact of this outbreak on those with HIV-infection and what could be done to prevent *Cryptosporidium* infections from occurring. Chronic diarrhea caused by *Cryptosporidium* is an AIDS-defining condition, and the massive exposure to *Cryptosporidium* among the HIV-infected community in Milwaukee could result in many new AIDS cases with substantial suffering because of the lack of an effective treatment. This outbreak occurrence provided an opportunity to survey a large community of HIV-infected individuals exposed to a point source of *Cryptosporidium* contaminated water to examine epidemiologic features and severity of clinical illness.

A group headed by Holly Frisby, DVM, an epidemiologist in the DOH AIDS/HIV Program, conducted a case control study incorporating a randomized sample of 263 among 703 HIV case-management clients in the five-county greater Milwaukee and one age- and gender-matched control selected from the general population using RDD methods. To facilitate participation and assure patient confidentiality, case patients were known only to their case managers. Case and control survey questions were similar. The survey participation among the sample of HIV-infected individuals was high (82%). During this outbreak, the attack rate of watery diarrhea among HIV-infected persons (32%) was less than among matched controls (51%); however, although HIV-infected individuals were not more likely to experience symptomatic *Cryptosporidium* infection than persons in the general population, once infected with *Cryptosporidium*, the duration and severity of illness were greater in HIV-infected individuals, particularly among those with CD4+ T-lymphocytes < 200 per mL.[20]

Mortality[21]

The media focused on severe and ultimately fatal *Cryptosporidium* infections in several individuals with previously diagnosed AIDS. During the first several weeks of our investigation, we were not aware of any deaths attributable to this outbreak that involved individuals who did not have immune compromise or some other serious underlying illness. We realized measurement of mortality attributed to this outbreak must be deferred because of delays inherent in obtaining accurate mortality data. When final state mortality data were available for 1993–1994, we were able to measure this. I was continually concerned regarding the arbitrary and unfortunate number of 100 deaths attributed to the outbreak and circulated in the media, as there were no data to support this, and we would be the ones to provide an accurate assessment. Our approach was to assess death certificate data that specifically indicated cryptosporidiosis as a cause of death that could conclusively be attributed to the outbreak and to measure the AIDS-related mortality during the first 6 months after the outbreak (the near term observed mortality that likely would be acutely associated with the outbreak) and compare that with expected AIDS-related mortality during this interval and to the AIDS-related expected mortality during the subsequent 6 months. We observed greater than expected AIDS-related mortality during the first 6-month interval and less than expected AIDS-related mortality during the subsequent 6-month interval. Thus, in addition to death certificate data (50 outbreak attributable deaths, 86% among persons with AIDS), we were able to measure premature mortality attributable to this outbreak among persons with AIDS with no death certificate mention of cryptosporidiosis (19 deaths).[21] The "official" outbreak-related attributable mortality was 69 deaths, of which 93% occurred in persons with AIDS.

Detection of Cryptosporidium in the Water Supply

Another of our objectives was to demonstrate *Cryptosporidium* in water or other material sampled during the actual outbreak interval. Our first lead was a company that manufactured very fine absolute pore-size filters. The company was located close to the South Plant. For many days in a row, their test filters were discolored by an apparent water impurity. Fortunately, the filters were dated and saved by the company and available to us.

Perhaps the most fortuitous opportunity involved a call from an ice manufacturing company to Greg Carmichael, a quality assurance officer who worked for the City of Milwaukee. The company, located near the South Plant, manufactured large (50 gallon) blocks of ice for sculpture. During March 25 through April 9, impurities in the ice spoiled its color and clarity; however, representative blocks were saved! A tremendous opportunity existed, and we generated a plan to use these slabs. Under Dave's supervision, each block of ice would be melted separately, and the resulting water would be divided into two aliquots, one of which would be filtered using a standard, nominal spun polypropylene cartridge filter, which was notoriously unwieldy to use and assay and crude in accuracy of results. The other aliquot would be filtered using a large (11.5 inch) Millipore membrane filter with a 0.45-micron fixed pore size that was suspected to be superior. Unfortunately, despite these elegant plans, there was confusion within the company, and all but the blocks of ice made on March 25 and April 9 were discarded. Nonetheless, the manufacturing dates of the remaining blocks were well timed for our purposes, and the study was completed according to plan.[2] Dave reported that the concentration of *Cryptosporidium* oocysts in ice produced March 25 and April 9 and filtered using the membrane filter was 13.2 and 6.7 oocysts per 100 liters compared with 2.6 and 0.7 oocysts per 100 liters, respectively, using the spun cartridge filter. Regardless of the filter used, *Cryptosporidium* was confirmed to be present in each block at substantial concentrations even though freezing reduces the recovery of oocysts. The March 25 data were notable as the peak turbidity of South plant water that day was 0.5 NTU, which was substantially less than the NTU peak days later when the measurable concentration of oocysts would be projected to be considerably higher. As expected, the submicron membrane filter was functionally far superior to the standard spun cartridge filter.

Investigation of the Milwaukee Water Works South Plant

During my first conversation with Dennis Juranek of the CDC regarding the outbreak, he provided me with the names of raw water and drinking water experts: Walt Jakubowski (EPA-Cincinnati), Stig Regli (EPA, Washington, DC), Joan Rose (University of South Florida), Mark LeChevalier (American Water Works Association [AWWA]), and others. I called each of these individuals shortly after my initial review of the finished water quality and the invoking of the boiled water order. One aspect of the conversation with Walt was the need to conduct an in-plant inspection of both of the MWW plants by an EPA engineer who was expert in all aspects of the drinking water treatment process. Walt mentioned that Kim Fox would be particularly skilled to conduct this aspect of the investigation. Kim and an EPA colleague Darren Lytle arrived in Milwaukee on April 12 and began their investigation by reviewing detailed operational and water-quality data from both plants followed by in-depth onsite inspections of the South and North plants and extensive interviewing of plant and other MWW personnel. In the report of this investigation, Kim noted that the South Plant received a highly variable quality of raw water from Lake Michigan (the influent) for processing and noted that during March 18–April 9, 1993, the raw water turbidity levels ranged from 1.5 to 44 NTU (usually 3 to 4 NTU in prior months), and raw water coliform concentrations were also quite variable. Specific deficiencies that may have contributed either to a delay in recognition of a problem or the inability to bring finished water turbidity to plant baseline values included the lack of historical use records for the coagulant used (PAC was used only since September, 1992). Also, the residence time for the water in the plant was relatively short, and the time required to see a result in treated water quality after chemical adjustment was relatively long. These factors contributed to difficulty in optimizing the coagulant dose. In addition, the finished water turbidity was measured in the clearwell rather than as the water left each filter. The clearwell was the massive receptacle where water from all the filters was pooled before it was released as effluent from the treatment plant. Also, although the filters were frequently backwashed to remove impurities and maintain optimal filtering capability, the backwash water was recycled through the plant instead of being discarded.

Comparison of the Efficacy of Different Surveillance Methods Used in this Outbreak Investigation[15]

The availability of a rich array of surveillance data from seven categories of data source provided us with an opportunity to compare the efficacies of using each category of surveillance data during this waterborne outbreak investigation. Mary Proctor took the lead on this project. We found that surveillance systems that could be easily linked with laboratory data were flexible in adding new variables, and those that demonstrated low baseline variability were most useful. Notably, geographically fixed nursing home residents served as an ideal population with nonconfounded exposures; however, the signals that were most timely (i.e., the shortest interval needed to learn about the peak) were consumer complaints to the South Plant utility (the best) and aberrant and peak finished water turbidity (Figure 13-4). Although not indicators of disease, these signals can be effectively used in stimulating heightened surveillance for human illness and generating timely messages to the public and persons at greater risk of water related illness and help reduce potential outbreak-related morbidity. This would be particularly helpful to implement in communities with populations greater than 100,000 with water supplies derived from surface water.

Unusual Clusters and Anecdotes

There were several unusual clusters. The Finals (Frozen Four) of the NCAA hockey tournament were held in Milwaukee April 1–3. We conducted a follow-up with cooperation from respective state epidemiologists to determine whether diarrhea illnesses occurred in any team or entourage members. Indeed, cases occurred among members or associates of three teams, but not among the team from the University of Maine that brought its own bottled water supply as a standard practice, and they won the NCAA championship. Bottled water generally should not be viewed as a panacea, but it sure was healthful in this instance. A large number of individuals with watery diarrhea illness were seen in the clinic facility at the speedway in North Wilkesboro, NC during a NASCAR event. All ill individuals had attended the funeral of the beloved NASCAR driver and Milwaukee resident Allen Kulwicki (killed in a crash of a private airplane) in Milwaukee 1 week previously. An outbreak of *Cryptosporidium* infections investigated in Michigan occurred among a Coast Guard crew on a boat that had its potable water supply tank filled in Milwaukee.

Professional sports were not spared. Several Milwaukee professional athletes became ill, and there were concerns raised among teams that had recently traveled or would be traveling to Milwaukee. The largest event of concern for which numerous special precautions were taken was the Milwaukee Brewers home season opening game that occurred before the boil water advisory was lifted. Of course, the beer was safe to drink.

Invoking and Lifting the Boil Water Advisory

When boil water advisories are enacted, it is important to envision the terms and conditions needed to discontinue (lift) them. After becoming familiar with water testing processes and having numerous phone conversations with experts at the AWWA, EPA, CDC, and the Wisconsin DNR and in academia, I began the process of generating a Delphi survey that involved the repeated interviewing of these experts regarding what they felt the standard should be for lifting the boil water order. The South Plant was closed, and thus, all of our attention was on the North Plant. We needed to demonstrate that the North Plant water was safe. This would involve repeated measurement of *Cryptosporidium* oocysts in samples of North Plant effluent water and representative samples of water obtained from distal sites in the municipal water distribution system. Also, spun cartridge filters, the standard at that time, would be used to filter samples of finished water and would then be tested for the presence of *Cryptosporidium* oocysts. The filters were sent to the AWWA laboratory in Belleville, Illinois. Mark LeChevallier and his colleagues in Belleville provided exceptional expertise and service during this outbreak.

After several rounds of calls, the Delphi process ultimately focused on the demonstration of less than one *Cryptosporidium* oocyst per 100 liters of filtered water at each of the sampling sites (one central and four distal) and in two consecutive samples at each of the central and distal sites. The samples would involve 12-hour collections at each site. With shipping, the cycle to process each filter took 2 to 3 days. I realized that it would probably take a minimum of 5 days to have the data needed to lift the advisory, and one sample from any site with results that exceeded the threshold could add another 3 days to the process. Sometimes my patience in waiting for test results wore rather thin.

Finally, the boil water advisory was lifted on the evening of April 14 after receipt late on April 14 of the results of processing samples collected during the third round on April 13. The city was served exclusively by the North Plant until June, when the water filters replacement and refurbishing was completed at the South Plant.

Additional Investigations and Studies

Protection from Point-of-Use Filters[22]

During a press conference in the early phases of the outbreak, I requested that individuals who had point-of-use (filters that were installed in homes or workplace settings) water filters installed in their homes before the outbreak contact us because we were interested in evaluating whether they were effective in preventing diarrhea illness during this outbreak. The response to this request was overwhelming, and many individuals volunteered to actually donate their filter if needed. Bob Pond, an Atlanta-based EIS officer, joined Dave Addiss and me in Milwaukee to conduct this evaluation. We surveyed 155 filter owners and 99 completed the self-administered questionnaire. Among residents and users of water in the southern or central Milwaukee, we found users of submicron (pore size less than one micron) point-of-use filters during the outbreak were significantly less likely to experience watery diarrhea than those who consumed unfiltered tap water in a public building and those who had home water filters with pore sizes greater than 1 micron. Being conservative in interpreting our data, we concluded that (even in these extraordinarily adverse field conditions) submicron point-of-use water filters may reduce the risk of waterborne cryptosporidiosis.[22]

Postoutbreak Transmission of Cryptosporidium[23]

Surveillance for new infections was sustained for many months. Postoutbreak secondary transmission of *Cryptosporidium* was expected to occur; however, of great concern was the potential of sustained waterborne transmission of *Cryptosporidium* that could be occurring with clinical muting of symptomatic illness related to the widespread emerging immunity to

Cryptosporidium. In a follow-up investigation of 33 individuals with onsets of laboratory-confirmed *Cryptosporidium* infection during May 1 to June 23 and neighborhood and household control subjects, we found water-borne transmission was not associated with these late illnesses. Risk factors for postoutbreak illness included immune compromise and living in a household with one or more children less than 5 years old suggesting person-to-person transmission. Despite biases introduced by the greater likelihood that immune-compromised individuals would be tested during the postout-break period, this study provided reassurance that new *Cryptosporidium* infections were not occurring as a result of drinking MWW water.[23]

Swimming Pool-Related Outbreaks

We were mindful that chains of transmission could be sustained as *Cryptosporidium* can be transmitted from person to person or an infected individual can contaminate a new, more limited water supply. Shortly after the Milwaukee outbreak and throughout the summer of 1993, outbreaks of *Cryptosporidium* infection among users of public or hotel pools were reported from several counties.[24,25] The earliest such outbreak north of Milwaukee could be directly attributed to the Milwaukee outbreak; however, the phenomenon continued through the summer as additional pools in Wisconsin and elsewhere were seeded with the chlorine-resistant *Cryptosporidium* oocysts and pool users became infected and then contributors to multiple generations of illness. The optimal concentration of chlorine in swimming pools was not sufficiently high to kill the oocysts before an unsuspecting swimmer ingested a small volume of pool water.

Genotyping

Speciation and further characterization of the outbreak strain of *Cryptosporidium* were another objective of this investigation. To accomplish this, three volunteers who had been ill during the outbreak and had labo-ratory-confirmed infections were recruited to donate large volumes of stool. To our disappointment, after shipment to and maintenance of these specimens at a CDC laboratory, the *Cryptosporidium* in these specimens became nonviable. These specimens still proved useful because they were ultimately (more than a year later) used to test the *Cryptosporidium parvum* DNA to determine genotype of the strains. An important goal of the geno-typing was to determine the source of the *Cryptosporidium*. Although lim-ited, genotype information provides clues regarding whether the source strain was human or bovine. In Milwaukee, the source strain was suggested to be human based on the genotype testing[26]; however, I believe the extremely small number of specimens from the Milwaukee outbreak used in the genotype investigation and perhaps the sources of stool specimens tested make these observations more conjectural. The suggestion of a human source is supported by the limited data available, but I do not believe that it is proven. Conceivably multiple genotypes were circulating.

Serologic Studies

We were very interested in the prospect of testing banked sera from ill and well individuals during this outbreak to assess immune responses when a reliable assay became available at some unspecified time in the future. More than 5 years after the outbreak, plasma samples obtained from 553 Milwaukee children aged 6 months to 12 years old who were being tested for lead exposure during the time of the outbreak were tested at CDC laboratories for *Cryptosporidium* antibodies[27] using an enzyme-linked immunosorbent assay to detect IgG to two immunodominant antigens of *C. parvum*. Samples were obtained during five distinct periods in a 5-week interval between March 1993 and May 1993. Each child was bled once, but the prevalence of antibody among children bled during each distinct period could be measured. Data were also available to compare antibody prevalence by region of residence in Milwaukee. The prevalence of antibodies increased from about 16% to 85% during the 5-week interval among children from southern Milwaukee ZIP codes and from about 21% to 45% during the 5-week interval among children from northern Milwaukee ZIP codes. Median antibody reactivity was also substantially greater among the children from southern ZIP codes compared with northern ZIP codes. In addition to corroborating our earlier epidemiologic observations, these data suggest that *C. parvum* infection was more widespread than initially measured based on our RDD studies.[27] Because the samples were obtained without accompanying clinical information, it is not known what the proportions were of subclinical or asymptomatic infection.[27]

Theories on Why This Massive Outbreak Occurred: A Perfect Storm[2,3]

Outbreaks of great magnitude are generally not easily explained, nor was this one; however, a confluence of likely contributing factors and events during March and April 1993 was exceptionally compelling and provided unique opportunities to dramatically amplify case occurrence.

The South Plant Intake Grid Location and Unusual Weather Conditions

The placement of the South Plant intake grid was unfortunate at best. As previously noted, the three rivers flowing through Milwaukee County join together to flow into a bay and harbor along the Lake Michigan shore. This harbor is protected by a large breakfront. The breakfront has three large outer gaps through which water can flow in and out of the harbor. As previously noted, the ambient current in the harbor contained within the large breakfront was southerly. Water flowing out the south fair weather gap typically flowed directly toward the South Plant intake grid. During and after rainy and other high-flow periods when increases in runoff and storm sewer overflow in the rivers are noted, the discharges of dirt and particulate matter into the harbor can be striking (Figure 13-6). This was

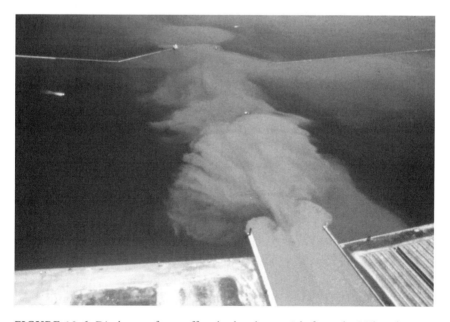

FIGURE 13-6 Discharge of run-off and related materials from the Milwaukee River into the Lake Michigan Harbor during or following a period of high flow, Milwaukee, Wisconsin, 1993.

occurring during a prolonged, intense high flow period compounded by unusual weather conditions:

- There was a high snow pack during the winter that melted rapidly while the frost line was still high. The runoff was excessive, and its impact was likely compounded by runoff manure spread onto the snow by farm workers intent on getting rid of it and concurrently enriching their fields.
- There was record setting rainfall in March and early April that contributed to runoff within the river watersheds. Within the City of Milwaukee, this rainfall contributed to widespread storm sewer overflows resulting in vast volumes of sewage that could be disinfected but otherwise bypassed treatment in the Milwaukee Metropolitan Sewage District facility before it drained into the bay that was protected by the breakfront.
- The wind conditions and direction were highly unusual. There was a prolonged period of northeasterly winds occurring in late March and early April. During this time, there was likely accentuation of the southerly flow of water within the breakfront with more flow of water in the bay out the south fair weather gap, which likely amplified plumes flowing directly toward the South Plant intake grid. Prevailing winds in other directions would have facilitated their dispersal.
- These conditions would have enhanced the transport of *Cryptosporidium* oocysts toward the South Plant water intake.

Cross Connection Between a Sanitary Sewer and a Storm Sewer

In early March 1993, during the construction of soccer fields near the Menomonee River and close to downtown Milwaukee, a linkage of a storm sewer draining the fields with a central main sewer was being created when a large volume of impacted contents was noted in the main sewer. The contents included animal material, particularly animal intestines. In addition, there were many rubber rings that were used to prevent spillage of enteric contents when bovines were slaughtered and eviscerated. Further investigation by local officials resulted in the detection of a cross connection between an abattoir kill floor sanitary sewer and the storm sewer. After elimination of this cross connection and correction of sewage flow, the storm sewer was cleaned during a multiple week process. The cross connection was estimated to have existed for years. Material from the abattoir kill floor that impacted in the storm sewer or flowed directly to the river via the cross connection would now travel through the sanitary sewer and be treated at the sewage treatment plant or be disinfected and bypass treatment during periods of high flow (heavy rains). It is not known whether *Cryptosporidium* oocysts were released directly through the storm sewer into the Menomonee River during or preceding these events or whether a bolus of oocysts properly flowing through the sanitary sewer during cleanup procedures may have bypassed sewage treatment during a period of high flow.

Change in Coagulant

The change in coagulant routinely used in both the North and South Plants 6 months before the outbreak and the difficulty in coagulant dosing during a period of abnormal turbidity to bring the turbidity under control were factors. Furthermore, the Milwaukee Water Works interpretation of finished water turbidity as an aesthetic indicator may have contributed to late recognition of the difficulties (or later recognition of the importance of the difficulties) they were having with water treatment. The occurrence of this outbreak provided a focus on the importance of turbidity as a water quality indicator.

Human Amplification

The amplification of the burden of *Cryptosporidium* oocysts among residents of the greater Milwaukee area was a critical factor. In humans, the infectious dose of *C. parvum* that can result in illness is small. Among healthy adult volunteers with no serologic evidence of past infection with *C. parvum*, the median infectious dose has been determined to be 132 oocysts[28]; however, billions of oocysts are excreted each day in the stools of symptomatic individuals, and excretion of oocysts typically continues for several weeks after symptoms resolve. Shedding can be more prolonged in those who are immune compromised. Additionally, the oocysts can remain infective in moist environments for 2 to 6 months. Thus, the opportunity for infection in this outbreak was extraordinarily, perhaps incomprehensibly, high. This was compounded by the aforementioned rainy, high-flow conditions when storm sewers typically overflowed and, other than disinfection, most sewage was not treated before discharge into the harbor. This all contributed to a sustained vicious cycle of oocyst and illness amplification.

Limited Testing Prior to Outbreak Recognition

There was some delay in recognition of this outbreak. Based on the sporadic occurrences of diarrhea illnesses weeks prior to the outbreak peak, the outbreak probably began in early March but was initially recognized on April 5. This delay can in part be explained by understanding that testing stool specimens for *Cryptosporidium* was not commonplace in medical practice at the time of this outbreak. Typically, testing for *Cryptosporidium* infection was requested in individuals with HIV infection who were experiencing diarrhea. The number of tests requested per month was relatively small, and most healthcare providers would not readily have suspected this diagnosis in healthy patients with brief or even prolonged diarrhea disease. If they requested obtaining a stool specimen to test for parasites, *Cryptosporidium* was not a pathogen routinely looked for. Tests for *Cryptosporidium* required an additional requisition. Indeed, a major factor in the limited number of test requisitions was the complexity caused by the additional pelleting and staining procedures and the attendant greater expense of testing. These factors may have contributed to this insufficient testing demand with consequent delay in ascertainment of an outbreak.

Policy Impacts and Infrastructure Improvements

Standards

The massive Milwaukee cryptosporidiosis outbreak was historic. It is the largest known outbreak of waterborne disease ever documented in the United States and possibly in the developed world. The magnitude of this outbreak coupled with the direct association of illness with a municipal water treatment plant that was operating within existing state and federal regulatory standards at that time had an immediate powerful impact that focused widespread public concern on the quality of drinking water, underscored the need to have far more stringent regulatory standards, and raised awareness of cryptosporidiosis as a diarrheal illness. A specific need to create specific regulatory standards for *Cryptosporidium* in drinking water was apparent.

The Milwaukee Water Works expeditiously adopted standards and quality indices that were maximally stringent and far more stringent than state or federal standards. Wisconsin state standards were also strengthened and clarified. The antiquated and confusing use of monthly or other interval averages in turbidity as a threshold standard was eliminated.

The EPA was in the process of generating and releasing its Information Collection Rule, which provided water treatment facilities with a list of laboratory tests and measures that would be needed to ultimately generate a final set of standards. The occurrence of this massive outbreak in the midst of this process had bearing on the content of the Information Collection Rule.

Infrastructure Improvements

Virtually immediately after the boil water order was invoked and with the assistance of many experts, officials began planning to make extensive changes to the Milwaukee water treatment infrastructure. Nearer term improvements included the revision of filters and filter beds (removal of all media, sandblasting all filter beds, structural changes, installation of new media) and installation of particle counters and automatic alarms for each filter (when very low threshold turbidity or particle counts are exceeded, there is automatic filter shutdown and diversion of affected water so that it did not enter the clear well). Longer term projects that took several years to complete included the construction of ozonation facilities at each treatment plant. Because *Cryptosporidium* oocysts are highly chlorine resistant, standard disinfection procedures are not sufficient to inactivate them. Ozonation as an adjunct to disinfection is effective because it inactivates oocysts by disrupting their cell walls and it is effective in disrupting other microorganisms found in raw water. The North and South Plants are now state of the art facilities and have been visited by utility related personnel from many states and countries.

CONCLUDING REFLECTIONS

The Milwaukee outbreak, the results of our collective investigations and the local and state responses were of great interest to drinking water related regulators, utility (public and private) administrators, and municipalities throughout the United States, Canada, Europe, Japan, Australia, and elsewhere. Although fear of such a large outbreak is a great motivator, the significant and tangible improvements in water treatment authorized by the City of Milwaukee administration has had substantial impact on voluntary and required improvements in water processing and in water quality in communities in many states and countries. The transparency of these processes has improved as have communications between the water treatment and public health communities. These efforts were certainly apparent throughout Wisconsin when communities recognized that Lake Michigan turbidity events were not limited to Milwaukee (Wisconsin DPH, unpublished data). Clearly, we learned the importance of the need for improved surveillance for infections that may result from waterborne pathogens and for aberrations in water quality. This requires cooperation, coordination, and communication among public health agency and water utility staffs.

The high level of civic resolve to focus on solutions to rapidly control this massive outbreak and prevent even teeny ones from occurring in the future was extraordinary. As a native of Milwaukee County, I was deeply moved and very proud of this enormous yet efficient effort. Our team was very impressed with the exceptional cooperation received from local government, businesses large and small, and private citizens. We could not have accomplished as much as we did without the degree of cooperation and collaboration that we experienced. As expected, the greater Milwaukee community did this with a great sense of humor, at times magnificently sharp and self-deprecating, and civic pride. In one photograph featured in the newspaper at that time, an illuminated sign from a pharmacy-food mart says simply, "We have Immodium AD. Open Easter." In another photo of a man walking to the front of a bar, the sign overhead says simply, "Mexican vacation? Why bother. Stay here."

Without question, application of the lessons learned from this outbreak has had a sustained impact on preventing subsequent outbreaks in the United States and other developed countries.

REFERENCES

1. Hayes EB, Matte TD, O'Brien TR, et al. Large community outbreak of cryptosporidiosis due to contamination of a filtered public water supply. *N Engl J Med* 1989;320:1372–1376.
2. Mac Kenzie WR, Hoxie NJ, Proctor ME, et al. A massive outbreak in Milwaukee of Cryptosporidium infection transmitted through the public water supply. *N Engl J Med* 1994;331:161–167.
3. Addiss DG, Mac Kenzie WR, Hoxie NJ, et al. Epidemiologic features and implications of the Milwaukee cryptosporidiosis outbreak. In Betts WB, Casemore D, Fricker C, Smith H, Watkins J, eds. *Protozoan Parasites and Water.* Cambridge, England: The Royal Society of Chemistry, 1995:19–25.
4. Marchione M. Detective story: Skill, luck come to fore. *Milwaukee J* 1993;April 11:1, 12.

5. Nime FA, Burek JD, Page DL, Holscher MA, Yardley JH. Acute enterocolitis in a human being infected with the protozoan *Cryptosporidium*. *Gastroenterology* 1976;70:592–598.

6. Jokipii L, Jokipii AMM. Timing of symptoms and oocyst excretion in human cryptosporidiosis. *N Engl J Med* 1986;315:1643–1647.

7. Wolfson JS, Richter JM, Waldron MA, Weber DJ, McCarthy DM, Hopkins CC, Cryptosporidiosis in immunocompetent patients. *N Engl J Med* 1985;312:1278–1282.

8. Meisel JL, Perera DR, Meligro C, Rubin CE. Overwhelming watery diarrhea associated with cryptosporidium in an immunosuppressed patient. *Gastroenterology* 1976;70:1156–1160.

9. Current WL, Reese NC, Ernst JV, Bailey WS, Heyman MB, Weinstein WM. Human cryptosporidiosis in immunocompetent and immunodeficient persons: studies of an outbreak and experimental transmission. *N Engl J Med* 1983;308:1252–1257.

10. D'Antonio RG, Winn RE, Taylor JP, et al. A waterborne outbreak of cryptosporidiosis in normal hosts. *Ann Intern Med* 1985;103:886–888.

11. Gallagher MM, Herndon JL, Nims IJ, Sterling CR, Grabowski DJ, Hull HF. Cryptosporidiosis and surface water. *Am J Public Health* 1989;79:39–42.

12. Richardson AJ, Frankenberg RA, Buck AC, et al. An outbreak of waterborne cryptosporidiosis in Swindon and Oxfordshire. *Epidemiol Infect* 1991;107:485–495.

13. Joseph C, Hamilton G, O'Connor M, et al. Cryptosporidiosis in the Isle of Thanet: an outbreak associated with local drinking water. *Epidemiol Infect* 1991;107:509–519.

14. Leland D, McAnulty J, Keene W, Sterens G. A cryptosporidiosis outbreak in a filtered-water supply. *J Am Water Works Assoc* 1993;85:34–42.

15. Proctor ME, Blair KA, Davis JP. Surveillance data for waterborne illness: an assessment following a massive waterborne outbreak of Cryptosporidium infection. *Epidemiol Infect* 1998;20:43–54.

16. Corso PS, Kramer MH, Blair KA, Addiss DG, Davis JP, Haddix AC. The cost of illness associated with the massive waterborne outbreak of Cryptosporidium infections in 1993 in Milwaukee, Wisconsin. *Emerg Infect Dis* 2003;9:426–431.

17. Mac Kenzie WR, Schell WL, Blair KA, et al. Massive outbreak of waterborne Cryptosporidium infection in Milwaukee, Wisconsin: Recurrence of illness and risk of secondary transmission. *Clin Infect Dis* 1995;21:57–62.

18. Cordell RL, Thor PM, Addiss DG, et al. Impact of a massive waterborne cryptosporidiosis outbreak on child care facilities in Metropolitan Milwaukee, Wisconsin. *Pediatr Infect Dis J* 1997;16:639–644.

19. Cicirello HG, Kehl KS, Addiss DG, et al. Cryptosporidiosis in children during a massive waterborne outbreak, Milwaukee, Wisconsin: clinical, laboratory, and epidemiologic findings. *Epidemiol Infect* 1997; 119:53–60.

20. Frisby HR, Addiss DG, Reiser WJ, et al. Clinical and epidemiologic features of a massive waterborne outbreak of cryptosporidiosis among persons with human

immunodeficiency virus (HIV) infection. *J Acq Immun Defic Syndr Hum Retrovirol* 1997;16:367–373.

21. Hoxie NJ, Davis JP, Vergeront JM, Nashold RD, Blair KA. Cryptosporidiosis-associated mortality following a massive waterborne outbreak in Milwaukee, Wisconsin. *Am J Public Health* 1997;87:2032–2038.

22. Addiss DG, Pond RS, Remshak M, Juranek D, Stokes S, Davis JP. Reduction of risk of watery diarrhea with point-of-use water filters during a massive outbreak of waterborne Cryptosporidium infection in Milwaukee, 1993. *Am J Trop Med Hyg* 1996;54:549–553.

23. Osewe P, Addiss DG, Blair KA, Hightower A, Kamb ML, Davis JP. Cryptosporidiosis in Wisconsin: a case-control study of post-outbreak transmission. *Epidemiol Infect* 1996;117:297–304.

24. Mac Kenzie WR, Kazmierczak JJ, Davis JP. Cryptosporidiosis associated with a resort swimming pool. *Epidemiol Infect* 1995; 115:545–553.

25. Cryptosporidium infections associated with swimming pools—Dane County, Wisconsin, 1993. *MMWR* 1994;43:561–563.

26. Sulaiman IM, Xiao L, Yang C, et al. Differentiating human from animal solates of Cryptosporidium parvum. *Emerg Infect Dis* 1998;4:681–685.

27. McDonald AC, Mac Kenzie WR, Addiss DG, et al. Cryptosporidium parvum-specific antibody responses among children residing in Milwaukee during the 1993 waterborne outbreak. *J Infect Dis* 2001;183:1373–1379.

28. Du Pont HL, Chappell, Sterling CR, Okhuysen PC, Rose JB, Jakubowski. The infectivity of Cryptosporidium parvum in healthy volunteers. *N Engl J Med* 1995;332:855–859.

CHAPTER 14

A Community Outbreak of Hepatitis A Involving Cooperation Between Public Health, the Media, and Law Enforcement, Iowa, 1997

Patricia Quinlisk, MD, MPH, Yvan Hutin, MD, Ken Carter, Tom Carney, and Kevin Teale

INTRODUCTION

When an outbreak of hepatitis A occurred in Iowa during 1996 and 1997, Yvan Hutin was an Epidemic Intelligence Service (EIS) officer with the Centers for Disease Control (CDC). Patricia Quinlisk was the state epidemiologist in Iowa. Ken Carter was the state's director of the Division of Narcotics Enforcement. Kevin Teale was the communications director for the state health department, and Tom Carney was a reporter for the Des Moines Register. In this chapter, they share the actions they took, while shedding light on their unique perspectives and how they interacted with each other while they were trying to understand and control an outbreak of hepatitis A in methamphetamine users. Although several counties were involved in the 1997 hepatitis A epidemic, the chapter focuses on Polk County, where Des Moines, the capital, is located (Figure 14-1).

Hepatitis A is a virus that can cause no symptoms at all or it may lead to jaundice, severe fatigue, tea colored urine, loss of appetite, diarrhea, and rarely death.[1] The virus is excreted in the feces, and is spread from one person to another via fecal contamination of water or food from unwashed hands. It is found in humans worldwide, but it is especially common where sanitation is poor. Where it is most common, outbreaks are less likely to occur because sporadic human-to-human transmission can maintain a relatively high level of exposure among the population. As a result, most of the population would be immune because long-term immunity occurs after infection, and much of the transmission occurs in a developing country during childhood. Many studies have shown that the seroprevalence of hepatitis A increases with increasing age, indicating that the longer one lives in an endemic region, the greater the likelihood one will become exposed and subsequently infected.

Sanitary conditions, in a developed country like the United States, minimize the risk of person to person and waterborne transmission of hepatitis A; however, American child care centers are often foci of spread because of attendance by diapered children who easily spread diseases via feces. Food-borne outbreaks occur sporadically but are not a major source of transmission. As recently as 2006, the Advisory Committee on Immunization Practices recommended that all children should receive hepatitis A vaccine at age 1 year. In addition, the hepatitis A vaccine has been administered to many U.S. citizens because of compliance with a variety of public health recommendations, including efforts to immunize groups where the epidemiology has demonstrated increased risk of either being exposed to the disease or of developing complications if disease occurs, such as travelers, men who have sex with men, persons with clotting-factor disorders, person is working with nonhuman primates, and users of injection and noninjection drugs.

Health departments determine when a hepatitis A exposure has occurred (such as with a restaurant food handler who works while infectious and potentially may have exposed hundreds of customers). Then, applying knowledge of the relatively long incubation period for hepatitis A (ranging from 15 to 50 days), the health department determines who can still be protected with immune globulin (IG) (i.e., up until what date

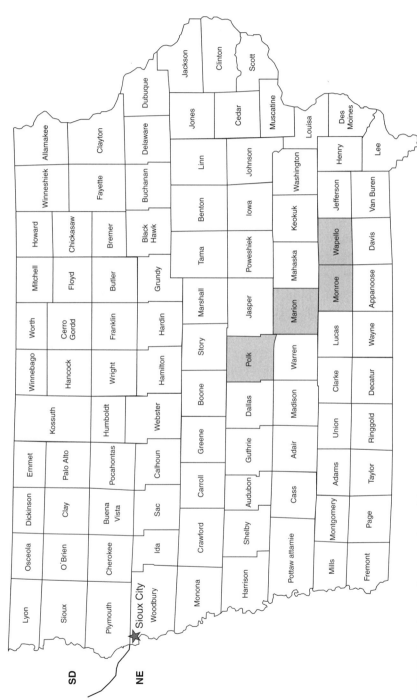

FIGURE 14-1 Areas of Iowa and Neighboring States Involved with the Hepatitis A Outbreak.

could those who were exposed be offered IG as an effective disease prevention measure). The usual time from exposure until it is too late to give IG is 14 days.[2]

Drug use is not the first risk factor one might think of when considering hepatitis A. In fact, when considering drugs, especially injection drugs, one is much more likely to think of hepatitis B or hepatitis C because they are transmitted primarily via blood and blood products. Activities like sharing needles or other blood-contaminated drug paraphernalia fit nicely into the understanding of transmission of hepatitis B and C. Thus, an outbreak of hepatitis A among methamphetamine users is unique.

An infectious disease outbreak involving collaboration with the media and law enforcement without a bioterrorism angle is even more unique. This investigation also demonstrates how the incubation period of an infectious disease can influence policy decision. This investigation also illustrates that health departments must sometimes act based on their interest in protecting the public even though they cannot predict with certainty what would happen if they did not act. For example, here the health department took action to warn of potential exposure to a food handler at a restaurant, even though it was too late to offer IG. They decided to reveal the name of the restaurant to the public so that the people could determine whether they had been potentially exposed. This message was accompanied by information on how to protect those with whom they have contact, for example, with good hand hygiene, in case they developed the disease. In the end, they did not learn of hepatitis A cases associated with eating at this restaurant. It was a difficult decision, and it had economic and personal consequences for the restaurant and food handler; however, it was a reasonable action to take given the public's need to information that could protect it from disease.

Many features of outbreak investigation are nicely displayed in the presentation of this outbreak: (1) the importance of good communication, (2) coordination between involved governmental entities, (3) community involvement in controlling an epidemic, and (4) the use of an epidemiologic study's findings to intervene and control an outbreak. The health department was challenged with a hard to reach population (drug users), a disease with prevention activities that need to be performed within a specific time frame to be effective (such as administration of vaccine and IG), information that needed to be handled very delicately to keep a clear message, and intense media and public interest.

The voices in the chapter include the following:

CDC: Yvan Hutin, EIS officer, CDC
Narcotics: Ken Carter, director, Division of Narcotics Enforcement, Department of Public Safety
Newspaper: Tom Carney, Science Writer, *Des Moines Register*
Press Liaison: Kevin Teale, Communications Director, Iowa Department of Public Health (IDPH)
State Epidemiologist: Patricia Quinlisk, State Epidemiologist, IDPH

State Epidemiologist: Historically, Iowa has had relatively low rates of hepatitis A, punctuated by occasional small outbreaks[3]; however, in the first few months of 1996, hepatitis A began to increase in the "Siouxland" area (around the Sioux City, Iowa, including parts of Nebraska and South Dakota), resulting in a community-wide outbreak that lasted about 1 year. A case-control study was performed during that time in collaboration with the local Siouxland District Health Department, the IDPH, and the federal CDC. This study identified three population groups at increased risk for hepatitis A; those who injected methamphetamine, those who used emergency rooms more than other health care facilities, and those who participated in the WIC (Women, Infants, and Children) program. Prevention and control interventions were expanded, and by the end of 1996, this community outbreak had essentially ended.[4]

Hepatitis A is a reportable disease in the state of Iowa. Thus, health care professionals, including laboratorians, are required to report any disease that the Iowa Board of Health determines to be significant because of public health importance, like hepatitis A. Usually diseases are made reportable if they can spread from one person to another (or from an animal to a human) and/or when public health intervention will modify the transmission or course of disease.

Press Liaison: For at least 3 years prior to 1996, no public health announcements concerning hepatitis A had occurred. Then, in February of 1996, media coverage about the outbreak in the Siouxland area began. At the same time, both the *Sioux City Journal* (the local paper) and the *Des Moines Register* (located in central Iowa, but with statewide readership) did stories about the sharp increase in the number of cases. Although the *Sioux City Journal* article stressed prevention, the *Register* article focused on the possibility the outbreak might have been tied to drug use. Siouxland health officials expressed concerns that the mention of a drug connection may hamper efforts to control the outbreak.

When press releases or information are released about a health concern, the media often asks many questions. With the exception of large media markets that may have trained health reporters, most news items are handled by general assignment reporters who do not have a background in health or science. Additionally, reporters are trained to produce stories with a reading level of third or fourth grade. It is sometimes difficult to work in the basic facts of a health concern (who, what, when, where, and why) and also work in medical information in a simple form. A delicate balance needs to be struck between keeping the media message uncomplicated and not missing important facts for simplicity's sake.

Also, the number of questions asked or time spent by a reporter with informants may not be an indication of how large a story will be published or the placement (front page or back page) of the story. The same story may get very different placement in different outlets on the same day because of other stories that the media outlet may be working on.

Sometimes public health officials will ask that key information or issues be contained in a story to address a specific concern, but we really have to rely on the media's cooperation for this to happen. That is why it is important to establish good relationships between the public health community and media outlets before a crisis situation erupts. We are fortunate in Iowa to have a media that understands health issues and very often will oblige our requests.

CDC: In recent outbreaks in the Midwest and the Northwest, a high proportion of the case patients with hepatitis A had reported use of illicit drugs, mostly injected drugs such as methamphetamine. Attempts had been made to determine why these drug users were at increased risk for hepatitis A, but the reason(s) continued to be unclear. These previous investigations had attempted to determine the risk factors for acquiring hepatitis A, but this had necessitated interviewing drug users, who were understandably reluctant to tell "the government" about their drug habits; however, Iowans are notorious for being cooperative, and thus, it was thought that a study there might be successful.

Narcotics: The Iowa Division of Narcotics Enforcement's (DNE) primary responsibility is to be the lead agency, by Chapter 80 of the Code of Iowa, in the investigation of major drug organizations, both within Iowa and in areas that have direct ties to Iowa. This mission is carried out within DNE through specialized enforcement, to include general narcotics, financial conspiracy, diversion, clandestine laboratories, marijuana eradication, and gang-related investigations

Methamphetamine (or "meth") use had dramatically increased in Iowa in the 3 years before 1997. Although only two clandestine meth laboratories had been seized in 1994 (neither in Polk County where Des Moines, the state capital, is located), by 1997, 63 laboratories were seized, 28 of which were in Polk County. Additionally, in 1994, only 26 people had been arrested in Iowa related to methamphetamine or amphetamine, but by 1997, 234 were arrested. Finally, in 1994, only 11,433 grams of methamphetamine or amphetamine were seized, but during 1997, 52,472 grams were seized.

Meth is a central nervous system stimulant and allows users to go for days without sleep or food. When users are "coming off" the drug, acute paranoia and violent behavior are quite common. This is when child or spousal abuse occurs and when behavior can be very unpredictable and explosive.

In Iowa, about 85% of meth comes from Mexico or the United States–Mexico border area; however, the number of meth laboratories in Iowa was exploding. With information about how to manufacture meth readily available (e.g., on the web), people are setting up "laboratories" (i.e., manufacturing facilities) in homes, hotel rooms, and farm outbuildings. Meth is produced from commonly available materials such as anhydrous ammonia (a farm fertilizer) and sinus/cold medication that was available over the counter at that time. Combining these components can be dangerous; for the short term, they can explode, but for long term, they can be carcinogenic.

State Epidemiologist: In early 1997, a truck stop food handler developed hepatitis A and was reported to us by the laboratory that did the serologic test. We investigated and found that there was potential for the spread of the virus to the public. We also found that his exposure to hepatitis A may have been linked to use of drugs that had been obtained in the Des Moines area. He prepared foods in such a way that he could have contaminated ready to serve foods with his hands that were carrying specks of feces laden with hepatitis A virus. Because the only tool the health department has to prevent disease in those who might have been exposed to hepatitis A via eating this contaminated food is by "going public," we put out a press release recommending those who had eaten at the truck stop to get IG shots. We also announced where the shots were available and clinics were opened at the local health departments.

The potential for spread of the hepatitis A virus to the public from an infectious food handler has four main components. We determine (1) whether the food handler had diarrhea while handling the food (high risk for transmission since the virus is found in the feces), (2) whether the food handler neglected to wash his/her hands after using the restroom (increased risk for transmission even if no diarrhea), (3) what foods the food handler handled (wet, rough, uncooked foods, such as salads, are highest risk, foods cooked thoroughly after handling are no risk), and (4) how many times a patron might have been exposed (increased "dosage" or amount of exposure to contaminated food may increase the risk of becoming ill).

In situations like this, we have to weigh the restaurant's need to be protected from bad publicity against the public's need to be able to protect themselves from disease. If there is a possibility of disease transmission, we feel that the public's needs far outweigh the restaurant's concerns; therefore, we put out a press release to notify those who may have been exposed to hepatitis A. We do try to minimize the damage to the restaurant, however, by stating that remedial steps have been taken, that it is safe to eat there now (if this is true), and how well they are cooperating. We do not release the food handler's name, as no purpose would be served by doing so.

Newspaper: The readers of the *Des Moines Register* became better acquainted with hepatitis A in February of 1997, when the state health department announced that a food handler at a truck stop had potentially exposed the public to hepatitis A. This was worrisome because the truck stop was located on Interstate 80, near the intersection with Interstate 29, one of the major crossroads of mid-America. The location raised the possibility that the disease could have been spread all over the Midwest, or even all over the country.

At this point, we published a straightforward news story about a foodborne illness. Although the story was important because of the potential for the spread of infection, we were simply following our most basic mission of publishing news reports on occurrences around the state. One of the criteria news organizations have for determining what constitutes "news" is impact. We consistently ask ourselves what has the greatest impact on the greatest number of people. This story had potential for great impact.

State Epidemiologist: After alerting the public to the potential exposure to hepatitis A at the truck stop, public health clinics provided several hundred people in Iowa and neighboring states with IG shots to prevent the disease. Luckily, no further cases of hepatitis A were reported related to this incident.

There are three main ways to prevent hepatitis A. The first and most obvious is to prevent exposure by having ill persons not handle anyone else's food, and for everyone to wash his or her hands, especially after going to the bathroom and before preparing food. The next method is to vaccinate a person who is at high risk of being exposed to hepatitis A. Before Iowa's epidemics, travelers to developing countries were the most commonly vaccinated Iowans. Today, many states require hepatitis A vaccination before school entry. The last method, and the only one that can be used after an exposure has occurred, is to give an injection of IG as soon as possible (usually within 14 days of the exposure because IG probably does not provide much protection if given more than 14 days after exposure). IG is a blood product that contains preformed antibodies to hepatitis A. Because antibodies are proteins (formed by the blood donor's immune system), they are eventually degraded by the receiver's metabolic system; thus, protection only lasts a few months. In contrast, vaccines stimulate the receiver's own immune system, thus that person is protected for a long time, perhaps even for the rest of their life.

In March of 1997, routine public health surveillance demonstrated that the number of hepatitis A cases was increasing in Polk County (Des Moines is in Polk County and has a population of about 400,000 in the metro area). In 1996, only between zero to three cases had been reported per month in the county; however, in March of 1997, 12 cases were reported, and that was obviously more than expected.

Meetings were held between the Polk County Health Department and the IDPH to determine appropriate actions. There was concern that this was the beginning of a community-wide outbreak. We suspected that drug use might be a risk factor (because of what had happened in the Siouxland area), and we thus began discussing community interventions, such as education of jailed persons (many of whom use drugs), persons attending substance abuse treatment centers, and a media campaign targeted at young adults. Also, we gave a "heads up" to restaurants and day care centers (since hepatitis A can be spread easily in these settings). In addition, in April, public health and substance abuse professionals in Iowa discussed two very important issues: the increase in hepatitis A cases possibly associated with substance abuse and potential strategies to address the current situation. We reviewed what had been tried in the Siouxland area and what had worked, and the kind of general strategies that are usually done when hepatitis A begins to spread in a community.

On April 1, however, before these measures could be implemented to any great extent, the great nationwide 1997 "hepatitis A in frozen strawberries" situation began.[5] Frozen strawberries that had potentially been contaminated with hepatitis A virus had been distributed to schools around the country, including Iowa, via the U.S. Department of Agriculture surplus food program (Exhibit 14-1). These berries were incorrectly labeled as grown in United States when actually from Mexico. Thus, children at many of Iowa's schools had potentially been exposed to hepatitis A. Although the schools had received the strawberries in January, after discussion with the Iowa Department of Education, it was believed that the majority of the strawberries had either not been served until recently in celebration of the spring holidays (i.e., on the Friday before Easter or before spring break starts) or were still in the school's freezers.

A "quick and dirty" epidemiologic investigation was performed. "Quick and dirty" refers to a type of preliminary survey that is usually done by interviewing those who have become ill or who have been exposed. It is "quick" because if can be completed in a few hours and considered "dirty" because open-ended questions are asked and sometimes opinions are elicited. The data obtained in this way are not considered "clean" nor "precise." The main benefit of this method is that information is quickly obtained that can be used to act on for an emergency response or provide guidance for designing a more precise and scientific survey or study. This type of study can also be used for hypothesis generation.

Exhibit 14-1   Headline

Hepatitis Prognosis: No Cause For Alarm

This headline was published by *USA Today* on April 3, 1997.

If the "quick and dirty" investigation had supported a hypothesis that students and teachers were getting hepatitis A from strawberry exposure, then to protect those who had been exposed, but not yet ill, IG shots would have been given to stop development of diseases. This would have been an important public health intervention. The risk from an intramuscular injection of IG (a sterile preparation of antibodies made from human plasma) is minimal. Usually soreness at the site of the injection is all that is noted among recipients with rare exception.

The "quick and dirty" epidemiologic investigation led to a very quick but formal survey of all schools that had received the strawberries. This survey found that only a few students or teachers in Iowa schools had any illnesses consistent with hepatitis A after eating the strawberries, and thus, we conducted emergency hepatitis A testing of the ill people to determine whether they had had hepatitis A. These laboratory tests showed no sign of recent hepatitis A infection. Thus, it was highly unlikely that the lots of strawberries distributed in Iowa were contaminated with the hepatitis A virus; therefore, the decision was made *not* to give any IG to any Iowa students or teachers, as we felt the risk from getting IG shots (i.e., soreness) was greater than the risk of getting hepatitis A from eating the strawberries.

Iowa's recommendation was in contrast to the CDC's recommendations that were released that same day, which said that all school children and school staff who had eaten any of the strawberries should be given an injection of IG. We quickly discussed with the experts at the Hepatitis Branch of CDC that we were not going to follow their recommendations and the rationale for our course of action. They understood our position and agreed that we had sufficient proof that the specific lots of frozen strawberries served in Iowa were not contaminated. Thus, Iowa was the only state in the United States that did not provide IG to its students and teachers. The remaining frozen strawberries were destroyed just in case.

In the end, no cases of hepatitis A associated with these strawberries occurred in Iowa; however, there was major media attention on this situation, both nationally and in Iowa, that continued to increase the public's awareness of hepatitis A.

Newspaper: In the "contaminated strawberries" story, the epidemiologists at the state health department reported that no students or school staff, who had consumed the strawberries, had become ill. Thus, the strawberries in Iowa were most likely not contaminated, and the IG shots were not needed. We reported that the risks from the shots were probably greater than the risk of getting hepatitis A from the strawberries. Apart from the news value, the *Register's* story presumably helped to calm the fears of parents, students, and staff members about their risks of infection and the usefulness of the shots in this situation.

My principal interest was in reporting the news in as comprehensive a way as possible, helping readers understand the situation, and providing information on what action, if any, they should take. In this case, getting the IG shots was not among actions recommended by the state epidemiologist—who for me, my newspaper and readers was the principal authority on the issue.

State Epidemiologist: This was a good example of the immense help the media can offer by immediately distributing information in situations that are rapidly evolving. There is no other way the health department can quickly educate large segments of the population. These articles really helped to answer questions from people all around the state and to help explain why IG shots were not being recommended or offered.

After all of the press attention to the Iowa truck stop situation where IG was given and all the front page articles in national papers, like the *USA Today*, about schools being given IG, we had started to create the impression in the public's mind that IG is always the answer to potential exposures to hepatitis A. These media stories helped the health department to explain why the shots were not recommended in this situation, where the risk of disease was so low.

In dealing with the media, having your SOCO in mind is very helpful. A SOCO is your "single overriding communication objective," that is, what exactly is the main point you want to get across to the reporter and therefore to the public. In this situation, my SOCO was "shots aren't needed because the risk of getting hepatitis from the strawberries in Iowa was nil." Everything else was extraneous.

Press Liaison: We worked with the media to insure that the correct information was available to the public. Although the "SOCO" was relatively simple, the reasoning behind it was not.

Relationships with the media must be a constant part of the work of public health. In times of a health crisis, there is no other realistic way to get information out to a large number of people without the cooperation of the media. That means responding to all media inquires in a timely factual manner, no matter how obscure the request may be or how busy we are. Working with the media in a noncrisis situation promotes good relationships and allows the health community to practice delivering a concise uncomplicated message about health issues, while "educating" the media about science and public health.

Newspaper: A few days after the strawberry story, I noticed a full-page advertisement in the *Register* by a pharmaceutical company. The ad urged readers to see their doctors and "ask about getting vaccinated against hepatitis A." Because at this time the vaccine was considered only useful prior to exposure (see note at end of the chapter), it was therefore too late to be used to prevent illness in those who had eaten strawberries, even if their strawberries were contaminated with hepatitis A. I contacted a family practitioner, who stated that the vaccine was good but would not be useful for people concerned about the strawberries. We then ran an editorial about this situation; we felt that a vaccine manufacturer had used the public's concerns to promote the use of a vaccine that was not appropriate.

Having educated myself and readers about the hepatitis A vaccine, I was surprised by the ad and wondered whether I had misunderstood the vaccine's usefulness in this situation or whether the pharmaceutical company was being overzealous in promotion of its product. Either way, it was new information on the "contaminated strawberries" story and needed to be checked out and reported. I presented the case by the pharmaceutical company and response from the health department, and—to expand the scope of authority in this case—I referred to a family practitioner who had some familiarity with the vaccine. Believing that the pharmaceutical company was presenting false information, I informed our editorial department, whose staff did its own research and wrote an editorial trying to clarify the issues (even though the pharmaceutical company had paid a great deal of money to place a full-page ad in our newspaper).

State Epidemiologist: A few days before Memorial Day weekend (May 24–26, 1997), concerns about a hepatitis A epidemic exponentially increased when the salad maker at a busy, landmark Des Moines restaurant was diagnosed with hepatitis A. Unfortunately, misleading information was given to the emergency room personnel where he had sought medical care and been tested for hepatitis A, resulting in a delay in the public health officials locating and interviewing him (and finding out that he was a food handler!). It was then realized that he had potentially exposed thousands of people to hepatitis A. The amount of time since the last day of this exposure to the public was determined, but because it was more than 14 days, it was too late to give IG to the exposed persons (and prevent them from becoming ill). Thus, at this point, there was major concern that these exposed persons would develop hepatitis A and potentially transmit it to others before realizing the cause of their illness.

A person with hepatitis A becomes infectious about 1 week before symptoms begin and can remain infectious for a week or two after symptoms start. Those with diarrhea are more likely to spread the disease because their hands can become so contaminated with fecal material (and therefore hepatitis A viruses) that washing may not clean them completely; however, anyone with hepatitis A who does not wash their hands after using the bathroom can spread this disease, regardless of the symptoms they have at the time.

When a food handler at a restaurant gets hepatitis A, it can become a public health disaster if appropriate control measures are not undertaken. In our outbreak, the control measure was to educate the public with a very unusual message: People eating at this landmark restaurant had been exposed, but it was too late to prevent them from becoming ill; however, we explained that if they took appropriate precautions, they could prevent spreading it to their family and friends.

Press Liaison: One of the difficulties with the possible outbreak from this restaurant was that our normal hepatitis A message had to be changed. Instead of a simple message of "get IG," the message here was complicated: "It is too late to protect the customers at this restaurant. But if those people become ill, they need to know what action to take to protect their family and friends." A substantial amount of media attention began after the press release with its complex message. The media stories after this ranged from a theme of "if it can happen here, it can happen anywhere," to the historical link to drug use, to the training sessions planned by the county health department for day-care centers and restaurants. We were fortunate to have the full cooperation of the landmark restaurant's owner, when we went public with the news of this possible exposure of the dining public.

Newspaper: At the press conference announcing that consumers had been exposed at the restaurant, the restaurant owner showed obvious signs of stress about what this announcement would do to his business, but it was obvious that the health officials considered this a serious threat to the public health, warranting the risk to a prominent business and business owner.

The landmark restaurant's owner was unusually frank, saying that the salad maker had told him that he had been hospitalized simply for an "infected liver." Despite comments by the health officials that such an infection didn't mean the restaurant had bad sanitary conditions, his business plummeted. In a Memorial Day interview at his home, he said his business, in the days since the press conference, had been only about 10% of normal. "I'm a victim," he said. "I tried to do right to protect my customers. I'm sure I'm a laughingstock among restaurateurs." Since this episode, the owner has been seen by the community as a very responsible restaurateur and is praised for his action; however, he did suffer a temporary decline in business because of his forthrightness.

Once again, the *Register* provided information to readers about how hepatitis A is transmitted. It published the recommendations that these restaurant goers be especially careful when handling food and to wash their hands often. "Wash, wash, wash," Dr. Julius Connor, medical director of the Polk County Health Department, was quoted as saying. It was apparent that health officials were beginning to worry about the increasing number of cases. Up to that point in 1997, 36 cases had been reported in Polk county, compared with only three during the same period of the previous year, and over 50% of cases in 1997 were occurring in people between the ages of 25 and 44, a very different age group than in the past when child care centers were the focal points of transmission.

I was pleasantly surprised that public health officials had named the restaurant, not because I was interested in jeopardizing the restaurant's business but because that famous name was a major part of the story. Here is where the interests of the media and those of public health officials sometimes part. The reporter considers those familiar names to be part of the public record and by law available to the public—no matter the consequences to the restaurant or the impact on other restaurants that come forward with such information. I was interested in presenting as much accurate information as possible, acting on the traditional press value that information is power. Public health officials often want to protect the identities of sources of outbreaks to help assure their cooperation in future outbreaks. (In my opinion, this position is not supported by Iowa law, which calls for openness unless some specific Iowa law precludes it.) Nonetheless, in this case, there was no conflict, and the interest of the press and public health officials coincided.

State Epidemiologist: Over the Memorial Day weekend, the Polk County Health Department established a hot line number for people to call if they had questions about hepatitis A. Between Friday evening and Tuesday, they reported receiving about 240 calls. The hotline continued service until late June 1997. As the outbreak continued, the hotline number was widely published, and the county health department became a reliable source of quality information.

Getting out the correct information during times of crisis can sometimes be as important as the other interventions. If a community is left without information, rumors can get started, often complicating the situation, and public health officials end up spending more time trying to correct false information than they would have if they had been proactive. (You may hear the voice of experience here!) Thus, I have come to the belief the more information given the better, and at times, I probably release more information than needed. I also believe in being "up front" with the media. If I get asked something that I know the answer to, but don't want to release, I say just that. I have found that this is better than trying to evade the question.

Some information, however, is considered confidential such as an individual's medical information (i.e., the name of the people who have hepatitis A) and, at least under Iowa law, entities (i.e., restaurant names) associated with outbreaks. We do not violate this confidentiality unless it is necessary to protect the public's health.

Narcotics: The DNE initial exposure to the hepatitis outbreak resulted from the press conference concerning the people who may have been exposed at the restaurant. The Polk County Health Department discussed with the DNE the possible connection between the use, distribution, and manufacture of methamphetamine and the outbreak of hepatitis A in Polk County. After the phone conversation, DNE was invited to attend a meeting at the Polk County Health Department a couple days before Memorial Day 1997. The Coordinator of the Governor's Alliance on Substance Abuse also attended this meeting. The meeting discussed the increasing number of hepatitis A cases and the increasing number of illegal methamphetamine laboratories being seized in the central Iowa area. Information was also shared about the manufacturing procedures, to understand how meth was made, thus allowing for determining whether and at what point could hepatitis A contaminate the product. At this meeting, several participants expressed concern over law enforcement being involved as a potential barrier to those that might seek treatment or prophylaxis for hepatitis A.

At this point, we were not interested in obtaining information about individuals with hepatitis A who might have used meth. Also, we understood the need for public health intervention in this group to stop the spread of hepatitis A. Our concern about the health risks to our narcotics agents was also discussed, and determinations were made of actions that could be taken to lower their risk.

The potential for meth to become contaminated with feces via dirty hands is quite extensive. For example, after drying the meth crystals, it is crumbled by hand prior to weighing and packaging it for sale; however, meth is quite acidic, and thus, the virus may not be able to survive on the meth crystals for long. As another interesting tidbit, meth is often colored by the "manufacturer" with food coloring for marketing purposes—that is, a user might prefer "purple" meth over "brown" meth.

State Epidemiologist: As we started to address the drug user link to disease, we were very concerned about the drug-using community having confidence in the health department's code of confidentiality. If we needed to do public health interventions in this community, we would need their cooperation, which we felt we would not get if they did not trust us. Thus, we were careful to maintain a distance from law enforcement, while accepting their assistance. The narcotics enforcement people understood our concerns and always acted professionally.

Outbreaks can make for strange bedfellows, and this can be one of the more interesting aspects of investigating outbreaks. I must admit that I never thought I would learn how to make methamphetamine, but the narcotics agents spent an afternoon teaching us not only how meth was made but how it was used so that we could understand how someone using meth might become infected with the hepatitis A virus.

Press Liaison: One media complication surrounding the situation at the restaurant was that a food handler came forward and declared that he was the one with hepatitis A but that he was not a drug user. Even though this man had "gone public" about his identity, because of the state health departments policy on medical confidentiality (and the state law), we could not, and never will, confirm or deny if this man was the restaurant worker with hepatitis A.

The issue of confidentiality overshadows media/public health relations. Media outlets want to personalize a story as much as possible, while breeches of confidence can undermine the ability of public health workers to investigate health issues. It is difficult to draft a black and white rule for confidentiality, other than to say that no personal identifying information should be released without the consent of the patient except in extreme situations. Sometimes the best action is to have the patient go directly to the media if they are interested in being identified publicly, thus taking the health department and our concerns of confidentiality "out of the loop."

Other information release "rules" vary based on the situation (see http://www.idph.state.ia.us/adper/common/pdf/cade/disclosure_reportable_diseases.pdf). Describing a patient as being an 11-year-old Hispanic male is obviously of less concern in a Southern California county than it is in a rural Iowa county (where there may only be one 11-year-old Hispanic male, thus allowing the individual to be identified). The decision to name a restaurant that has a worker who may have spread hepatitis A infection is driven by the need to communicate information about an ongoing health risk to a specific population where there is no other way of identifying that population. In the case of a food borne outbreak at a private gathering where a complete guest list was maintained, there may not be a need to communicate news of the outbreak to the general public, as we would already know who was potentially exposed. In other situations, such as a follow-up to an industrial injury, it may not be necessary to identify the specific location or business involved, if the circumstances that lead to the risk have been eliminated. One option that can be tried, if time and circumstances permit, is to have the public health community act as a go-between to approach the patient or institution to see whether they are willing to "go public" and then giving them the reporter's phone number that they can then call. The primary reason for doing so is to educate in the hope that this prevents others from going through the same experience.

Newspaper: On May 29, 1997, we ran a front-page story "Ex-worker at *landmark restaurant* is Sorry for Health Risk." In this article, the food handler with hepatitis A identified himself and was quoted as saying, "I would never have knowingly hurt anyone. I probably have infected some-one or their family or their loved one or their significant other. That hurts me, and I can't say sorry enough. It's not like I'm some drug addict or street junkie." He admitted that he told hospital officials that he was not working at the time but said that he had given them a series of addresses where he had been staying. He said that he had decided to come forward, even though his name had not been made public, because of a man's kind-ness at the unemployment office. "When I went in, he asked me my last employer, I said *landmark restaurant.* Then he asked my last position. I said a salad bar worker. The man just looked at me and I hung my head. He told me 'you don't have to hang your head.'" At the end of the article, we quoted him as stating, "I'm a victim too." In this article, a manager at the restaurant stated that they "are the ones who forced him to go to the doctors. We wouldn't let him work until he did."

A companion article in the same issue had the headline of "Doctors to Dine at *landmark restaurant* to Assure Public of Safety" for a story on local doctors having dinner at the restaurant to demonstrate their support and confidence in the safety of the restaurant's food. The food worker's public apology and the visit of local doctors to the restaurant were both important follow-up pieces in the hepatitis A story. It added more "human" elements to a story that was becoming as much about the effects disease has on patients, their families, and society as about the epidemiology.

THE FIELD EPIDEMIOLOGIC INVESTIGATION BEGINS: LATE MAY 1997

State Epidemiologist: When we realized that we had another outbreak to bring under control and another opportunity to study the modes of trans-mission of hepatitis A, we called CDC and asked for an "Epi-Aid."

Epi-Aids are called when a state has a health event occurring that has (or may have) national impact and when the state needs assistance in order to investigate it fully. Because the CDC has investigators looking for events to investigate, expert consultants available and laboratories with capacity to perform large numbers of tests, we felt that Iowans would be best served by collaboration between the state health department, the local health departments, and the CDC. Together we might not only be able to stop the outbreak but might be able to learn something that could prevent or help control future outbreaks.

We were particularly concerned about the link of spread of hepatitis A to methamphetamine use for several reasons. Iowa had recently experienced a community-wide outbreak of hepatitis A in Siouxland and the epidemiological investigation revealed a statistically significant correlation to drug use. Also, by this time we had two recent case reports of hepatitis A in restaurant workers that may have been using drugs obtained in the Des Moines area. In addition, nationally, methamphetamine use was being linked to hepatitis A transmission.

CDC: In May of 1997, when this request came in, I was at the end of my first year as an EIS officer working in the Hepatitis Branch of the CDC. EIS is described as a "unique 2-year post graduate program of service and on-the-job training for health professionals interested in the practice of epidemiology." One of the core functions is to help in epidemiologic investigations, and in this capacity, I had already been to Iowa once.

The previous fall (of 1996), during the outbreak of hepatitis A in Siouxland, I had investigated the causes. In that outbreak, a high proportion of cases had reported injecting drug use, particularly methamphetamine. A case-control study had been done in Sioux City, Iowa to identify what population group could be identified at highest risk and targeted for intervention.[4]

Even after the study, the methods of hepatitis A transmission among illicit drug users remained unclear. The Siouxland study had been started after the outbreak had been occurring in that greater community for several months. This meant that the outbreak had expanded by then and new subpopulations were involved that had different modes of transmission than had originally occurred. Therefore, when the central Iowa outbreak first started, it was recognized that this was a great chance to study transmission of the virus in its early phases and perhaps better determine the primary and initial routes of transmission.

State Epidemiologist: When we were told that Dr. Yvan Hutin would be sent as the CDC primary investigator, we were thrilled. We knew Yvan quite well from the Sioux City outbreak and were very impressed by his abilities. Thus, we were in good spirits as we geared up for the intensive investigation. We also used the arrival of the two CDC investigators (Dr. Hutin and Dr. Keith Sabin) to generate more publicity that might help continue the effort to educate the public. We felt that the more the community knew about the situation, the better chance public health had in getting it under control. With diseases like hepatitis A, it is the community that has to take the definitive action (such as good hand washing and seeing a physician for diagnostic evaluation early in the course of illness). Public health's responsibility is to make that action as easy as possible for the public to achieve.

Newspaper: On June 3, Iowa's health officials announced that they had asked federal investigators to help unravel the mystery of the hepatitis A outbreak in central Iowa. When interviewed about the arrival of the CDC's investigator, the state epidemiologist replied, "We said, 'Great, we'd like to have some help.'" The CDC spokesperson said that their investigators typically work along side the state epidemiologists and state health care providers to help identify a source.

We reported that it was not clear yet what was causing the increase of hepatitis A cases in Iowa but that hand washing was critical, particularly after using the bathroom, after changing an infant's diaper, and before preparing food. We also reminded people to go immediately to a doctor if they had been exposed to hepatitis A and to go to a doctor if they were having symptoms of hepatitis A, because as the state epidemiologist said, "If you already have hepatitis A, there's not much we can do for you, but there are things we can do at that point to protect your family and friends." By this time, our goal at the newspaper was to provide any new information about what had become an ongoing story.

CDC/State Epidemiologist: After the CDC investigators arrived in Iowa, we met with them, and the local health department's epidemiologists to discuss the outbreak, interventions, and investigations. At this meeting, it was decided that one of the most critical items was to determine the way that hepatitis was being transmitted; therefore, between June and July of 1997, a case-control study was conducted to identify specific modes of hepatitis A transmission among persons using methamphetamine. The first step was to identify all persons reported with hepatitis A having onset dates between April 1 and July 24, 1997, the dates from when the outbreak started and when the study needed to end. Then, in early June, a pilot study involving 13 of the people with hepatitis A, also known as case-patients, was performed to help generate hypotheses about potential modes of transmission. Pilot studies are often done to test the feasibility of the study design, including the patient questionnaire, and for a quick check of the hypotheses. If you have time, performing a pilot study can be indispensable for fine-tuning your investigation.

Narcotics: On June 4, 1997, the DNE was contacted by the CDC to notify us that they had an individual en route to Polk County per the request of IDPH. On June 12, personnel from CDC, IDPH, and the Polk County Department of Health met at the DNE headquarters in Des Moines for further information on the increasing number of clandestine meth labs and how this substance was illicitly produced. This allowed the epidemiologists more insights into the possible points during production and distribution of meth that contamination with hepatitis A virus could occur.

From information gathered by us at this meeting, it was decided that hepatitis A shots would be provided to all members of the Division of Narcotics Enforcement because of the high potential of coming in contact with law violators who are infectious with hepatitis A. Divisional agents have a large number of undercover investigators who have contact with potential and known methamphetamine distributors. During the months of June and July, all DNE Special Agents received the first of the two doses in the hepatitis vaccine series.

CDC: In the pilot study, the 13 case-patients were asked both open-ended and close-ended questions about meth use, practices associated with meth usage, paraphernalia use, and injection practices. Open-ended questions have no set answers, such as "What did you do last night?" Close-ended questions, however, such as "Did you eat the potato salad last night?" have limited answers (i.e., yes or no). This information was used to generate an appropriate questionnaire. Of the 13 case-patients, 10 identified using the emergency room as their primary health care source. This was important because the emergency room had been found to be an important source of health care for the hepatitis A cases in the Sioux City outbreak and it provided a contact point for case ascertainment (finding people that have or had hepatitis A) and for possible intervention.

We then put together our primary team of investigators consisting of two CDC investigators and two epidemiology students (doing rotations at the state and Polk County health departments). With additional assistance from other professionals at the health departments, we began our main study. Then we had to find people who were like the case-patients except that they were not ill with hepatitis A. These would serve as our control patients.

Because the pilot study identified the emergency room as the primary source of health care for the meth users, controls were recruited prospectively from patients seeking medical care at two emergency rooms in the area (in Polk and Wapello counties) and at a clinic associated with the public hospital in Polk County. During the study period, the triage nurse in each facility asked all patients between 15 and 45 years of age about methamphetamine use in the last 12 months. Patients who admitted to use during this time period were recruited as controls.

We did have exclusion criteria for controls. Each was asked to give a blood sample for hepatitis A testing, and if found positive for IgM (evidence of acute disease), they were excluded from the study. Potential controls who could not or would not be tested were also excluded.

The investigation team trained interviewers, from both the state and local health departments, to administer the questionnaires to study participants, collecting data on demographic characteristics, living conditions, use of social and public assistance services, exposure to day care centers, contact with a hepatitis A case, international travel, sexual activity, history of substance abuse, behaviors associated with methamphetamine used during the 2 to 6 weeks before illness, quantity and routes of administration of each type of meth used, paraphernalia use, and injection practices.

If the persons who design the questionnaire are using others to administer it, it is important to train the interviewers. This ensures consistency in asking questions and in recording answers. It can be surprising how many ways someone can answer even simple questions such as this: "Did you eat the potato salad?"

There were 95 case patients with onset dates after April 1, 1997; of these, 75 were interviewed. Of the remainder, 19 could not be located; only one refused to participate (and she suggested that the interviewer return when she was feeling better).

When performing studies like this, when the CDC investigators take the lead role, it is critical to have the support of state and local public health personnel. In this situation, both the state and local health departments provided logistic and personnel support, which allowed the study to be so successful. Also, it is the local health department people who knew the community partners that became involved in the study. For example, in this study, the local health department personnel helped us to contact and coordinate with the hospitals and emergency rooms to help us to identify potential cases of hepatitis A and vaccinate those at high risk.

State Epidemiologist: We had a running joke in the office about how cooperative Iowans were, even the illicit drug users. In the study, 75 out of the 76 hepatitis A cases (99%) contacted agreed to participate in the study. It was my understanding that a similar study had been tried in other parts of the county with little success, because the drug users were unwilling to cooperate, to the point of meeting interviewers at the door with guns!

I'm happy to report that none of our interviewers felt unsafe while doing this study, although this was a concern when the investigation began, especially because some of the interviewers were young female students, inexperienced in public health interventions or working with this population; however, the drug users were willing to tell interviewers about their health and drug use. The only piece of information that we were not able to get was from whom they bought their drugs. It would have been nice to trace back the drugs to the production point to evaluate potential "bad batches" and types of potential contamination, but it was not absolutely necessary for the investigation.

While the CDC study was getting started, the health departments stepped up efforts to control the outbreak. In general, a two-pronged approach was used: to try to prevent disease in the groups at highest risk for becoming infected (e.g., those using meth) and to prevent transmission from groups at highest risk for spreading the virus (primarily food handlers and those associated with day care centers). Thus, in June, both on weekdays and on weekends, the local and state health department personnel provided seminars for restaurants, other food serving establishments, and day care centers, with instruction on how to reduce their risk of transmitting hepatitis A. Food establishments are at high risk because of the potential of exposing large numbers of people via contaminated food or, in the case of day care centers, because their children are often in diapers, allowing for fecal contamination of the environment with easy spread to other children.

These seminars were very well attended. In fact, some national chain restaurants sent managers from regional offices to attend. There was also extensive media coverage of the seminars, reinforcing for the public what needed to be done to decrease the transmission of the virus (Exhibit 14-2). Also, many handouts such as brochures and fact sheets were either developed or modified for distribution to the public, parents, day care center employees, and food handlers.

Exhibit 14-2   Headline

Huge Hepatitis Outbreak Feared

"We are asking for your help and cooperation so that we don't end up with hundreds, if not thousands, of people infected in Polk County."

Dr. Patricia Quinlisk, addressing restaurant owners

This was quoted in the *Des Moines Register*.

Newspaper: On June 4, we ran a story on the "prevention" seminars being offered to child care providers and restaurant workers in Des Moines. In this story, we reported on the briefing that had occurred that day, and we helped advertise the sites and times of these future briefings. The article focused on children and child-care facilities, and why they were of such concern, that is, that children often had no symptoms but still spread the disease, that children in diapers and those still being potty trained can spread the disease more easily than others, and why hand washing was so important. The side bar to this article listed pertinent facts on hepatitis A. Providing information about the response, including prevention seminars, was considered part of our mission to keep our readers informed about the outbreak.

Narcotics: After discussions about the potential for methamphetamine to transmit the hepatitis A virus, we were asked whether it might be possible to obtain some meth, confiscated in a raid or arrest, for testing for the virus. Thus, the Division of Narcotics Enforcement attempted to obtain samples during the execution of search warrants on clandestine meth laboratory sites. Coordination was accomplished with the United States Attorney's office in Des Moines to permit the DNE to immediately release evidentiary samples to the IDPH for analysis. Appropriate storage containers and packing materials were also purchased to preserve any samples for future analysis. Unfortunately, with the exception of one laboratory site, syringes possibly containing meth were not located. The one syringe that was obtained was not fit for analysis because of improper storage.

State Epidemiologist: We appreciated the narcotics staff's willingness to go to such lengths to help us obtain some drug samples for hepatitis A virus testing. It was not easy for them to get permission to give us illegal drugs for testing. If we had been able to obtain some and test it, it would have allowed us to "close the circle" of the outbreak. Unfortunately, this was not possible in this situation.

The preliminary public health surveillance information suggested that injecting drug users and men who have sex with men were the groups at highest risk for developing hepatitis A in central Iowa, and because the Advisory Committee of Immunization Practices (the committee that recommends how vaccines should be used in the United States) already recommended hepatitis A vaccination for these risk groups, it was decided in early June (before the study was started) to go ahead with a vaccination campaign. It was estimated that over 3,000 people would need to be vaccinated and that approximately 5,000 doses of vaccine would be needed. Although two doses of vaccine are recommended for full protection, from experience we only expected about 50% to return for the second dose of vaccine 6 months later.

Several barriers existed to a successful vaccination campaign: (1) difficulty in getting the vaccine to a population that may not want to be identified (e.g., running an ad in the newspaper asking all illicit drug users to come to health department on Thursday for shots would probably not work), (2) most of the population that needed the vaccine would not have the resources or perhaps the willingness to pay for a $50+ per dose vaccine, (3) the hepatitis A vaccine requires two doses over a 6-month period for full protection, and (4) the health departments did not have money in their budgets to pay for the amount of vaccine needed.

One of these barriers was addressed politically. On June 12, 1997, after discussions with the state health department and the CDC, U.S. Senator Tom Harkin (D-Iowa) announced that the CDC had agreed to provide Iowa with a "significant amount" of vaccine. He stated in his press release, "I am grateful to the CDC for their prompt and dedicated assistance to our state in dealing with this public health problem."

Newspaper: Out of our Washington bureau, we ran an article that the CDC would pay for 5,000 doses of hepatitis A vaccine to head off the outbreak in Iowa. We also reported that the CDC had committed about $160,000 to the vaccine effort and had sent two investigators to Iowa in the wake of reports of 140 cases of hepatitis A in the state since January. In addition, the CDC action was important because of the potential for a community-wide outbreak to develop involving hundreds of thousands of people.

We wanted to provide information on the outbreak from any and every source, and a reporter in our Washington bureau had an angle—the activities of the CDC in the outbreak—that I didn't hear about in Des Moines.

CDC/State Epidemiologist: Now that we had the vaccine, we needed to decide how best to get it to those at highest risk. It was decided to focus on the four counties in central Iowa with the highest rates of hepatitis A— Marion, Monroe, Polk and Wapello—and to use various access points, such as health departments, emergency rooms, jails, drug treatment centers, sexually transmitted disease clinics, malls, churches, and HIV screening sites. We also ran a clinic in the lobby of the local gambling casino in the middle of the night on the advice of the Narcotics Enforcement people that this was a good place and time to find meth users.

Believe it or not, there are a few places to go in Des Moines in the middle of the night if you are unable to sleep. The local casino is open all night long and with meth being a stimulant drug, it makes sense one might find some meth users in this environment late at night. We ended up vaccinating quite a few people there.

A variety of techniques were used to get the word out to those who needed to be vaccinated (or possibly be given IG because of a recent exposure), including health department personnel speaking about the issue whenever possible. Pamphlets were widely distributed in places where drug users and/or men who have sex with men might congregate, such as gay bars and drug treatment centers. Educational cards were given to those diagnosed with hepatitis A to distribute to their drug sharing partners, friends, and families who they might have exposed to hepatitis A. These cards could then be presented at a vaccination site, at which time they could be vaccinated without having to answer any questions. This was done to encourage anyone who might be in a risk group for hepatitis A or may have been exposed to the case patient to be vaccinated and/or be given IG.

In mid June, the state health department developed a "Recommended Protocol for Hepatitis A Vaccination Programs for Targeted Populations." It addressed issues such as administration costs, standing orders for vaccination, informed consent, vaccine ordering and handling, and patient recall (for the second dose). This packet also contained a sample letter for ordering the vaccine, a consent form, a fact sheet for the patient, and a report form to send back to IDPH on the number of doses of vaccine administered by month. This was distributed to all appropriate local health departments and vaccination sites.

Developing clear guidance, including the protocol and forms, was an important coordinating function for the state health department to perform, especially when multiple jurisdictions and agencies get involved as happened here. It helped to organize the vaccination efforts, ensured consistency in procedures across the counties, and helped to track efforts. Consistency is especially important because different protocols in different counties can cause the public to become concerned. "What does that county know that my county doesn't know?" Inconsistency can undermine the credibility of a health department's efforts and interfere with control of an outbreak.

Even with all of the efforts everyone was making in June, we knew that it would be several months before we would know whether the rates of hepatitis A were decreasing since the incubation period—time from exposure to the virus to the onset of symptoms—can be up to 6 weeks. Throughout this time we remained very concerned that it would spread to the general population.

Newspaper: On June 9, 1997, we reported that the Blood Center of Central Iowa had sent letters to 5,300 blood donors asking whether they ate a meal at the landmark restaurant between April 21 and May 5, when they might have been exposed to hepatitis A. If they had, they were asked to contact the blood center. The center would then destroy the donated blood to reduce any risk of transmitting hepatitis A to blood recipients. Our report also noted that all persons attempting to donate blood were being deferred from donating if they had been exposed to hepatitis A at the restaurant.

Once again, our intent was to provide any new information about the continuing story.

State Epidemiologist: Although much of our communication efforts were aimed at a general audience, in early June, we were pretty confident that illicit drug users were one of the major, if not *the* major group, spreading the disease. We were hesitant to go public with this information at this time for several reasons: (1) During the Sioux City outbreak the previous year, the drug use connection had been made public, but local public health officials felt this had made their jobs more difficult and had possibly stopped some people from being diagnosed. (2) We were doing a study to determine the modes of transmission, and thus, we wanted to be able to document this connection and determine some way of addressing this issue before making it public, and (3) we were not absolutely confident that drug use was the real risk factor. Thus, when we went public with the vaccination clinics, we recommended it for all the high-risk groups identified in the national recommendations (for hepatitis A vaccine use), which included drug users.

The public health departments, however, had already began a targeted education program for drug (primarily methamphetamine) users and men who have sex with men, as these two groups appeared to be a highest risk, but may not be getting information through regular channels such as the media. Thus, pamphlets with target population specific information were also handed out at drug treatment centers, gay bars, sexually transmitted disease clinics, and so forth.

Newspaper: On June 23rd, we reported the opening of free hepatitis A vaccination clinics. We also reported that the shots were being recommended for (1) anyone who has injected illicit drugs or used meth in the last year, (2) men who are having sex with men, (3) friends and families of these two risk groups, (4) friends and family members of those who have hepatitis A, (5) persons with chronic liver disease, and (6) persons with blood-clotting disorders. To encourage acceptance, it was reported that those seeking vaccination would not be asked about lifestyles or drug use.

The article also reported concerns about the outbreak spreading to the general community and that if it did it would be almost impossible to stop. If a community outbreak did occur, health officials stated that it could take up to 2 years and hundreds, if not thousands, of cases before it ended.

We wanted to report the latest development in this story and without overstating it; we wanted to inform readers about the risks of the outbreak spreading to the general population. To convey these risks, we depended on the state epidemiologist, who helped us put it all in perspective.

State Epidemiologist: We had watched the reports of cases of hepatitis A carefully for any cases reporting exposure to the landmark restaurant. By the beginning of July it became apparent that this had not occurred. In the end, there were no cases of hepatitis A that we could directly link to exposure to food at this restaurant.

Even though there was no spread, we were comfortable with our actions the month before (going public about the potential transmission of the virus from the food handler and the subsequent outbreak that could occur). It would be great if we could predict the future, but this is obviously not possible. Thus, we prepare for the worst and hope for the best.

Newspaper: On July 3, we reported "Hepatitis Epidemic Apparently Avoided" but that central Iowans weren't in the clear yet. Health officials reported that there had not been a community-wide outbreak from the food handler at the landmark restaurant with hepatitis A and attributed part of this to the "incredible" public response to the warnings and recommendations.

It was reported that most cases were occurring in 23 to 38 year old adults, although health officials declined to speculate why the disease is prevalent in that age group. Dr. Connor, the Polk County medical director, was quoted as stating that the health officials hadn't determined how the virus had been spreading in Polk County, but that it had been decided to recommend the vaccine to high-risk groups.

On July 10, an article titled "Hepatitis A Still Rising Among the Young" was published. It reported that health officials were increasingly concerned about the continuing rise in the number of cases. A possible second case of hepatitis A in a Polk County food handler was also noted.

We were still interested at this point in continuing to inform the public about developments, being careful to make distinctions in the July 3 and July 10 stories to avoid the perception of a contradiction. The epidemic had *not* spread to the general population on the one hand; on the other, the incidence of the disease was still rising among the young. Our thinking in this and other health messages, such as the results of current research, is that we would present information as clearly and succinctly as possible, having confidence that the majority of readers get the true picture.

CDC: By late July, the investigation of the modes of transmission had definitively identified that the groups at increased risk included meth users and injecting drug users. The case control study found that, among meth users, having used meth with someone who had hepatitis A and injecting meth with a syringe were the two factors statistically associated with getting hepatitis A. Not all the meth users who got hepatitis A reported injecting the drugs, indicating that at least some fecal–oral transmission probably occurred. Among injectors, only half reported sharing needles. Sharing paraphernalia such as spoons, cotton (for filtering the drug solution), and cups was common among the injectors, even if they did not share needles. We concluded that the injecting paraphernalia was probably becoming contaminated by handling during use and then shared with others, infecting them. We termed this mode of transmission "fecal–percutaneous."

State Epidemiologist: Yvan Hutin, Dr. Julius Connor, and I had a press conference to announce these results on July 23. We were concerned that the general public hearing these results might do a couple things: "blame" the outbreak on the drug users and think themselves safe and thus relax precautions such as careful hand washing. We stressed that those at risk were victims of this disease and should not be blamed and that there could still be a community-wide outbreak if everyone didn't continue to do their bit. The importance of those at risk getting vaccinated was reinforced as an important public health intervention and that those at risk should seek vaccination. It was announced that more vaccine clinics would be held at health departments, emergency rooms, substance abuse treatment centers, and sexually transmitted disease clinics. Polk County Health Department helped staff some of these clinics.

When setting up these clinics, there was a lot of discussion about how to encourage drug users to come in for vaccinations—for example, how to allow a person to remain anonymous, how to use those that came in for vaccination to encourage their families and fellow drug users to come in, how to overcome the distrust of government agencies that many drug users have, and whether or not we should use this opportunity to address other health risks in this group of people (i.e. HIV and hepatitis B and C). It was decided that hepatitis A prevention was our first priority, and if there was time and opportunity for other issues, they could be addressed.

At the press conference, it was emphasized that those using drugs should stop. If they were going to continue to use drugs, they needed to wash their hands prior to drug use and not share drug paraphernalia, and if a drug user's drug-sharing partner develops hepatitis A, the user should get an IG shot immediately.

There was also concern about how we would be able to deliver the second dose of the two-dose hepatitis A vaccine 6 months after the first. It was felt that we were morally obligated to try to encourage those that obtained the first dose to get the second. Usually, the vaccinee would be contacted and reminded by a "reminder postcard" or a phone call; however, many of these vaccinees might be reluctant to give identifying information about themselves, and we had promised that the vaccine could be obtained anonymously. Thus, we ended up explaining about the need for a second dose and offered to remind them if they would leave us a way in which to contact them.

Narcotics: On July 24, the drug czar of Iowa publicly applauded the decision by health officials to seek out meth users for hepatitis A vaccinations. He stated that he hoped the attention would heighten public awareness about the serious consequences of the drug's increased prevalence in Iowa. "It should open some eyes," he said, to the dangers associated with using meth. ". . . It's going to spread to the community beyond the drug users and spread in the family to the younger, innocent family members."

State Epidemiologist: By July 29, Polk County Health Department alone had vaccinated over 1,200 people. The clinics were so successful, partially because of all of the publicity the outbreak was receiving, that they were extended. In late July, other counties in central Iowa, such as Wapello, had started vaccination campaigns also. By August 9, over 1,540 doses had been given in Polk County alone.

Unfortunately, but not unexpected because of the lengthy incubation period, the number of cases continued to rise. For the month of July, Polk County reported 79 cases (compared with 9 in the same time period the year before), and Wapallo County reported 45 (compared with 1 the year before).

Because of the epidemic, Polk County Health Department found themselves in need of extra staff. This resulted in the Polk County Board of Supervisors appropriating funds to hire more nurses and program aids to assist in this effort (Exhibit 14-3). This action allowed Polk County Health Department to continue to address the problem aggressively and fully implement the interventions needed to stop the outbreak.

Exhibit 14-3   Headline

Hepatitis Outbreak Spreads

Cases in August were the highest in Polk County this year, and the county health chief should seek help.

This was quoted from the *Des Moines Register*.

CDC: By the end of July, our study was coming to an end in Iowa, although some laboratory results and quite a bit of analysis still needed to be done. This part of the study would be completed after we returned to the CDC.[6]

We concluded that methamphetamine users in Iowa, especially injecting drug users, were at increased risk for hepatitis A. Hepatitis A was being transmitted from person to person through multiple routes among drug users, including sharing of drug paraphernalia. Also, a common source cluster of cases associated with a contaminated batch of "brown" methamphetamine may have occurred.

The benefits of our investigation included that it provided scientific data on the modes of hepatitis A transmission among drug users and that it provided information to support nationwide recommendations on vaccine use and prevention of hepatitis A transmission.

Narcotics: During the outbreak period, I constantly updated my colleagues at the division, as well as the four other states in the Midwest High Intensity Drug Trafficking Area (Midwest HIDTA), which combats the continuing rise of methamphetamine use. None of the other states reported outbreaks of hepatitis A in their areas. In mid January 1998, divisional agents received their second hepatitis A shots.

Newspaper: As a journalist, my role in all of this was to report what I heard and saw from health officials and other sources and develop any other related stories that would help readers understand the subject and the players. Fortunately for the public, other journalists, and myself, there are good relationships between the media and those at the state and local health departments. As the state epidemiologist was once quoted as saying, "Getting information to the public is a huge piece of the job, and we couldn't do it without the media."

State Epidemiologist: As steps were taken to control the outbreak, the CDC investigation was completed, and the media attention dissipated, we watched the case numbers carefully. By early fall, they began to decline, and although the numbers briefly increased again later, the outbreak was over by the spring of 1998.

In 1997, 1,574 doses of hepatitis A vaccine were given in Polk County. Of these, 78 were given anonymously. The rest provided names and addresses to facilitate sending second dose reminders, of which 1,496 were sent. Just over 250 of these reminders were returned by the post office for reasons that included insufficient address or resident no longer at that address. Although no response was received from 720 people, 492 persons did return to the local health department to receive the second dose of hepatitis A vaccine.

The fact that so many people gave their names and addresses to the local health department for the second shot reminder demonstrates the confidence that the people in these risk groups (e.g., the drug users) had in public health to keep this information confidential. It says a lot about how comfortable this community felt in working with the local public health workers, especially the nurses.

In the end, a lot of resources were used to investigate and control this outbreak, but hepatitis A never expanded to a community-wide outbreak. We felt we had been successful.

CONCLUSION

Epidemic investigations are never done in isolation. As you can see by the previously mentioned example, many people, organizations, and the public participate in stopping an outbreak. By definition, epidemics occur in a community or a portion of a community, and ultimately, it is the community's actions that contain or stop an outbreak. Public health's main role is to determine the cause(s) of the outbreak and then to assist the community in implementing the actions that would be most effective in halting the epidemic. If the community is not behind the public health efforts, it is unlikely that the epidemic will be controlled.

REFERENCES

1. Heymann DL. Viral hepatitis A. In Heymann DL, ed. *Control of Communicable Diseases Manual*, 18th ed. Washington, D.C. American Public Health Association, 2004:247–253.
2. Centers for Disease Control and Prevention. Prevention of hepatitis A through active or passive immunization. *MMWR Morb Mortal Wkly Rep* 2006;55:1–23.
3. Iowa Department of Public Health. Reportable Diseases by Year. 1930 to Present. Retrieved April 20, 2007, from http://www.idph.state.ia.us/adper/common/pdf/cade/decades.pdf.
4. Hutin YJF, Bell BP, Marshall KLE, et al. Identifying target groups for a potential vaccination program during a hepatitis A community-wide outbreak. *Am J Public Health* 1999;89:918–921.

5. Centers for Disease Control and Prevention. Hepatitis A associated with consumption of frozen strawberries—Michigan, March 1997. *MMWR Morb Mortal Wkly Rep* 1997;46:288.
6. Hutin YJF, Sabin KM, Hutwagner LC, et al. Multiple modes of hepatitis A virus transmission among methamphetamine users. *Am J Epidemiol* 2000;152:186–192.

Note: In 2007, the Advisory Committee on Immunization Practices (ACIP) revised the national guidelines to include the use of hepatitis A vaccine postexposure. See http://www.cdc.gov/mmwr/preview/mmwrhtml/mm5641a3.html/.

CHAPTER 15

Tracking a Syphilis Outbreak Through Cyberspace

Jeffrey D. Klausner, MD, MPH

INTRODUCTION

It was April 1999. I was less than a year into my new job as deputy health officer and director of the Sexually Transmitted Disease (STD) Prevention Section in San Francisco. At that time, the section had about 70 staff members, operated the municipal STD clinic, and conducted surveillance, epidemiology, disease intervention and sexual health education and promotion with a budget of about $4 million. Whenever I mention my job title, folks always comment how tough it must be to have such a role in San Francisco. It seems that "Baghdad by the Bay" continues to have a reputation of unbridled sexual expression, resulting in the unmanageable consequences of the spread of sexually transmitted infections. Trying to control such diseases in San Francisco must be a Sisyphean task, they think.

Fortunately, I was well trained. I attended Cornell University for my undergraduate and medical school education, completed an internship and residency in internal medicine at Bellevue Hospital in New York City, and received a Master of Public Health degree from Harvard University. After all that, I became a member of the Center for Disease Control and Prevention's (CDC) Epidemic Intelligence Service, the nation's premier investigators of disease outbreaks, and was posted in the local health department in San Francisco. Finally, I completed a fellowship in infectious diseases at the University of Washington in Seattle to be certain that I'd be able to get a great job in public health.

In this new position as a public health official—my first "real job"—having finished 12 years of postgraduate education, I was seriously concerned that I would lose touch with patients and the care of sick individuals. To reduce that likelihood, I volunteered weekly at the San Francisco municipal STD clinic every Monday morning. It was a great way to start the week, meeting men and women who have waited all weekend for the STD clinic to open and get treated for the various bumps, sores, ulcers, and discharges emanating from their genitalia.

One Monday morning in the spring of 1999, I was interviewing a new patient at the STD clinic about his sexual behavior. When asked how many new sex partners he had in the past 6 months, he said 14. When asked how many new sex partners he had in the past 2 months, he said 14. Nonplussed, I asked him what happened 2 months ago. He paused, smiled and replied, "I got online."

I was curious and allowed my training as a COC investigator to manifest itself and asked the patient to tell me more. The story he related I will never forget. That story has become the foundation for an entire new field in sexual and reproductive health promotion and disease control—using the Internet to promote healthful behaviors, conduct disease investigations and partner notification, and offer screening and treatment for STDs.

Bill (whose name has been changed) told me that he went every day to America Online (AOL) to a specific chatroom named "SFM4M." In that chatroom, men looked for an immediate "hookup" (an in-person sexual encounter). When I looked at the screen for this chatroom, it showed that all the city sites were full—each had a capacity of 23 members at a single time. AOL members initiated a conversation through "instant messaging" and gave their "stats" such as age, hair and eye color, height, weight, and chest, arm, and penis size or provided a link to a webpage with photographs and additional specifics such as preferred sexual activity or meeting place.

Bill described how he—a self-described HIV-positive, balding, overweight man in his late 40s who had been finding it difficult to meet new sex partners lately—could now go online, meet a potential new sex partner in just a few minutes, and speak to them on the telephone. If he liked their voice, he'd invite them to his house. Peering through his living room window, he'd check them out and decide whether to let them in. Once inside his home, often verbal communication stopped, and he and his new partner had sex. Whether they had sex again or not was of little interest to him. He was just amazed at how easy and quick it was to find a new partner. Bill said that on some occasions hookups could be initiated and realized in less than 15 minutes. He seemed quite pleased with his recent discovery. I, however, felt much different. My emotions shifted from cool clinical detachment to an acute sense of epidemiologic foreboding.

THE OUTBREAK

In the summer of 1999, the CDC launched the fourth effort in the history of the United States to eliminate syphilis. Syphilis cases were approaching an all time low, and Congress had allocated $30 million a year in new funding to help the CDC reach that goal. Locally, we formed a syphilis elimination team with health department staff members, including the syphilis disease control investigators and representatives from a variety of community-based organizations. We drafted an outbreak response plan and met biweekly to review and improve current syphilis control efforts. In addition, I personally reviewed each and every new case to assure adequate treatment and to try to identify additional opportunities for the interruption of disease transmission.

Before the AIDS epidemic, syphilis was common in San Francisco, in particular among gay men and other men who have sex with men. Case counts hovered at about 2,000 cases a year in the 1970s, making San Francisco the nation's leader in new cases of syphilis. With the advent of the AIDS epidemic and the profound fear surrounding that untreatable and deadly disease, sexual behavior changed dramatically, and the number of cases of syphilis in San Francisco dropped substantially from over 2,200 cases in the early 1980s to a few dozen by the late 1990s. More importantly, there were only eight cases in gay men and other men who have sex with men in 1998, the lowest number ever recorded in San Francisco. It was perfect timing to eliminate syphilis. All of the conditions required for potential disease eradication were in place—only human-to-human transmission, low case counts, an easy and accurate test, and highly effective treatment that both prevented and cured infection. In the spring and summer of 1999, we were hypervigilant trying to detect the early signs of an outbreak—an increase in the number of cases over the expected rate. We performed a team review of every new case and carefully tried to rule out any evidence of sustained person-to-person transmission. Because the number of baseline cases was so few, any cluster of cases could be considered a potential outbreak.

Upon hearing Bill's story, I requested the syphilis team to inquire about Internet use and subsequent sex partnering or "hookups" among new cases of syphilis. I asked them to ask new syphilis cases who had used the Internet to meet sex partners what specific Internet sites they used and where they met—at someone's house, public space, or bar. In July, just 1 month later, we had two cases that reported meeting partners on AOL at SFM4M. One patient had met partners at that site only. Bingo! To identify additional cases, the investigators went back and reinterviewed persons with prior cases of syphilis infection acquired in the past year reported to the health department in 1999. The investigators found that all but one new syphilis case who used the Internet to find sex partners used AOL and the specific AOL chatroom SFM4M. I asked the disease-control investigators to collect "handles" or the screen names that AOL members use when they log in and use the chatrooms. I thought that we might be able to link cases through their screen names, as many case patients did not know the names or have other personal identifying information about their partners.

Based on our initial investigation of syphilis cases in gay men and other men who have sex with men in San Francisco, we were able to create a sexual network of interconnected cases. Figure 15-1 shows that network, the early cases, and subsequent secondary cases. That one AOL chatroom linked all of the cases.[1] We defined cases as "early-stage syphilis among gay men reported to the San Francisco Department of Public Health in July and August 1999." (Early syphilis is defined as a patient who has acquired syphilis in the past year). Examining the sexual network demonstrated that the cases were all linked through the use of the chatroom and revealed the increased number of sex partners reported by some cases. One case reported 47 partners in the past 6 months. A moderate proportion (42%) of the contacts identified by the case patients had confirmed clinical evaluations (Figure 15-1). Overall, however, that moderate proportion of contacts receiving evaluation would make syphilis control in this population very difficult.

From case identification and confirmation of the outbreak, we had to move to a very important stage of our outbreak investigation—public health response. That was going to be tricky, as this was completely new territory,

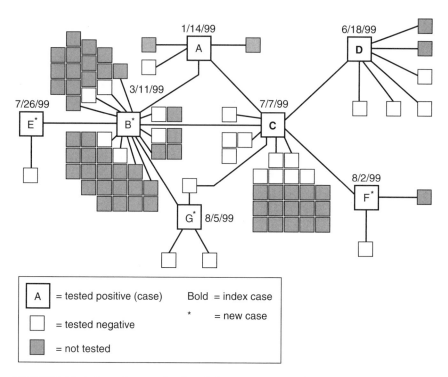

FIGURE 15-1 Sexual network of syphilis cases associated with Internet use, San Francisco, 1999.

Adapted from Klausner JD, Wolf W, Fischer-Ponce L, Zolt I, Katz MH. Tracing a syphilis outbreak through cyberspace. *JAMA* 2000;284:447–9. Copyright © 2000 American Medical Association. All rights reserved.

uncharted by prior epidemiologists and unknown to the CDC. This was cyberspace. We needed to act in parallel to warn users of the chatroom of their increased risk and determine the extent of their risk. I knew that the network diagram would be insufficient evidence for some, in particular for some fringe but outspoken gay men who were concerned at that time that the health department was falsely reporting increases in STDs in gay men and other men who have sex with men in its efforts to stigmatize gay sex further. (By 2001, my family and I received death threats that resulted in felony charges and prolonged jail time for two renegade gay male activists—but that is another story for another time.)[2] In addition, we needed very strong evidence because a multinational corporation such as AOL could try to refute the potential damaging association of syphilis and chatroom use. A nay sayer would argue that the frequency of Internet sex partnering is very common such that seven syphilis cases from one chat-room would not be beyond what might be expected.

Fortunately, after that discussion with Bill in April, I had immediately thought of the need to understand more about the use of the Internet and its role in sexual health at the population level. I collaborated with a PhD candidate at the University of California–Berkeley, Andrea Kim, who was looking for additional projects related to her thesis about the epidemiology of sexually transmitted diseases. We initiated a voluntary confidential sur-vey in gay men and other men who have sex with men attending the munic-ipal STD clinic to learn about the characteristics of men who used the Internet and measured the frequency of Internet use to find sex partners. Those survey results were linked to each participating patient's STD test-ing results, and I could easily identify a control population—a group of somewhat similar patients who were tested for syphilis and who were unin-fected.[3] I then could do a case-control study and compare the frequency of recent Internet use (the exposure) among those control patients from the survey with the frequency of recent Internet use among case patients. For the case-control study, I defined case patients as San Francisco residents with reported early syphilis infection (syphilis acquired in the prior year) from July to August 1999. I chose early syphilis as the disease classification because early syphilis is recently acquired—persons are infected by defini-tion in the past 12 months—and did not include patients with late syphilis or syphilis of unknown duration to reduce misclassification. In addition, I restricted the case population to gay men and other men who have sex with men to match the surveyed population of control patients.

Using standard epidemiologic analytic techniques, I made a 2×2 con-tingency table comparing the frequency of exposure in case-patients: 4 of 6 (67%) used the Internet to meet sex partners versus 6 of 32 (19%) who used the Internet to meet sex partners among control patients. The odds ratio or measure of association between the odds of being a syphilis case and recent use of the Internet to meet sex partners was 8.7. That value was statistically significant ($P = 0.03$) and thus was very unlikely to be due to chance. In other words, syphilis cases were nearly nine times more likely to have used the Internet to find a new sex partner than patients without syphilis. I had the evidence I needed. The evidence was irrefutable in the court of epidemiology.

Because of the strong and significant association between men using the Internet to meet sex partners and the fact that five of the six cases reported using the AOL chatroom SFM4M, my next steps were to inform AOL and alert the community and medical providers in San Francisco. As part of our outbreak response plan, we had a list of contact information for key community leaders, community-based organizations, local newspapers, and medical care providers, including those who took care of patients with HIV-infection and dermatologists—skin specialists who often see patients with diseases such as syphilis. We sent out a letter through the mail and facsimile stating that we had identified an increase in the number of syphilis cases in gay men and other men who have sex with men that were linked to meeting in a chatroom, AOL SFM4M. We informed readers of the basic signs and symptoms of syphilis and provided treatment and management recommendations and a link to our website (www.sfcityclinic.org) with more information.

Reaching someone at AOL who would collaborate in our investigation and public health response was a significant challenge. How many of us have tried to reach an Internet service provider and were successful in speaking with a live person? I was no different and had no special access. I went to the AOL website and tried to identify the location of the corporate headquarters (Virginia) and attempted to call someone who would work with me to inform AOL members and handle the gathering media storm. Realizing that this was as much about public relations as anything else, I asked to speak with someone in public relations who might provide some assistance. My main aim, initially, in working with AOL was to gather additional locating information for cases of which I only had screen names. AOL certainly had personal and contact information such as name, home address, electronic mail, and various telephone numbers, including likely cellular telephone number. With that information, I could have the investigators contact AOL SFM4M users, directly notify them of their potential exposure, and encourage them to get tested and treated for a possible exposure to syphilis.

Because the incubation of syphilis is on average 3 weeks, if a person is given preventive treatment after exposure with injectable penicillin, the syphilis infection can be aborted. Fortunately, the same dose of penicillin used for preventive treatment is used for the treatment of early syphilis; therefore, even if treatment is delayed in exposed patients, it is still adequate.

My second aim was to convince AOL to work toward proactively preventing future outbreaks of STDs associated with its members meeting sex partners in chatrooms. I suggested they post advertisements in the chatroom about the syphilis increase, promote regular STD and HIV testing, provide links to further information about safer sex practices, and create a chatroom environment that was conducive to healthful sexual encounters.

Reaching anyone within AOL who would collaborate with me proved very difficult, however. No one would return my calls. Because the headquarters of AOL was in Virginia, I contacted the Virginia Department of Health and asked them to help me. Although not definitely obstructive, the state epidemiologist in Virginia at the time did not agree with me about the urgency to contact AOL. He had spoken to others at the CDC who seemed to agree and were reluctant to exercise their public health authority in the response to the outbreak. I don't think that they appreciated my unique perspective here in San Francisco where Internet partnering was rapidly increasing and the Internet was becoming a very popular place to meet sex partners. Over time, my concern was validated, and Internet sites have become the most commonly cited place where new cases of syphilis in California report meeting sex partners (Figure 15-2). Finally, as the news of the outbreak began to be covered in the media, I did reach an AOL public relations executive, Peter (whose name has been changed). The power of the media is an important lesson that I have learned in public health. When the media calls a company or institution,

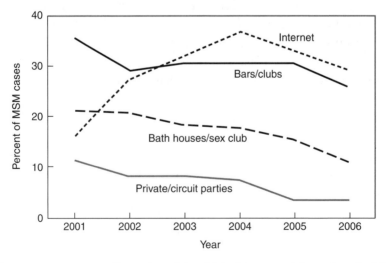

FIGURE 15-2 Percent of Interviewed Gay Male Primary and Secondary Syphilis Cases.

someone has to comment, and the person making those comments is often a senior executive within the company. After that person's name is associated with the issue in public, that person owns, at least partly owns, the problem; however, Peter was not willing to facilitate my getting further contact information on AOL members who used the SFM4M chatroom. Members' information was private. I became frustrated but soon obtained a lucky break.

Through a personal contact in San Francisco—a friend's sister worked at AOL corporate headquarters—I learned the name of an AOL corporate attorney in Virginia. I sent her e-mail, facsimiles, and certified letters by the U.S. postal service making sure that she was aware—and there was ample documentation of my communications—of the serious nature of the current situation. Through other contacts, I learned that a former high-level gay male governmental official in the Clinton Administration was now working as a senior executive for AOL-Time Warner in New York City—the parent corporation of AOL—and thinking that he might be sympathetic to such issues in gay men's health sought his advice and cooperation. With the continued pressure that I applied, I was ultimately and officially informed that such personal contact information of AOL members could only be released on Federal subpoena or in the case of an imminent grave danger—such as homicide or suicide. I could not justify that syphilis infection posed an immediate and life-threatening danger (with the advent of penicillin and other antibiotics, death due to syphilis infection had become rare in the latter half of the 20th century, and I had never seen a patient die of syphilis infection). A Federal subpoena seemed possible but would take a long time and be expensive and not by any means a guaranteed success.

Of course, I had informed my colleagues at CDC at the Division of STD Prevention and even further up the hierarchy to include the Director of the National Center for STD, HIV, and TB Prevention. Again, I sent e-mails and facsimiles and mailed letters to the CDC. Although personally sympathetic, various persons at the CDC felt it could not directly intervene with AOL, did not want to make a "federal case" out of it, and would leave things to me in San Francisco. It seemed to me that leaders at the CDC failed to recognize the significance of the outbreak as a harbinger of much larger things to come.

Fortunately, the public relations executive from AOL, in his never ending quest to get rid of me and delegate what only could be a massive headache and public relations disaster for him, put me in touch with Ted (name has been changed), the Chief Executive Officer of PlanetOut, an online community for gay, bisexual, lesbian, and transgender persons headquartered in my hometown in San Francisco. The PlanetOut website offered a range of services, including travel, news, weather, and an online community and was partly owned or supported at that time by AOL. Ted was what I needed. He was a tall, gregarious man with the "can do" "24/7" attitude working in the midst of the 20th century Internet gold rush of 1999 building his great profit machine in cyberspace. Media attention was what he needed and wanted most. Ted detailed a dozen of his staff—various programmers, writers, and marketing personnel—to go online to AOL SFM4M for 2 continuous weeks and inform users about the syphilis outbreak, offer syphilis education, and encourage users to get tested. Because of the privacy concerns of both of the companies, we don't have data about the number or frequency of users who were informed, got tested, or received preventive therapy. Based on chatroom usage patterns, we estimated that thousands were made aware of the outbreak and learned about syphilis, and many of those sought medical care. To evaluate those prevention efforts, we polled a sample of users of SFM4M about the appropriateness of the information campaign. The online survey revealed that 25 of 35 respondents (71%) thought that the awareness campaign on the Internet was useful and appropriate.

To enhance community awareness further and further persuade AOL into being more cooperative, the San Francisco Department of Public Health issued a press release in August of 1999 identifying the direct link between use of the AOL chatroom to meet sex partners and the increase in syphilis cases. In that press release, we also highlighted the lack of willingness of AOL to inform its members but the welcome assistance of staff from PlanetOut. I felt that shaming AOL in view of the general public might prompt them into action. Using the media to confront corporations is a potentially useful but dangerous tactic. No one likes to be embarrassed in the media, particularly public companies. It is a tactic, however, that I have witnessed to be very effective in certain areas of AIDS activism. It is necessary to avoid hyperbole and let the reader or viewer draw his or her own conclusions. Because the media is neutral and is primarily interested in selling newspapers or advertising time, the media does not really care whether the story is about an overzealous local government or an uncaring corporation. The media will go where the most provocative story is. In my case, because my main goal was to raise awareness about the outbreak, any local media I could generate would be beneficial. National media would not help local persons at risk for syphilis but could sway AOL into action. At the minimum, the CDC could not deny its awareness of the situation and might also be pushed into action.

Steve Case, the founder of AOL, had attributed the rapid and sustained success of AOL to its use by the gay community. In public comments, Mr. Case stated that the gay community's use of features like electronic mail, chatrooms, and instant messages unique to AOL at the time was key to AOL's success. He went on to thank the gay community for their early support and allegiance to AOL. "The gay community was a godsend for the company," wrote *Wall Street Journal* technology reporter Kara Swisher in her book *AOL.com: How Steve Case Beat Bill Gates, Nailed the Netheads, and Made Millions in the War for the Web.*[4] "AOL offered a 'live and let live' online space and gays responded by generating huge amounts of revenue for the company." Steve Case said, "Thank God for the gays and lesbians," according to Swisher, noting that use of the online service by gays was particularly heavy in sexually themed chat rooms.

Privacy concerns among Internet users became an issue of national debate. Many national newspapers, including a lead front-page article in the *New York Times* ("Privacy Questions Raised in Cases of Syphilis Linked to Chat Room"),[5] reported on the varied opinions of privacy experts and public health advocates regarding an individual's right to privacy and the government's mandate to protect public health.

In addition to collaborating with Ted at PlanetOut to conduct specific awareness to the potentially exposed population identified through our outbreak investigation, we developed new protocols for public health disease control investigators on how to use the Internet to conduct online partner notification.[6] It is hard to believe that in 1999 many county and state health departments in the United States did not have Internet access or use electronic mail. For those that did, some could not access Internet sites on the World Wide Web outside of their own local network. Many localities had administrative policies specifically stating that personnel could not access the World Wide Web and used firewalls and other techniques to block staff from such use.

By late Fall 1999, the number of new syphilis cases who reported meeting sex partners on AOL SFM4M declined. Unfortunately, that was not the end of increases in syphilis among gay men and other men who have sex with men in the United States. Over the next several years, San Francisco experienced an increase in syphilis from that low in 1998 of 8 cases in gay men and other men who have sex with men to over 550 cases by 2004. Other cities such as Seattle, Los Angeles, San Diego, Chicago, Houston, Atlanta, Miami, Fort Lauderdale, and New York have experienced similar increases. In many cities, those increases continue today. Similar increases have been seen internationally in major cities of Australia, Canada, and Western Europe. The use of the Internet by gay men and other men who have sex with men to meet sex partners has helped to let the syphilis "genie" out of the bottle.

Currently, asking whether new cases of syphilis have met recent partners on the Internet is a routine component of syphilis surveillance. In California, the frequency of meeting partners on the Internet among syphilis cases increased from about 10% in 2000 to over 40% in 2005, making it more common than traditional sites such as bars/clubs, sex clubs, or parks (Figure 15-1). The Internet has become the bathhouse of the 21st century.

Chatrooms have given way to entire Internet sites that exist for the expressed purpose of linking sex partners. Persons can post photos, maintain a record of prior contacts, and search and sort by a variety of sexual preferences. Sites such as Manhunt and Adam4adam have replaced AOL as the most frequently reported venue for new syphilis cases to report meeting sex partners. Sites such as Craigslist that have city-specific sites like CraigslistSF.org allow for persons traveling to certain cities to identify and plan sexual encounters in advance. To its credit, Craigslist has allowed its site to host online sexual health message boards and provides a routine warning to users of categories such as "men seeking men" about the increases in syphilis transmission associated with meeting partners online.

IMPLICATIONS

Recognizing that the Internet has become the most common venue for gay men and other men who have sex with men at risk for sexually transmitted diseases, including HIV infection, required me to develop a new approach to sexual health promotion and disease prevention. With the additional resources for syphilis control made available in San Francisco by the CDC's effort for national syphilis elimination and the requirement that a proportion of those funds be directly allocated to community-based organizations, I helped stimulate the creation of a new organization called Internet Sexuality Information Services, Inc. (www.ISIS-Inc.org). ISIS-Inc. provides a variety of Internet-based prevention services targeting gay men and other men who have sex with men. Originally focused on men in San Francisco, now ISIS-Inc. works with health departments and community-based organizations worldwide. Innovations developed by Deb Levine, the founder of ISIS-Inc. and I include an online syphilis testing program (STDTest.org) where the public can complete their own syphilis test requisition form, print it out, and bring it to a private laboratory for a free syphilis test. Test results are available securely online. The health department contacts all testers with syphilis and assures timely and adequate treatment. Currently, about 10 to 20 persons a week use the testing service, and the rate of syphilis positivity is about 5% (much higher than any other screening program in San Francisco).[7]

Another innovation includes a site called inSPOT.org, which allows cases of STDs (any STD including HIV infection) to notify a recent sex partner either anonymously or confidentially of exposure to that infection through an electronic postcard with embedded links to more information about the disease, referral information for testing. In the specific case of chlamydia and gonorrhea, inSPOT.org provides access to a free online prescription for treatment. Partners can print out the prescription and take it to a local pharmacy in San Francisco. This augmented peer-to-peer effort for partner notification empowers the user and the community and allows those who wish to take personal responsibility for partner notification an easy opportunity to conduct this important task. Anywhere from 10 to 100 notifications are made monthly in San Francisco, with the highest number of notifications occurring for cases of chlamydia and gonorrhea.

Further Internet-based prevention efforts include banner advertising on major websites named by recent cases of syphilis or HIV infection. These advertisements promote testing or other websites with information about STDs and safer sex practices. By monitoring the frequency of the display of these banner advertisements and the number of click-throughs to the site advertised, one can calculate the cost to the health department per click-through. We have measured a range of costs from less than 5 cents to over $10 per click-through, depending on the site and advertisement. "Ask Dr. K" at AskDrk.org (I am "Dr. K") is a website with honest and evidence-based answers to common questions about sex, sexual health, and sexually transmitted diseases. Although it has limited promotion, over 100 new questions are submitted each week. Frequently asked questions are posted to provide readers with ready and searchable answers.[8]

Other researchers and health officials have also developed Internet-based prevention interventions. Basic services like websites allow users to access sexual health information and clinic operating hours and see sites like Californiamen.net where users can download an electronic black book to record contact information of recent sexual encounters and follow the personal blogs of newly identified HIV-infected men. In 2007, the CDC funded the first Internet-based prevention research center at the Denver Department of Public Health, whose mission is to evaluate and promote effective Internet-based interventions. Scientists at the University of Washington-Seattle have developed and evaluated computer-based personal risk-reduction interventions. If adopted, promoted, and scaled to Internet users at risk for STDs and HIV infection, this intervention has the potential to have a profound impact on sexual risk behavior.[9]

Finally, Internet sex partnering sites run by health organizations that serve to facilitate both sex partnering and safer sex are in development. The move from the old model of bathhouses of the 1970s to 1980s that had no focus on sexual health to the new model of current bathhouses that supply safer sex materials (condoms, lubrication, educational pamphlets) enforce no sex without condom policies, restrict substance use on site, and make STD or HIV screening available is similarly and rapidly occurring on the Internet in its own context. Such sites have online health educators, links to information about sexual health, STDs and HIV infection, links to sites with testing information, and policies mitigating substance use and trafficking of illicit drugs such as methamphetamine.

Perhaps the most exciting aspects of Internet-based sexual or reproductive health promotion and disease prevention are its widespread availability, ease of use, and broad applicability to a range of health issues, in particular those health disparities affected by access to health care. In its first few months of operations, an online service in San Francisco for increased access to Plan B, the age-restricted over-the-counter medication for emergency contraception, has rapidly become a common site for adolescents—those under age 18 years of age who have limited access to Plan B—to obtain information and a free prescription, which they can use at any pharmacy in San Francisco.

CONCLUSIONS

What my patient relayed to me that Monday morning in the spring of 1999 set the stage for the identification and control of the first infectious disease outbreak associated with the use of the Internet to meet sex partners. Furthermore, with broad training in medicine, infectious diseases, and public health, as well as the availability of flexible resources and a highly supportive department director, I was able learn from the outbreak and stimulate the creation of a new field of health promotion and disease prevention. I am often asked to lecture in the United States and across the globe (e.g., Canada, England, Germany, Peru, Brazil, India) about the Internet, the outbreak of syphilis, and disease prevention. People seem fascinated by the combination of technology and sex. To update the old adage "sex sells," today I'd say "sex and the Internet" sells. Every new successful technological advance—printing press, photography, telephone, cinema, television, and the Internet—seems to have one thing in common, its ability to enhance life's sexual experiences.

Actively investigating outbreaks, including incorporating and even acquiring new knowledge during fieldwork, is what the term in the CDC's Epidemic Intelligence Service "shoe leather epidemiology" is all about. It is where the rubber meets the road. I hope this brief description of my experience in tracking a syphilis outbreak in cyberspace will allow future practitioners and policy makers to apply similar lessons in public health and observational epidemiology to improve the community's health and the conditions in which we all live.

REFERENCES

1. Klausner JD, Wolf W, Fischer-Ponce L, Zolt I, Katz MH. Tracing a syphilis outbreak through cyberspace. *JAMA* 2000;284:447–449.
2. Winter G. San Francisco AIDS debate leads to criminal charges. *New York Times*, December 24, 2001:A10.
3. Kim AA, Kent C, McFarland W, Klausner JD. Cruising on the internet highway. *J AIDS* 2001;28:89–93.
4. Swisher K. *AOL.com: How Steve Case Beat Bill Gates, Nailed the Netheads, and Made Millions in the War for the Web.* New York: Random House, 1998.
5. Nieves E. Privacy questions raised in cases of syphilis linked to chat room. *The New York Times*, August 25, 1999:A1.

6. Kent CK, Wolf W, Nieri G, Wong W, Klausner JD, Peterman TA. Internet use and early syphilis infection among men who have sex with men—San Francisco, California, 1999—2003. *Morb Mortal Wkly Rep* 2003;52:1229–1232.
7. Levine DK, Scott KC, Klausner JD. Online syphilis testing—confidential and convenient. *Sex Transm Dis* 2005;32:139–141.
8. Klausner JD, Levine DK, Kent CK. Internet-based site-specific interventions for syphilis prevention among gay and bisexual men. *AIDS Care* 2004;16:964–970.
9. Mackenzie SL, Kurth AE, Spielberg F, Severynen A, Malotte CK, St Lawrence J. Patient and staff perspectives on the use of a computer counseling tool for HIV and sexually transmitted infection risk reduction. *J Adolesc Health* 2007;40: 572.e9–16.

CHAPTER 16

Eschar: The Story of the New York City Department of Health 2001 Anthrax Investigation

Don Weiss MD, MPH, and Marci Layton, MD

INTRODUCTION

Definition:

> Eschar (es´kär)
> Greek eschara, a fireplace, a scab caused by burning]. A dark scab, coagulated crust or slough resulting from the destruction of living tissue following a burn, the bite of a mite or as a result of anthrax infection (adapted from the Oxford English Dictionary).

(The term anthrax is used here to describe clinical disease caused by infection with *Bacillus anthracis*. The terms *Bacillus anthracis* and *B. anthracis* are used when referring to the bacterium).

Late on the afternoon of October 4, 2001, Marci Layton, Assistant Commissioner of the Bureau of Communicable Disease, New York City Department of Health (DOH) called us into her cramped office. She wouldn't call it cramped, but if more than three people met with her at the same time, one had to squeeze into a chair wedged between the bookshelf and the table. I moved to that seat in anticipation of Joel Ackelsberg and Annie Fine joining Sharon Balter, Mike Phillips, and myself. Joel, Annie, Sharon, and I were the bureau's core of medical epidemiologists, and Mike was our first-year Epidemic Intelligence Service (EIS) officer. Marci, as assistant commissioner, ran the operation. Sharon and I and a legion of others who certainly wouldn't fit into Marci's office had just spent the weeks following the destruction of the World Trade Center (WTC) towers setting up a new disease surveillance system in New York City. This system was implemented to bolster detection of unusual disease events, specifically bioterrorism, and relied on placing an EIS Officer in each of 15 sentinel emergency departments. We worked 12- to 18-hour days, doing everything from playing den mother to the 40 EIS officers to investigating unusual clustering of patients with febrile and other illnesses.

Just a few days before the meeting in Marci's office, we'd returned to our 125 Worth Street offices. The damage at the WTC had affected the local power grid and phone service in the area, and this, along with the pungent air, forced a 2.5-week relocation uptown. Although power was restored, most phone service remained out. My cluttered cubicle looked as foreign to me as a time capsule opened after 50 years of internment. The Centers for Disease Control (CDC) wanted their EIS officers back, and thus, our task was to convert the mostly manual system to an exclusively electronic one, all while trying to get back to our usual and long-neglected tasks such as investigating cases of typhoid fever, meningococcal disease, and West Nile virus. Thus, we exhaled deeply as we moved into Marci's office and prepared for the news.

A high-level epidemiologist in the CDC's bioterrorism response program, stationed in New York City since 9/11, had pulled Marci aside to tell her that the Florida Health Department and CDC were about to announce a case of inhalational anthrax in a 63-year-old man who worked as a photo editor. His disease onset was September 30; he had evidence of meningitis as well as mediastinitis and was doing poorly. The investigation was examining possible natural exposures, as the individual was reportedly an avid outdoorsman with a recent fishing trip to North Carolina. In the initial public comment about the case, Secretary of Health and Human Services, Tommy Thompson, offered the conjecture that the patient acquired anthrax from drinking spring water contaminated by a dead animal carcass. We are, by nature and experience, a skeptical lot. Although we all immediately considered this bioterrorism until proven otherwise, a photo editor and the Florida location seemed an unlikely choice of a terrorist. There was a rumor about an airport near the patient's home that may have been used as a training location for the 9/11 hijackers. Rather than indulge in debate, our oft and wanton pastime, we began constructing a plan for enhanced surveillance for inhalational anthrax in New York City. Over the next 2 days we made what would become the first of several rounds of active surveillance calls. Concerned that there might be an undiagnosed anthrax case, we called every hospital and laboratory operating in New York City to inquire about possible anthrax and to remind the medical community to report suspect cases.

The disease anthrax is caused by infection with the spore-forming bacterium *Bacillus anthracis*. Named for the coal-black scab (eschar), which forms at the site of skin invasion, it is mostly a disease of animals but has plagued humans since antiquity. It can be found worldwide and persists in soil in the dormant spore form. Several clinical syndromes are recognized and differ by the route of entry into the human body. Cutaneous anthrax occurs when *B. anthracis* enters through a breach in the skin's protective barrier. A pimple forms which progresses to an ulcer and heals with the characteristic black scab. Cutaneous infections mostly remain limited to the skin and area lymph glands; however, bloodborne infection can occur. Although the mildest form, untreated cutaneous anthrax may kill up to one fifth of its victims. Gastrointestinal anthrax occurs when the bacteria are ingested. This form usually occurs by consumption of contaminated meat from animals that died of anthrax. After a period of abdominal pain, fever, and vomiting, bloody diarrhea and sepsis may ensue, claiming half of those infected. Inhalational or pulmonary anthrax occurs when spores are inhaled. The most serious form of anthrax, it is fortunately rare and in the modern era has mostly occurred in workers exposed to aerosols generated during the commercial processing of animal hair and hides. An infection in the lung's lymph nodes and surrounding tissue, known as mediastinitis, is the major clinical finding. The bacteria then enter the blood where released *B. anthracis* toxins cause a rapid collapse of the circulatory system. Once in the blood stream, *B. anthracis* can travel to other locations, causing multiorgan failure and meningitis. Death is the usual outcome in inhalational anthrax cases. The vast majority of anthrax cases are the cutaneous form and the disease is quite rare in the United States.

THE OUTBREAK AND INVESTIGATION

I couldn't help thinking, as we organized staff to make the enhanced surveillance calls, that we had only just returned to our offices and had begun reconstituting routine surveillance activities. One thing we didn't do very well during 9/11 was involve enough of the DOH workforce. Now we needed to get people back to work. Resuming normalcy was one way to try and put the horror of September behind us. Thus, while getting staff involved in making the calls to hospitals and labs wasn't exactly their normal activities, it did bring them into the investigation. We targeted emergency departments, intensive care units, infectious disease department chair persons, infection control practitioners, and laboratorians. We told them what we knew of the Florida case and asked them to be particularly observant. Should a previously well person come in with sepsis, respiratory failure, or meningitis, he or she should keep anthrax in their differential diagnosis. Should a Gram-positive rod appear in a culture broth, don't discount it as a contaminant; instead, look into it further, and above all, call us. They could expect a medical alert from Marci soon explaining all of this in detail. We also conducted retrospective surveillance asking clinicians whether they had seen any patients going back to September 11th that fit the symptoms of inhalational, meningeal, or gastrointestinal anthrax. Four to five calls to 70 plus hospitals and labs kept staff occupied. I figured typhoid fever could and would have to wait a bit longer. To handle incoming calls after hours, we divided up the city giving the Poison Control Center, which received after-hours calls from clinicians, our cell phone numbers. Marci took all calls from Manhattan hospitals. Sharon got Queens. Annie took Brooklyn, and I took the Bronx and Staten Island. It wasn't long before our phones began ringing at all hours.

Meanwhile, Marci prepared a medical alert. The medical alert system was her own creation and had served DOH well during the West Nile virus outbreak of 1999. At the time, it was relatively low-tech, blast faxes sent to hospitals and laboratories with information, instructions, and specific requests for assistance. Hospital-based health care providers had come to expect these alerts and trusted that if there was something going on the DOH would communicate it to them in all due haste.

What several of us didn't know at the time was that Joel had evaluated a white powder threat letter and suspicious cutaneous anthrax case on October 1. As our bioterrorism readiness coordinator and intra-agency liaison, he regularly responded to such incidents, a dozen or more since joining the department the previous summer. All of the incidents had turned out to be hoaxes. The woman in question was Tom Brokaw's assistant at NBC News, and she noticed on September 25th a flesh-colored bump about the size of a pea just below her left collar bone and rimmed by scant erythema (redness). Over the next few days, it enlarged and became a fluid-filled vesicle. The surrounding skin became more inflamed and swollen, resembling an oblong cigarette burn. The weekend passed fitfully for her; she experienced headache and malaise, and after repeated urgings from her husband to see a doctor, she began taking leftover antibiotic that she had at home. That Monday, October 1st, the erythema increased, and the normal contour of her collarbone was obscured by the swelling. She showed it to the physician at NBC. Recalling the unusual threat letter containing powder that spilled on her chest the previous week, she raised the possibility of anthrax.

When Joel heard her story, he followed the protocol he had written. The FBI retrieved the threat letter and powder, which were tested at the New York City Public Health Laboratory (PHL). The powder was negative for *B. anthracis* by direct fluorescent antibody and culture. Direct fluorescent antibody is a staining technique in which antibodies specific to the *B. anthracis* cell wall are linked to chemical that glows when exposed to a certain wavelength of light. It is an extremely powerful tool for identifying *B. anthracis*, as it can be used on powders as well as clinical specimens. A routine swab of the wound for bacterial culture was negative, not surprising because the patient had been on antibiotics. Based on these results and that she was improving on treatment, there appeared little reason to perform a biopsy, the excision of a small amount of wound tissue to examine for *B. anthracis*. The patient's unusual skin lesion was attributed to the bite of a Brown Recluse spider that had ventured far from its normal range. NBC, as we were soon to learn, received these types of letters quite frequently.

We followed the Florida investigation like football fans watching the OJ Simpson trial, hoping it wasn't so. Secretary of Health and Human Services Thompson was again speaking publicly, emphasizing the isolated nature of the case. We remained dubious. The Florida patient died the next day, October 5th. Investigations in North Carolina and the patient's office had not turned up any clues. The EIS officers, now stationed in 12 New York City hospitals, kept looking for unusual cases, and we triaged calls from worried clinicians seeing patients who were ill and bore some distant connection to Florida. By October 7, the CDC and FBI knew that the Florida case was bioterrorism. People in Florida likely knew as well because the FBI had sealed off the America Media Inc. (AMI) building, where the patient had worked, as a crime scene. The next morning the rest of the country found out that environmental samples taken at AMI, from the work space of the Florida case, were positive for *B. anthracis* and that a second AMI worker had inhalational anthrax.

October 8th was Columbus Day, a holiday, although most of us worked anyway. Marci spent the morning evaluating a smallpox case that wasn't and the afternoon through evening at another white-powder incident at a British Company in midtown Manhattan. The rest of us were busy fielding an increase in anthrax calls from worried New Yorkers and the physicians caring for them that had been provoked by the breaking news from Florida. It was nearly 10:00 p.m. when Marci returned to an empty DOH building. Her momentary peace was interrupted by a call from the FBI agent who was with her at the white-powder hoax earlier that afternoon. The incident wasn't why he was calling. The sick NBC employee called him. She was following the news closely, and she wondered whether her unusual skin lesions could be anthrax after all. Marci called the NBC employee and the woman described to her in chronological detail the progression of her skin infection and then e-mailed Marci links to web images of cutaneous anthrax that looked like her own lesion. Over the next 24 hours she was seen by an infectious disease specialist who felt certain this was cutaneous anthrax and then by a dermatologist who concurred. Sharon met her at the dermatologist's office where a biopsy of her lesion and a blood sample for *B. anthracis* antibodies were obtained. Sharon next called CDC to ask that they test the tissue and blood. The emergency response center at CDC informed her that they were swamped with the Florida investigation and suggested that she try the New York State lab. This didn't sit well with Marci, who out of experience, or perhaps premonition, knew that this was an important sample that needed to go directly to CDC. Although the New York State Wadsworth Center was a very good laboratory, they lacked the experience with *B. anthracis* and would not be able to perform immunohistochemical staining (IHC) on the skin biopsy sample. IHC is a tissue-staining technique that uses antibodies specific to what you are looking for, in this case the anthrax bacillus. The antibodies are linked to a molecule that produces a color reaction, thereby highlighting the presence of the organism. Marci made a call to a high-level official at the CDC who she knew from her many interactions with them, from the 1996 Cyclospora in raspberries outbreak to initial U.S. outbreak of West Nile virus in 1999. He agreed to test the clinical specimens as well as the September 25th threat letter. Both were immediately flown to the CDC in Atlanta, GA by a special courier, who happened to be the same CDC staffer who first informed Marci of the Florida anthrax case. The specimens arrived contemporaneously with a power outage at CDC, which postponed testing until October 11. While awaiting the results, we stayed busy with phone calls and preparing for the worst case scenario.

One of the things that worked well during our response to 9/11 was computer and network access. Within hours of our relocation to the PHL back on September 12, 2001, the information technology team had us up and running. Their support throughout the anthrax investigation was to prove invaluable. Thus, when I arrived at my cubicle on October 9, I was unprepared to see the "blue screen of death," a well known sign of serious computer trouble. Perhaps it was an omen of what was to come because that very evening I found myself on Staten Island sorting through trash outside a suspect case's home, looking for a threat letter with powder reportedly postmarked from Florida (Figure 16-1). The recipient and his family had vague medical complaints but were not seriously ill. My

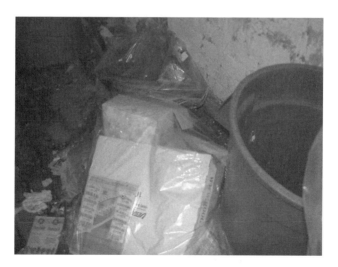

FIGURE 16-1 Sifting through trash for a threat letter on Staten Island. Courtesy of Don Weiss.

rumpled appearance and odd questions about tape and excessive postage on envelopes, possible signs of tainted letters, must have made me seem like Detective Columbo. The next day, October 10, I recorded in my notebook a heightened sense of anxiety at work. More calls were coming in from community physicians. The chief of staff's assistant stopped by to inquire about a rumor that the FBI had some tests results. This I could not confirm, and when I approached Marci, even she was uncharacteristically terse.

Another young woman, who regularly opened mail at NBC for Tom Brokaw and worked closely with his assistant, was herself ill in late September 2001. For her, it began with throat soreness, swollen glands, and a few papules on her face. She too experienced fever and fatigue and saw her doctor on the same day as her co-worker, October 1st. After a few days recuperating at home, she returned to work just as the news about the Florida inhalational anthrax case was breaking. She began to put it together. Brokaw, on learning of another of his staff with a suspicious skin lesion, arranged to have her seen by the same infectious disease specialist who had seen his assistant. On October 10, Sharon spoke with the doctor and then the young woman. Sharon learned that among the many "critic" letters there were actually two recent ones that had contained powder. The letter that arrived on September 25th and had tested negative for *B. anthracis* bore an uncanny similarity in penmanship in the eyes of NBC staff to the letter that had arrived a week earlier around September 18th. The first letter arrived a week after the WTC attacks and contained a crushed brownish material. Written on the enclosed note was, "Death to Israel, Allah is God." The powder she had discarded, but the letter was kept. When the second letter arrived, this time with a finer, white powder, security came to take it and instructed staff not to open these types of letters anymore. In retrospect, we might have decided to send in a team of moon-suited investigators to search for the September 18th letter. This would have most certainly disrupted operations at NBC and caused alarm among their staff and a nationwide media stir. We had no evidence yet of anthrax in New York City, and it seemed prudent not to move to this step before we had proof based on laboratory confirmation of human illness or environmental contamination.

Results from CDC on the skin biopsy from Tom Brokaw's assistant, as well as retesting of the envelope, came near midnight on October 11th. The September 25th NBC letter (the second one received) had again tested negative. Polymerase chain reaction (PCR) testing on the skin biopsy was also negative for *B. anthracis*. PCR is an extremely powerful laboratory method that can detect small quantities of DNA specific to a particular organism, in this case *B. anthracis*. I think the building breathed a sigh of relief; otherwise, I don't think Marci would have left work at all that night. What remained were the IHC and antibody results. Although some of us slept uneasily at best, senior epidemiologists and laboratorians at CDC met in the early morning hours and agonized over apparently conflicting results. Although PCR on the letter and biopsy were negative, the immunohistochemical stain of the biopsy was positive for *B. anthracis*. This stain targets specific proteins in the *B. anthracis* capsule, and it was "lighting up" under a microscope. Sherif Zaki, a seasoned CDC pathologist, read the slide and was convinced that it was real. The implications of anthrax from a mailed letter were staggering, and the CDC deliberated as dawn approached. The final test for antibodies in her blood sample wouldn't be ready for several more hours. Just before 3:00 a.m., CDC Director Jeffrey Copeland awoke Marci to tell her the news; they were considering this positive for *B. anthracis*. Marci next switched on the phone tree that jolted the rest of us out of our fitful slumbers. Anthrax was here, in New York City. Report for work at 6:00 a.m. Among the thoughts running through my mind was a line from the Robin Williams movie *Good Morning Vietnam*. Williams as disc jockey Adrian Cronauer crows on the radio, "It's oh-six hundred hours," and then pointedly adds that the "oh" stands for, "Oh my f-ing God its early." In as much as Cronauer's expletive was more a comment on the Vietnam war than the early hour of reveille, our churning stomachs cared less about the hour of our congress than its topic.

October 12th was the beginning of a massive public health mobilization and multipronged investigation that was to last through Thanksgiving. In addition to the cutaneous anthrax case at NBC, we would hear about other highly concerning cases at three more major media corporations as well as letters, illnesses, and environmental contaminations requiring investigation. Over the ensuing 3 weeks, we performed an average of three concurrent investigations each day with some days as many as six (Figure 16-2). The following pages describe the major investigations in the order in which we learned of them. Details for each investigation are given as they unfolded over several days. The chronology of the story then returns to October 12 to follow the thread of the next investigation. Unspoken, yet never far from the minds of all involved in the investigation, and likely the entire

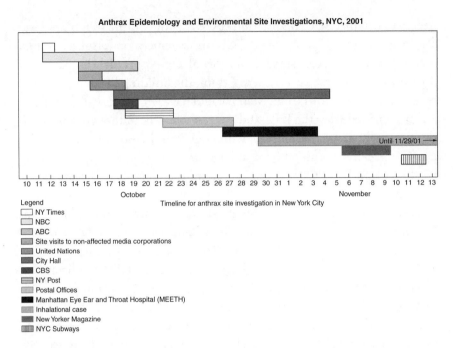

Anthrax Epidemiology and Environmental Site Investigations, NYC, 2001

Legend

Timeline for anthrax site investigation in New York City

☐ NY Times
☐ NBC
▨ ABC
▨ Site visits to non-affected media corporations
▨ United Nations
▨ City Hall
■ CBS
▤ NY Post
▨ Postal Offices
■ Manhattan Eye Ear and Throat Hospital (MEETH)
▨ Inhalational case
■ New Yorker Magazine
▥ NYC Subways

FIGURE 16-2   Timeline of anthrax investigations.

city, was the apprehension about inhalational anthrax. If cutaneous anthrax was in New York City, could inhalational be far behind?

A team was dispatched to NBC to interview workers in the same office as the index case. A point of distribution (POD) clinic was rapidly mobilized to dispense prophylactic antibiotics. A multiagency environmental assessment team was formed to create a *Bacillus anthracis* sampling plan. Mike and Marci went to 30 Rockefeller Plaza (the location of NBC offices), whereas Sharon stayed at our office to handle the deluge of provider calls. A medical alert was quickly drafted and distributed (Exhibit 16-1). It announced the case at NBC and added the clinical and diagnostic findings of cutaneous anthrax to the previously distributed descriptions of pulmonary and meningeal anthrax sent after 9/11 and again on October 5th. The alert reassured the medical community (and indirectly the public) that both traditional and syndromic surveillance systems had not uncovered any suspicious inhalational anthrax cases.

After the first case was verified, we actively sought out additional cases through interviews of co-workers and review of worksite employee health records. Surveillance was established for those currently ill, anyone whose

---

Exhibit 16-1   Medical Alert Announcing the First Cutaneous Anthrax Case in New York City

---

The City of New York

DEPARTMENT OF HEALTH

October 12, 2001

ALERT #8: 1—Case of cutaneous anthrax in an employee at 30 Rockefeller Center possibly exposed to a contaminated envelope.

[Correction: Prior communication that you may have received was inaccurate; at this time, NYC DOH is recommending prophylaxis and routine anthrax testing for *only* those who were on the 3rd floor of 30 Rockefeller Center on September 18th and 25th.]

The New York City Department of Health

- Requests Immediate Reporting of an Suspected Cases of Cutaneous, Pulmonary, Gastrointestinal, or Central Nervous System Anthrax (see Appendix I)
- Strongly Recommends Against Prescribing Prophylactic Antibiotics for anyone who was NOT on the 3rd floor of 30 Rockefeller Center on September 18th and 25th.
- Encourages Healthcare Providers to Remain Alert and Immediately Report any Unusual Disease Manifestations and Clusters

Please Share this Alert with All Medical, Pediatric, Nursing, Laboratory, Radiology, and Pharmacy Staff in Your Hospital

TO: Emergency Medicine Directors, Infection Control Practitioners and Infectious Disease Physicians, Laboratory Directors and Others on the NYCVDOH Broadcast Alert System

FROM: Marcelle Layton, MD, Assistant Commissioner

Communicable Disease Program

Case of cutaneous anthrax in New York City: On October 12, the New York City Department of Health was notified by the CDC that a specimen from a skin lesion was positive for *B. anthracis* by immunohistochemical stain. The patient is also serology positive.

Source: City of New York Department of Health.

illness in the past month met the case definition, and for future cases. At sites where threat letters were found, tracking the letter's path allowed us to focus the epidemiologic and environmental investigations on individuals at highest risk.

My assignment on October 12 was a stomach tossing, lights and sirens ride in an unmarked police car to the *New York Times* building, where a journalist had just opened a threat letter filled with powder. The target was a former Middle East correspondent who had recently written extensively on the risk of bioterrorism. She sliced open the letter at her desk in a large open room filled with work stations. Removing the single sheet, the pure white powder fell into her lap and onto the floor. The letter advised her to "go away for the next 4 weeks" and "watch the Sears tower come down." Witnesses described the powder as flour or talc-like with both a perfume and acrid odor. It turned out to be a hoax, but not before a long and tortuous journey to get the powder tested that involved the *New York Times* flying the specimen to the Massachusetts State laboratory in its own private jet. The journalist never did get her favorite sweater returned, which was submitted for testing.

At NBC, while Mayor Rudy Giuliani and Health Commissioner Neal Cohen announced the first anthrax case to the city from a hastily convened press conference, epidemiologists and law enforcement, alerted to the possibility of a second threat letter, began the search in parallel. When notes were compared, we learned the path that mail took through NBC. It was believed to have arrived on September 19th and was promptly x-rayed, as was the procedure for all mail. It was next taken to the 2nd-floor mailroom, where it was sorted into a pile destined for the 3rd, 4th, and 6th floors. It was further sorted to the 3rd-floor Nightly News offices, where it was given to a page, the woman Sharon had interviewed a few days earlier with suspicious skin lesions. She opened it just outside of the office of the first case, getting some of the crushed brown substance on her hands. The powder was dumped in the trash, the odd letter receiving no more notice than its mention of "Death to Israel," and "Allah is God." The envelope and letter were paper-clipped and given to Brokaw's assistant. It was then placed in a gray interoffice envelope and set aside, on her desk, next to the printer and forgotten. On October 9th, NBC security came and retrieved the gray envelope along with a stack of unopened, suspicious letters, placing them all in an ordinary plastic shopping bag. The bag was next brought to the 16th floor and left on a chair. Security moved the letter over the next several days to different offices, eventually returning it to the mailroom where the plan was to x-ray it again. Knowing the exact trail and possible contact with other mail would become important not only to make sense of the subsequent environmental findings but to understand transmission dynamics of the cases yet to come.

Thus, two threat letters with powder arrived at NBC in September 2001. One postmarked September 18th and the other September 25th. The letter of the 25th had already been tested and was negative at both the PHL and the CDC. The letter postmarked September 18th was located on the afternoon of October 12th in the 2nd-floor NBC mailroom and taken into evidence by a New York City Police Department detective and FBI agent. It was couriered to the PHL, where lab technologist Marie Wong was assigned to process the specimen. Inside a large, clear plastic Ziploc bag she found the folded gray interoffice envelope that contained the mailing envelope. A smaller Ziploc bag, also inside the larger one, contained the letter opened flat so that it could be read through the bag. Marie had been the laboratorian who tested the previous NBC letter (postmarked September 25th), which contained a copious amount of powder that was not *B. anthracis*. This letter looked different.

Taking the specimens into the biosafety hood for testing, she observed that the mailing envelope that had contained the threatening letter had very little powder. First, she delicately dug into each corner with a spatula, returning nothing. She slanted the envelope and tapped. Still nothing. Pausing for a moment, she noted that the handwritten address was slanted and looked like a child's writing. Peeling back the wrapper of a sterile swab, she applied a few drops of sterile saline and gently worked it into each corner of the envelope. When she pulled it out, stuck to the fuzzy tip were brown and black specks along with some sparkling white crystals. Pretty crystals, she thought. She prepared a wet mount and peered down into the microscope. She saw many large, oval structures lying on top of each other, packed like sardines. The entire slide was filled with them. Uh-oh, she thought, these look like spores. She called over two of her colleagues. They weren't sure but knew additional testing would answer the question. Marie promptly proceeded to set up the tests that within hours would confirm her initial observations that this was really *B. anthracis*.

Although the various law enforcement teams that routinely respond to powder threat incidents are usually exceptionally scrupulous about donning personal protective equipment and sealing off areas before entering a possible "hot zone," the chaos of that day, and perhaps concern over alarming NBC staff, disrupted standard operating procedures. The NBC letter had been stored in an ordinary, open plastic shopping bag and was transferred to the sealed plastic bag in open air. The gray interoffice envelope, which had for days contained the letter, was moved about without consideration that it too might be contaminated. Before testing occurred, the letter was photocopied down the hall from the bioterrorism lab, spreading *B. anthracis* spores throughout the copy room as well as the lab. This led to three PHL laboratorians and the detective courier testing positive on nasal or facial swabs. There may have been others contaminated by aerosolized spores, including myself, as the letter and bag made their way from NBC to the PHL, but no others were tested. I was in hallway outside the laboratory that evening to interview the detective and lab staff on what had transpired. The New York City bioterrorism lab was shut down because of *B. anthracis* spore contamination, just as the first batch of what would eventually number over 3,000 samples were arriving. While the PHL was prepared to respond to a bioterrorism event, consisting of one or a few samples, protocols and staffing were not designed to handle the daily influx of hundreds of environmental samples and nasal swabs from the media investigations, clinical specimens from hospitals, and items submitted from an increasingly unnerved general public. The loss of the primary laboratory served only to hasten the saturation point of laboratory capacity. What ensued has been termed "white powder hysteria" that not only affected New York City and the rest of the United States, but spread throughout the world. Anthrax scares disrupted government offices in Canada, England, France, Germany, and Australia in the week after the announcement of the NBC case. Powders closed newspaper offices, grounded planes, held people in quarantine for hours, and caused stocks to tumble.

Another of my assignments, along with our public health veterinarian Bryan Cherry and recent EIS alumnus Denis Nash, was to assist at the PHL with a specimen accession and result tracking system for environmental samples. The pressure for rapid reporting of results came from all sides—the mayor, the health commissioner, the CDC, media moguls, and the public. Their urgency clashed with antiquated laboratory information management systems. After the bioterrorism lab was closed, another lab was quickly outfitted, but the backlog of samples was immense. Some samples were shipped to other state laboratories whose own capacity was severely challenged by their own powder incidents. Although necessary, the use of these reference labs further compounded the problem of tracking results. Help also came in the form of laboratory teams from the CDC and the Department of Defense, but even with the extra hands there was really no keeping up with the influx of specimens, some of which were rather unusual.

The public was seeing threatening white powders where before they had seen ordinary items of their daily routines. Items such as parmesan cheese, Little Debbie Devil Creams, Apple Jacks, onion powder, and 40 fifty-dollar bills coated with a white substance were viewed with new suspicion and submitted for testing. Each panicked public call required the police or other law enforcement officers to evaluate, package, and transport the item(s) for testing. One prankster placed a small pile of talcum or the like on a sheet of toilet tissue in a common bathroom stall and then rolled it up so that the next patron got a very different puff than the one they had expected. Items clogged the storage area at the PHL and overflowed to the loading dock. Some items, like a sofa from Tom Brokaw's office, couldn't fit in the lab safety hood and presented additional challenges. PHL, CDC, and Department of Defense laboratory staff divided into teams and worked in shifts, 24 hours a day just to keep up, despite the implementation of a protocol to prioritize which specimens needed to be tested.

Specimens from a patient with a clinically worrisome illness consistent with any form of anthrax were given the highest priority. Incidents in which there was documented dispersal of powder with a possible risk to many came next, and the third level was for letters or packages in which law enforcement had determined a credible threat existed. Credible threats were those that appeared similar to letters already found, with one or more of the following characteristics: a threat letter mentioning anthrax or referencing 9/11; no return address, suspicious postmark, or handwriting; common word misspelling; excessive postage or securing materials such as tape; noticeable bulk; marked as "personal" or "confidential"; or sent to a high profile person such as Tom Brokaw. Other items were either not tested or testing was postponed. One FBI agent, who through his integrity and open communication had already earned the respect and admiration of many involved in the investigation, practically lived at the PHL triaging the incoming samples.

Returning to the swirl of events on October 12th, an interminably long day for those of us in the field and certainly equally exhausting for those left back at the home base to receive phone calls, we learned of other suspicious cutaneous cases at ABC, CBS, and the New York Post. These new reports fit the profile of a clinically compatible skin infection in a person who handled mail for a high-level media employee. In order to handle multiple investigations DOH re-activated its Incident Command System, which had precious few days to recover from responding to the World Trade Center attack. The Incident Command System was developed in order to coordinate the multiagency response to large forest fires and relied on a military-style structure of responsibility and reporting. An associate commissioner or comparable level staff was assigned to each media site to function as the direct link to the health department. His or her job was to oversee the teams dispatched to conduct epidemiology interviews, perform environmental sampling, assess risk exposure and distribute prophylactic antibiotics at point of distribution (POD) centers, and provide education about anthrax.

In the beginning, what we knew about anthrax all came from textbooks and expert consultants who like us had never dealt with a bioterrorism attack. Educational sessions at the media sites in the early days of the outbreak were daunting. Dr. Isaac Weisfuse, then associate commissioner for disease control and site liaison to NBC, faced an anxious and agitated crowd of investigative reporters on that first day, October 12th. Because of concerns of spore dissemination, the air conditioning system had been shut off. For what seemed like hours, they pummeled him with tough, unanswerable questions. The implacable Dr. Weisfuse realized the right thing to do was to acknowledge that we simply didn't know all the answers, rather than reassure the public based on insufficient data. The critical decisions of risk communication that emerged that day and over the course of the outbreak were deftly managed by the DOH communications director, Sandy Mullin. For Dr. Weisfuse, however, the temperature in the room wasn't the only thing broiling that afternoon.

The environmental investigation was complicated by the absence of existing protocols for *B. anthracis* environmental testing. What is the normal background rate of *B. anthracis* spores? What is the threshold limit that poses no human health threat? Conventional wisdom held that once spores fell to the ground, they would remain, pinned in place by electrostatic forces. Was this really true? If spores were tracked elsewhere, was there any risk to human health? Environmental testing occurred at all media sites in which a clinical case was detected as well as media sites without cases in order to detect exposure before disease occurred (Figure 16-3). The role of nasal swab testing for *B. anthracis* spores was purely to learn the location and expanse of exposure, not for individual patient treatment decisions; nevertheless, employees at the involved media sites, who learned of the swab test, had come to expect their noses to be swabbed and treatment decisions based on the results. We were in uncharted waters—icebergs seemed to be everywhere and safe port invisible beyond the horizon.

The next media site investigated was ABC. The call also came in on October 12 about a 7-month-old boy who was hospitalized with a skin infection. He attended a seemingly innocuous workplace birthday party,

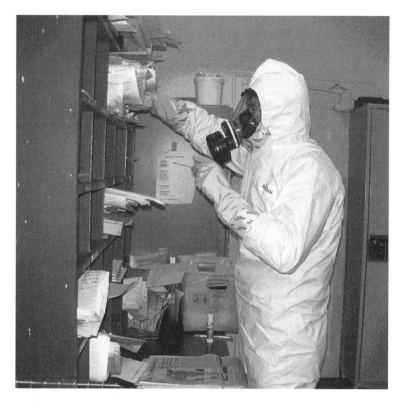

FIGURE 16-3 Swabbing mailboxes for *Bacillus anthracis* spores at a media site. Courtesy of Don Weiss.

held on September 28th at ABC's upper west side studio, with his mother, a producer at ABC World News Tonight. The next day he developed a weepy, silver-dollar size sore above his left elbow that oozed yellowish fluid through his shirt. The child appeared unfazed and the sore was initially regarded as an insect bite. The next day his pediatrician decided to treat the sore as cellulitis, a skin infection, and prescribed an oral antibiotic. The infant didn't tolerate the medication and was hospitalized on October 1. The wound continued to progress through stages: becoming purple with significant erythema and arm swelling and then ulcerating and finally forming a black eschar on the same day the Florida inhalational anthrax case was announced. Despite other complications, the child was well on the way to recovery when the news of the NBC cutaneous case first broke. The patient's mother immediately reminded physicians of her occupation and the call was made to DOH initiating the investigation that confirmed the child as another victim in the evolving outbreak of cutaneous anthrax. The site investigation at ABC officially began on October 15, a day after the child's diagnosis was confirmed at the CDC. Although no specific threat letter could be recalled by staff or was ever found, *B. anthracis* spores were detected in the mailroom and staff mail slots.

Sharon Balter had just joined the DOH 2 months before the attack at WTC and the subsequent anthrax outbreak. Fortified by her experiences as an EIS Officer and CDC epidemiologist, she possessed the requisite sense of humor and ability to take adversity in stride to do well at the DOH. She took to her position with the bureau like a duck to water, which was a good thing, not only because she was the head of our Waterborne Disease Program but because she was one of the few left in the office when yet another call came in late on October 12. The particulars were eerily familiar—this time the sick woman was the personal assistant to CBS anchorman Dan Rather, and as part of her job, she opened from 2,000 to 4,000 letters a day. She first noted two small red dots on her left cheek on October 1. These were accompanied by swelling that began beneath her eye and spread across her face. She was nauseated and light headed. By October 4 she was convinced this was a reaction to an insect bite, something she had experienced before in her life. Her physician prescribed antibiotics. After a few more rough days of feeling light headed, the swelling began to subside, and she was feeling better. A co-worker of the CBS case, on hearing the news about the NBC situation, decided to reach out to DOH through a mutual friend who was a medical epidemiologist with the bureau. Sharon was tasked to make the initial call to the patient and arranged to meet the woman at her doctor's office. Both patient and doctor were quite skeptical that this was anthrax. Sharon took a digital picture (Figure 16-4), and despite her urging, diagnostic testing didn't occur at that visit. Sharon arranged to meet the patient again, after the unfolding events convinced the woman that she should be tested. At Dan Rather's office on October 16th, Sharon drew more blood to check for *B. anthracis* antibodies (the initial sample had clotted). A day later at the patient's dermatologist office a skin biopsy was performed. Both the biopsy and blood test confirmed her as the fourth cutaneous anthrax case in New York City. The investigation at CBS began on October 18th, and with both the NBC and ABC investigations already underway, the resources of the DOH were severely stretched. Experiences from the first two investigations, however,

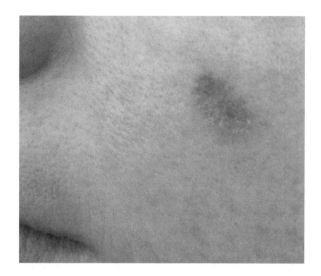

FIGURE 16-4 Cutaneous anthrax, 16 days after onset.
Courtesy of Sharon Balter.

proved valuable as the CBS investigation proceeded quickly. No one recalled a threat letter with powder and none was found. CBS president, Andrew Hayward, Dan Rather, and DOH staff did much to put the risk of disease into perspective for the CBS employees. Many had been overseas in war-torn nations. What was a little cutaneous anthrax compared to a Scud missile? Rather himself refused to take antibiotics despite spores being found on a desk he used. It was reassuring that in the 2-plus weeks since the patient's onset there had not been any further cases of any form of anthrax at CBS. As a result, many fewer employees had their noses swabbed, and none was put on long-term prophylactic antibiotics.

Before the sun had the chance to set on October 12th we were to hear about one more case. At yet another media organization, an editorial assistant at the New York Post had a suspicious blister on her middle finger. She first noted pus draining near the second joint of her right middle finger while at a friend's wedding on September 22nd. Her onset date, if confirmed, would make her the earliest case, the true index case of the outbreak. The progression was much as the preceding cases with swelling, ulcer formation, and the characteristic black eschar. She too received antibiotics with the addition of a surgical procedure to remove necrotic tissue and radiographs to exclude bone infection. A hospital guard noted the upward position of her bandaged right middle finger as she exited the emergency department and inquired whether it was a statement meant for Osama Bin Laden. A photograph of the same image was later published on the tabloid's front page above the exclamation, "Anthrax this!"

As the editorial assistant her job included opening mail. She explained that she opened several weird letters a day but none with powder stuck in her mind. She placed these letters in a box beneath her desk and thought that they had been thrown out by the time we interviewed her on October 12th. She too heard the news about the NBC case on October 12th prompting her to contact us and arrange a visit to an infectious disease specialist. As her infection was well along in the healing process, the biopsy did not find evidence of anthrax; however, her blood showed specific antibodies. This was evidence that she had fought off *B. anthracis*, not something a New York City newspaper woman should have coursing through her blood stream, unless her previous assignment was embedded with a troupe of African animal hide traders (naturally occurring anthrax has historically been associated with the handling of animal hides).

Fortunately, staff members at the New York Post were already suspicious about their worker's finger infection after hearing about the anthrax letter received by Tom Brokaw. Thus, they rounded up all the letters from the desks of editors into several U.S. Postal Service containers. The letters were reviewed to assure that no important correspondence was included, and the pile was transferred to a green garbage bag, which ended up at the bottom of the freight elevator. The FBI and New York City Police Department eventually located and searched the bag of letters on October 19th, finding one letter with the recognizable child-like, hand-written address and bearing a Trenton, NJ postmark. The letter had not been opened, perhaps explaining why the editorial assistant didn't recall it and tested positive for *B. anthracis*. It contained the identical five-line, three-words-per-line, 15-word message as did the NBC letter (Figure 16-5). *B. anthracis* spores were found in the mailroom and on desks of editorial staffers at the New York Post.

By the end of the third week of October, it appeared as though the outbreak might be drawing to a close. The media investigations at NBC, ABC, and CBS were in the environmental remediation stage, and the epidemiology component was winding down. Although two additional cutaneous anthrax cases subsequently came to light, they were both tied to the same exposure, the positive letter at the New York Post. The sixth New

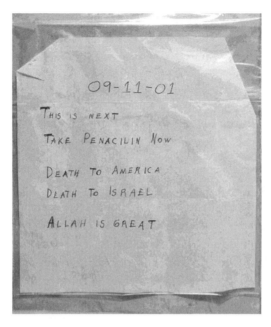

FIGURE 16-5 Image of the anthrax contaminated letter sent to NBC anchor Tom Brokaw.

Image by FBI.

York City case occurred in a 34-year-old New York Post mailroom worker, perhaps out of carelessness, and the seventh case in a 38-year-old editor out of curiosity, as they sorted through the boxes of suspicious mail after it was known that a tainted letter may lie therein. Both likely handled the letter postmarked September 18th from Trenton, NJ.

While we were immersed in prophylaxing hundreds of individuals in the face of cutaneous anthrax, another serious situation was unfolding in nearby states. Postal workers from New Jersey and Washington, DC mail distribution centers were in the initial throes of inhalational anthrax. It was on the afternoon of October 22 that I first heard the news that four postal workers from the same facility had inhalational anthrax; two were already dead. Within 40 minutes I was in a car headed uptown to the James A. Farley Post Office in Manhattan. In the car with me were two CDC physician epidemiologists, the double cell-phone toting Stephanie Factor, and the taciturn yet meticulous Tom Matte. Our tasks were to trace the path of the NBC and New York Post letters through the New York City mail grid, learn how mail was handled and where there were potential risks for spore exposure, and double check that no New York City postal workers were ill with symptoms of any form of anthrax. The James A. Farley building is the width of two city blocks and sits majestically on 8th Avenue across from Madison Square Garden and Pennsylvania station. Its familiar façade, inscription and Corinthian Colonnade are as familiar to New Yorkers as the Statue of Liberty or Empire State Building. Whenever I think of the place, I can't help seeing its immense stone blocks glimmering in a fusillade of snow with legions of "couriers" trudging great sacks of mail to and fro. In an elegant, richly wood-paneled conference room with enveloping chairs, we learned that mail entering the city first arrives at the Morgan Processing and Distribution Center (P&DC) stretching from 28th to 30th streets between 9th and 10th Avenues. After leaving the Morgan P&DC, mail headed to both NBC and the New York Post passed through a secondary post office, the Times Square post office. Mail to ABC passed through Ansonia post office and mail to CBS through the Radio City post office. On October 21, a contractor had done swab samples along the path the letters passed in the Morgan facility, and these were being processed at a commercial laboratory.

Next, we walked down the block to the workhorse of the New York City Postal Service, the equally immense, but minimally adorned Morgan P&DC. On the third floor we met the stalwart of the Morgan facility, the delivery bar code sorter machine. Mail from all over the country arrives by truck and is unloaded and placed in carts that transport it to conveyer belts that bring it up to the Area Distribution Center. Here the crates of mail for all the New York City zip codes are unloaded and wheeled to rows and rows of bar code sorter machines. One postal worker grabs a yard-width stack of mail and places it in a spring-loaded bin, jogging it to level the letter bottoms. The end holder snaps into place and guides the letters into the machine, which sucks each letter along a lengthy line of rollers, squeezing through a reader that picks up the bar code that had been imprinted by the originating post office. The letters are then expelled into bins, sequentially separating the letters into zip codes and then postal routes. Although the line of rollers was covered, dust and bits of letters could be seen above, behind, and all around the machine. Hanging from the ceiling was a compressed-air hose that was used to unclog the sorter machines by blowing out the dust at 70 lbs/in^2. A large fan stood nearby; it was evidently hot work. We could see lots of places where a letter carrying *B. anthracis* spores might release some of its contents. As we stood in the cavernous floor, looking at row after row of delivery bar code sorter machines an alarm went off. We followed our guide towards the stairs where a worker hurried over with news. A plastic bag filled with white powder had just been found near the time clock, on top of a wooden shelf. Hazmat was on the way; we'd have to evacuate the floor.

Back at our offices, staff members were again busy making calls. With the news breaking of postal workers in the District of Columbia and New Jersey ill with inhalational anthrax, we again called hospital emergency departments, intensive care units, and infection control practitioners. In addition to wanting to hear about previously well individuals with either sepsis, respiratory failure, or meningitis and clinical presentations that could be any of the various forms of anthrax, we now asked specifically about postal workers. The newly reported inhalational cases began their illnesses with vague, influenza-like symptoms of fever, chills, malaise and dry cough. Thus, we broadened our inquiry to include postal workers with any influenza or respiratory complaints. As influenza season was approaching, we began including in our medical alerts community influenza surveillance data, which at this point of the season was fortunately rare. To assist clinicians further in differentiating influenza from more worrisome illness in individuals at higher risk for inhalational anthrax as discovered in our epidemiology investigation, a guidance document on how to discriminate influenza from possible inhalational anthrax was also distributed.

It came as little surprise that several of the delivery bar code sorter machines from the third floor of the Morgan P&DC tested positive for *B. anthracis* spores because all of the contaminated mail with New York City destinations passed thorough this facility. The initial testing by the contractor was confirmed by samples taken by a National Institute of Occupational Safety and Health (NIOSH)/CDC team. What did seem unusual was that of the several "downstream" post offices of Rockefeller, Times Square, Radio City, and Ansonia, the intermediate recipients of actual and hypothesized letters to NBC, New York Post, CBS, and ABC, none was positive for *B. anthracis* on initial and repeat testing. Furthermore, nearly 300 nasal swabs of postal workers from these locations were also negative. There were no cases of anthrax, cutaneous or inhalational, in any New York City postal worker. Curiously, contamination could be found at Trenton, the letters' entrance into the mail system, at its next step, Morgan P&DC and at the destination sites. Perhaps there was something about the handling process at the *B. anthracis* negative facilities that differed, the absence of delivery bar code sorter machines to aerosolize spores, or perhaps we just didn't look hard enough. This is one of the many questions in the 2001 anthrax outbreak that remains unanswered.

The massive effort to administer prophylaxis to postal workers in New York City was performed by the CDC (as federal employees). From October 24 to 27, over 7,000 postal workers were given a 10-day supply of antibiotics at a POD held at the James A. Farley Building while awaiting the results of environmental testing. A second POD was held from November 2 to 6 for individuals who did not attend the first POD and to distribute the remainder of the recommended 60-day course to workers exposed to the positive sorter machines. Over 4,000 postal workers were seen at the second POD.

By the third week of October, the U.S. outbreak had expanded to include 20 cases of anthrax from an intentional act of bioterrorism, with 7 cases in NYC and 13 other cases in residents of five states (Florida, Maryland, New Jersey, Pennsylvania, and Virginia) plus Washington, DC. Eleven were the milder, cutaneous form, and nine the more deadly inhalational type. Three had died, all from inhalational anthrax. The deaths were in the photography editor exposed at the AMI building in Boca Raton, Florida and two postal workers from the Brentwood P&DC in Washington, DC. The presumed exposure for all of the cases was letters or packages laced with powdered *B. anthracis* spores. Some received or handled the tainted mail, whereas others breathed in the spores as they were aerosolized by mail sorting machines or the compressed air used to clean them. The simultaneous criminal investigation paralleled and intersected the public health one, until the two investigations eventually merged with the report on October 28 of an anthrax case of a different ilk.

Among the abundant facts and skills learned in medical training is microscopy. Pioneered by Van Leeuwenhoek in the late 1600s, the microscope is perhaps the oldest medical instrument still in use today. I remember fondly closing the door to the emergency department mini-laboratory during residency training in order to secure a few moments away from the chaos beyond. There, with the simple implements of glass slides, stains, and a trusty, if not rusty, Zeiss microscope, one could spend a few minutes in diagnostic bliss. Just after 6:00 p.m. on October 29, I found myself once again staring down the barrel of a microscope. The cell walls of certain bacteria absorbed the dye crystal violet and appeared purple-blue. I was seeing blue. Bacteria come in various shapes, sizes, and arrangements.

Most are either rods (oval) or cocci (round) and can appear in pairs, clusters, or chains. Large rods in short chains were on the slide before me. The hospital microbiology laboratory director had stayed late just to be there when I arrived, and he couldn't help from beaming at his staff's diagnostic acumen, despite its ominous implication. Was I looking at *B. anthracis*? The slide had been prepared from a culture of blood taken less than 18 hours earlier, unusually fast growth, but consistent with *B. anthracis*. I asked whether it was nonhemolytic and nonmotile, as these are discriminating characteristics of *B. anthracis*. It was nonhemolytic; however, motility testing was not yet complete. There was still a chance this wasn't anthrax after all. Before taking the culture to the PHL for confirmation, I was escorted to the intensive care unit to see the patient. She was on a ventilator and was heavily sedated; there would be no interview. I was shown the computerized tomography scan and saw the enlarged mediastinal nodes, a telltale feature of inhalational anthrax. No one in the intensive care unit seemed to believe it, yet none doubted what they were seeing.

The unfortunate source of that blood was a 61-year-old woman originally from Vietnam. Kathy Nguyen had come to America in 1976 as a refugee seeking a better life. She had worked for the last 12 years in the stockroom of a local specialty hospital, the Manhattan Eye, Ear, and Throat Hospital (MEETH). The hospital provided mostly outpatient services and same-day surgical procedures with few inpatient beds. She was well liked by all who knew her but precious few details were known of her life outside of work. Her illness began a few days earlier, on October 26, with muscle soreness, weakness, cough, and shortness of breath that progressively worsened. When she coughed, her phlegm was tinged pink. After 2 days at home without improvement, she arrived at the hospital at 11:00 a.m. breathing fast and shallow, signs of respiratory distress. Her oxygen test was low, and there was no fever. Kathy Nguyen told doctors that it hurt right below her breastbone and that she needed three pillows in order to sleep (three pillow orthopnea is a cardinal sign of heart failure). With a past medical history of hypertension, orthopnea, and a physical examination suggesting lung congestion, her initial diagnosis was pulmonary edema caused by heart failure (a noninfectious condition). The chest radiograph was consistent with this diagnosis showing bilateral pleural effusions (a collection of fluid in the spaces surrounding the lungs). Nothing in her initial laboratory tests indicated another diagnosis, but as a routine, a culture of her blood was taken. Treatment for pulmonary edema proved ineffective, and an echocardiogram of her heart failed to establish a cardiac cause for her respiratory distress. She remained without fever, but her pulse was increasing while her blood pressure fell. Her doctors had to look elsewhere to explain her rapidly deteriorating condition. The emergency department physician received his daily call from Dr. Michael Tapper, an infectious disease specialist and hospital epidemiologist. Since 9/11, Dr. Tapper made a practice of calling the emergency department at least once a day to learn about potentially worrisome cases. He was told about Kathy's illness and came down and saw a suggestion of mediastinal widening on the chest x-ray. He brought it to the radiologist, who concurred. Dr. Tapper instructed the emergency department physicians to begin antibiotics immediately to cover for the possibility of anthrax. Next, he dialed Dr. Layton to report his concerns. The computed tomography scan of the chest done later that night revealed the enlarged chest cavity lymph nodes and blood, both ominous evidence of hemorrhagic mediastinitis, a hallmark of inhalational anthrax. Early the next afternoon the Gram-positive rods were visible in Kathy Nguyen's blood that prompted my trip to the lab.

A team was quickly mobilized and dispatched to MEETH to begin the investigation. When Joel and Sharon arrived, they were met outside the hospital by the New York City Police Department chief of counterterrorism. All around them were police and emergency vehicles. Specially trained officers had donned their Tyvek protective suits, whereas others stood before the hospital entrance, not allowing anyone to leave or enter. New Yorkers cruised by on their hurried Monday afternoon commute home unconcerned with the goings on at the hospital. The chief was concerned for his officers' safety and explained that his men were not going into the building until DOH could assure them that it was safe to enter. Joel explained to the chief, in a calm, pedantic monologue, that he couldn't give him that assurance. For all he knew, there could be a dissemination device inside. An impasse arose. The chief was known for his passionate if not zealous approach to his work. He grew visibly impatient, and the fire in his eyes caused Joel to wonder whether the chief wasn't considering throwing him in jail for his honest yet blunt assessment. Sharon, out of exhaustion, frustration or both announced, "If there is anthrax in there, we'll just take antibiotics," and marched in. The New York City Police Department eventually followed, but the FBI set up across the street to conduct interviews. The scene typified both the difficulty in making decisions in the absence of precedent and scientific data, as well as the conflicting needs of public health and law enforcement; however, in contrast to this auspicious beginning, the New York City inhalational anthrax case investigation enjoyed the greatest integration of public health and law enforcement of any of the anthrax investigations. Joel would later remark, "It was like I was embedded within NYPD."

The first phase of the investigation focused on the hospital basement stockroom where the patient had worked. When I arrived near midnight that first evening, a POD was being set up, and the hospital staff members that had been forced to remain were clearly anxious and eager to leave. The few inpatients the hospital had were transferred and visitors prohibited. That night and into the next day, over 200 employees were interviewed and given antibiotics pending the results of environmental testing. Few of the patient's co-workers knew her regular routine. Her tasks did not include processing incoming mail, and none of the MEETH employees had seen or heard of any suspicious mail arriving at the hospital. A nurse recalled that sometime in the last week the patient had come to her requesting to have her eyes flushed, remarking about the dust down in the basement. It might have been on October 25. That would have been one day before onset, and if it occurred in the hospital, there should be a trail of spores. Hospital staff members that worked in the mailroom, stockroom, and basement were tested by nasal swab, and all were negative. On three separate occasions, the CDC, NIOSH, FBI, and New York City Police Department donned their protective gear and took environmental samples; first from the basement, the location of the stockroom and mailroom, then from multiple locations in the hospital; and then again from the basement. Items from the patient's locker were checked twice, the second time using a method to enhance the recovery of *B. anthracis* spores. All tests were negative. Surveillance of MEETH workers turned up several with recent respiratory and skin infections, but none with anthrax. The 1,500 patients and visitors to MEETH over the preceding weeks who had been started on antibiotics at the POD were instructed to stop. Kathy Nguyen became the fourth fatal victim of the intentional anthrax attack on October 31, 2001.

Ms. Nguyen had lived for more than 15 years in a largely Hispanic neighborhood located near the elevated subway in the Southeast Bronx. She lived alone and had infrequent visitors. Efforts to locate relatives were unsuccessful. She was described by neighbors and co-workers as friendly and generous, often buying gifts for others. She was reserved in social interactions and was said to have distrusted banks, choosing to pay her rent using postal money orders. She was reported to have enjoyed shopping. Her one bedroom apartment was neat and uncluttered, suggesting frugality. In her home the FBI took the lead on sampling. Greeting cards, her comb and brush, the television screen, a fluorescent light, a letter opener, her address book, towels, shoes, hats, her cell phone, receipts, and even her Chapstick lip balm were tested. When these results were negative, sampling expanded to other parts of her building—her mailbox and the elevator. Swabs of the mail found in her apartment were examined for *B. anthracis* spores, as were the local post offices serving her home and work. No spores were found. Items, such as her clothes, were vacuumed with a high-efficiency particulate air filter to trap items as small as 1 micron. This too failed to find any spores. Her neighbors were interviewed to learn information about her life that could lead to *B. anthracis* exposure and to search for possible cases. The DOH held a meeting for tenants with Spanish interpreters to answer questions and explain the investigation. One woman was identified with a suspicious skin lesion that tested negative for *B. anthracis*.

With nothing uncovered from the most likely locations, on November 3, the investigation turned toward more remote exposure possibilities. By using her New York City subway fare card (Metro card), credit card statements, receipts, and accounts from her co-workers, Kathy Nguyen's schedule in the weeks preceding her death was reconstructed. Each swipe of her credit card purchased Metro card recorded the date, time, and station of entry. The sum of her electronic footprints still didn't provide a comprehensive timeline of her activities, however; in the absence of a case interview, it was our best lead toward identifying possible exposures to *B. anthracis* spores.

Epidemiologists, using shopping receipts as guides, visited stores she frequented with her picture hoping to extract snapshots of her life to piece together how she encountered *B. anthracis*. She was said to have attended church, although the exact one was uncertain. EIS officers visited churches near her home and place of work, speaking to priests and parishioners, some who recalled her, most who did not. No leads were produced. Along the route she would have walked from the train station to her apartment were several stores and businesses. Other than clerks in the nearby laundromat and grocery stores, none knew her. The check cashing office in the neighborhood had a file for Ms. Nguyen, but it did not indicate any activity in several years. No receipts were found for postal money orders to trace back to a contaminated post office. On the off chance her exposure could have been along this route, store owners and staff were asked about recent illnesses; none was reported. Teams visited Macy's Department Store in the Bronx and various businesses in Chinatown, two locations she was known to frequent. Still, no leads were uncovered.

What remained was the unthinkable and the possibility was approached delicately. Kathy Nguyen took the subway nearly every day. Could she have been exposed on the platform or the train? The implication threatened to raise the anxiety level in New York City to a new fever pitch and extend anthrax surveillance indefinitely. Before the results on her home and work came back, a plan to test the New York City subway was drafted. Critical to the plan was consideration of how to respond to a positive finding. With over 4 million riders daily, any interruption in service would have major ramifications for people and business in the greater metropolitan New York area. The goal was simply to try and identify where Kathy Nguyen might have been exposed to *B. anthracis*, not to evaluate risk posed by riding the subway. It was reasoned that because there was only a single case among millions of riders and several weeks had passed without any other anthrax cases not directly connected to mail, a positive finding would represent little risk to the public health. Surveillance of Metropolitan Transportation Authority workers, which began shortly after the 9/11 attacks, had not identified any worrisome cases either that supported this response plan. Five stations used by Kathy Nguyen and four control stations whose trains did not intersect with the target stations were tested. Within the station, areas presumed to retain dust particles or be a possible risk area were tested. It was decided that in the absence of any evidence of disease, spores found in a station used as a control location represented very little risk to public health. Positive findings at a station visited by Kathy Nguyen would result in thorough cleaning. Such a finding did not indicate the need for nasal swabs of Metropolitan Transportation Authority workers or riders, nor would antibiotic prophylaxis be warranted.

When the results from the subway testing came back in early November, the Mayor and Health Commissioner discussed them at a press conference. Commissioner of Health Dr. Neal Cohen remarked straight faced that although no *B. anthracis* was found in the New York City subway system, "We can now conclude that the New York City subways are not a sterile environment." Injecting humor into what had otherwise been a dire conversation was much needed and a skillful use of risk communication. It helped to place in perspective both the results and massive effort put forth by DOH, the New York City Department of Environmental Protection, the federal Environmental Protection Agency, the CDC, NIOSH, the New York City Police Department, and the FBI to find how Kathy Nguyen was exposed to *B. anthracis.* When the leading hypothesis became cross-contamination of mail, I believe it was the open and communicative handling of the investigation that facilitated the public's acceptance of this theory. The truth remains that there were very few alternative hypotheses, and cross-contamination was the least improbable.

The final case in the multistate anthrax outbreak occurred in a 94-year-old Connecticut woman whose activities were quite limited. As with the Kathy Nguyen investigation, no *B. anthracis* spores were found anywhere that she had been in the immediate period before her illness, but unlike the NYC case investigation, spores were detected at the local post office that processed her mail. It was determined that a letter postmarked in Trenton, that passed through the delivery bar code sorter machine shortly after a known-to-be tainted letter, traveled through the Wallington Distribution Center in Connecticut and was delivered to a home in a neighboring town. That letter was found and tested positive for *B. anthracis.* No illness was associated with the letter, but it added much needed credibility to the prevailing cross-contamination theory.

If you hang around public health bioterrorism experts long enough, you'll invariably hear them all say something like this: "It isn't a question if another bioterrorism event will occur, it is when." For those of us on the ground in state and local health departments, the question is really how? Despite the numerous hoax letters that preceded the actual tainted ones, we didn't expect *B. anthracis* spores to be mailed because it wasn't believed to be an efficient method of dissemination. The letters sent to television icons and U.S. Senators dispelled this notion. We didn't consider that an ordinary sealed envelope, squeezed through the high-speed postal machinery, could spread spores. No one expected that letters, whose paths merely crossed with contaminated letters that became contaminated by passing through sorting machines after the tainted anthrax letters, would be able to cause inhalational disease. Evidence from the outbreak suggests that the minimum infective dose for inhalational anthrax is much lower than conventional wisdom held in 2001, perhaps as low as a few spores adhering to the surface of an envelope. We didn't expect cutaneous cases either. The ability to make or acquire weapons-grade *B. anthracis* spores was believed to be nearly impossible for all but the most accomplished bioweapons scientist. These former truths guided our initial approach to the investigation. Although much was learned during the anthrax investigation, we likely will not know the "how" in advance of another bioterrorism attack. This continues to be the crucial public health task upon which disease mitigation depends.

CONCLUSIONS

Doctors are trained to think of common ailments first when evaluating a patient's symptoms, not the rare ones. More than a few medical students have been admonished by the adage, "When you hear hoof beats, think horses, not zebras." In 1999, when West Nile virus made its first western hemisphere appearance in New York City, it was initially believed to be an outbreak of St. Louis encephalitis. The bird die-offs that preceded the outbreak were not thought to be linked to human illness; we were wrong on both counts. In public health, we've now come to replace the old adage with a new one: "Expect the unexpected." The anthrax ordeal lasted just over 2 months and resulted in 22 cases nationally, small when compared with such public health enemies as lung cancer or AIDS. More than 12 work sites, 8 confirmed cases, and well over a hundred suspect case reports were investigated in New York City (Figure 16-2). The anthrax mail attack was unprecedented, malignant, and shocked the nation. Although this chapter ends here, the story does not. Health departments across the country continue to plan and drill for the next act of bioterrorism. The criminal case remains unsolved, the FBI investigation open, and the perpetrator at large.

ACKNOWLEDGMENTS

The following current and former DOH staff graciously agreed to be interviewed for the project. They provided valuable recollections and insights from their experiences as part of the 2001 Anthrax Investigation team: Polly Thomas, Susan Blank, Hadi Maki, Andrew Tucker, Annie Fine, Sarah Perl, Tom Matte, Ben Mojica, John Kornblum, Laura Mascuch, Isaac Weisfuse, Sheila Palevsky, Jeannine Pru'dhomme, Sally Beatrice, Marie Wong, Denis Nash, Joel Ackelsberg, Marci Layton, Sharon Balter, Michael Phillips, Andrew Goodman, and Adam Karpati.

CHAPTER 17

Ebola Hemorrhagic Fever in Gabon: Chaos to Control

Daniel G. Bausch, MD, MPH&TM

INTRODUCTION

The Usual Inconvenient Beginning

Damn . . . did I screw up. I would have bet you a million dollars that that kid didn't have Ebola. Not fun—this feeling of incompetence. What am I doing here in Gabon making misdiagnoses? It was the usual inconvenient beginning: December 12, 2001. Christmas was approaching, and I had long-made plans to visit my fiancé in Switzerland for the holidays and then to help her move to London to begin the tropical medicine program at the London School. I'm in some routine meeting in Atlanta when Tom Ksiazek, chief of the Special Pathogens Branch of the Centers for Disease Control and Prevention (CDC), sticks his head in and points to me— "Can I see you for a minute?" Tom is not known for being the chatty touchy-feely type, so I knew he wasn't calling me out to wish me a Merry Christmas. In fact, before I even got out of the door, I knew that the holiday was gone—no Christmas in Switzerland, no visit with fiancé, no move to London. No, my Christmas would be spent attending to an Ebola outbreak in Gabon and the Republic of the Congo. By the way, for anyone aspiring to this kind of work, sudden calls to Ebola outbreaks that ruin your Christmas plans seem dramatic and exciting only once.

Why not just refuse? All of these plans that you've had for so long are ruined in just a second. It's not so much pressure from your boss or even machismo. It's more black and white; you're either in the outbreak business and attend to it when it happens (damn it), or you're not (although there are limits, as evidenced by my staying home to watch my son be born instead of heading to Angola for the 2005 epidemic of Marburg hemorrhagic fever).

Why me? I would like to think that it had something to do with my experience and expertise—an infectious disease doctor with degrees in public health and tropical medicine, having been at the CDC since 1996 and with experience in outbreak responses and control efforts for a number of different hemorrhagic fevers—Ebola and Marburg in Uganda and the Democratic Republic of the Congo, Lassa fever and yellow fever in various spots in West Africa, and dengue in El Salvador. True, all of that helps, but all of the medical training and field experience were more prerequisites than a deciding factor. In reality, I knew that there was an equally important reason, one that (fortunately) comes up frequently: I speak French—a lucky break brought about by required classes in junior high (in which I started out doing quite poorly), my parents' foresight in enrolling me in a summer exchange program in France as a teenager, and later on, a succession of fortunate professional opportunities. Thus, here is the first lesson for would-be international virus hunters: Leave the advanced molecular biology and volunteering at the hospital alone for a minute and learn a language. French is great for sub-Saharan Africa, but others will work too. It doesn't matter; pick an area of the world and a corresponding language that interests you, and sign up for conversational classes on Thursday nights at your local community college.

I never planned on a career in viral hemorrhagic fevers. In fact, after finishing my infectious disease fellowship and Master's of Public Health degree at Tulane University in New Orleans, I turned down a spot in the CDC's Epidemic Intelligence Service to take a position directing a community education and training project with a tiny nongovernmental organization (NGO) working in the Central America country of El Salvador—a place in which I had been very involved since medical school. The position entailed training community health workers and doing some clinical work in the rural area of Suchitoto half the week and, as a visiting professor, teaching infectious diseases to medical students and residents at the Universidad National de El Salvador in the capital the other half. The person who learned the most, however, was me. The major lesson was that, although I did and still do support it philosophically as an appropriate health care delivery strategy, I wasn't cut out for being the primary implementer of a community-based health care project.

After an often frustrating year and a half in El Salvador learning what I wasn't good at, I was ready to explore new opportunities elsewhere and mentioned this in a phone call to Barney Cline, one of my professors from Tulane and a key mentor and friend over the years. As it happened, C.J. Peters, then the chief of the CDC Special Pathogens Branch and a friend of Barney's, was coming to lecture at Tulane the following week. Barney offered to inquire with C.J. regarding possible opportunities with the CDC. I knew a little bit about C.J.; he lectured to our public health class at Tulane, and by chance (or was it fate?), I had recently read Richard Preston's *The Hot Zone*, which chronicles C.J.'s tussle with Ebola in a monkey facility in Reston, Virginia. Although I had never envisioned myself as anything close to a "virus hunter," I was intrigued enough to listen to any ideas he might have.

C.J. and Barney called me the next week. The initial discussion centered on the possibility of working with the CDC to analyze data collected on a disease called hemorrhagic fever with renal syndrome dating back to the Korean War. As this entailed primarily sitting in front of a computer in Atlanta, I wasn't too enthusiastic. We were just about to end the conversation when C.J. asked, "You don't speak French by chance?" Thus, the door opened to head up another project that C.J. had in mind: to establish a field station for research on Lassa fever in Guinea, a French-speaking country on the coast of West Africa. A year or so later I joined the CDC and started learning about and working on the viral hemorrhagic fevers.

EBOLA OUTBREAK RESPONSES

In the absence of effective vaccines and therapeutics, the response to Ebola outbreaks has relied almost solely on the classic measures of communicable disease control: case isolation and contact tracing. An outbreak team is assembled, almost always consisting of personnel from the Ministry of

Health of the involved country and local health care workers in the area of the outbreak, assisted by a diverse group of international partners from groups such as the World Health Organization (WHO, usually the coordinating body), the CDC, the National Institute for Communicable Diseases in South Africa, Health Canada, and Médecins Sans Frontières (MSF) and other NGOs.

The group is usually divided into teams, including the epidemiologists who work on case identification, contact tracing, and keeping the primary database; clinicians who establish and maintain isolation wards and treat patients; water-sanitation experts who are responsible for important aspects of the physical maintenance of the isolation wards; laboratory personnel who perform diagnostic testing, establishing field laboratories when necessary; community health workers who deal with social mobilization and prevention campaigns; and zoologists and ecologists who seek to identify the Ebola virus reservoir. Depending on the outbreak and the needs, I might be involved to some degree in virtually all these activities, although my primary roles, including in Gabon, were usually as part of the clinical and epidemiology teams, always with an eye for collecting useful research data in the course of these activities.

Excluding a few laboratory infections, human infection with Ebola virus has been exclusively noted in sub-Saharan Africa (Figure 17-1). Gabon and the neighboring Republic of the Congo were and are hotspots. This is not by chance. Being two of the few countries with large tracts of rainforest still intact, the critter that carries Ebola virus (a bat?) still has a habitat. Consequently, humans in the region are also bound to stumble into an Ebola virus now and then. At the CDC we were honestly not overly enthused about participating in Ebola response operations in Gabon and Congo. First, with their sparse populations, the number of cases was usually few and dispersed in remote, hard-to-reach areas, not easily amenable to control efforts or scientific study. Second, being former French colonies, the conventional wisdom is that this region is "French turf," where participation of the CDC (who sometimes carried a reputation, rightly or wrongly, of barging in and taking over) was less than enthusiastically welcomed; however, this particular time, rumor had it that Senator Kennedy heard that there was an Ebola outbreak in Gabon and wanted to know what the CDC was doing about it. So there was to be no Christmas in Switzerland for me. I was going to Gabon.

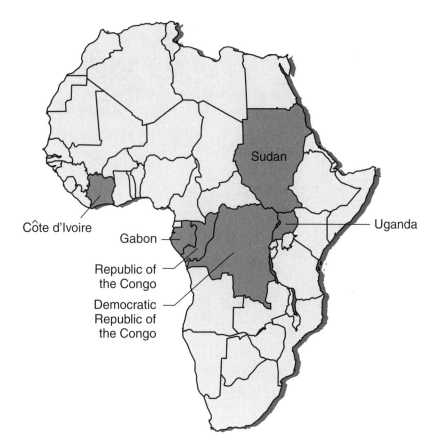

FIGURE 17-1 Countries in which human cases of Ebola hemorrhagic fever have been confirmed, excluding imported cases and laboratory infections.

OUTBREAK RECOGNITION AND LABORATORY CONFIRMATION

Recent reports had trickled in of cases of a febrile illness, often associated with bleeding, some of them in health care workers, in Gabon's remote Ogooué Ivindo Province, a heavily forested region bordering the Congo (Figures 17-1 and 17-2). As Ebola had been seen in Ogooué Ivindo before, this was the diagnosis until proven otherwise. In fact, the diagnosis of Ebola was not in doubt. A Gabonese research center, the Centre International de Recherches Medicales de Franceville (CIRMF), had already made

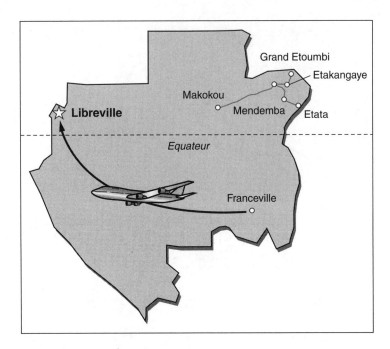

FIGURE 17-2 Geographic distribution of cases of Ebola hemorrhagic fever in Gabon, October 2001–March 2002.

Nkoghe D, Formenty P, Leroy EM, Nnegue S, Edou SY, Ba JI, et al. Multiple Ebola virus haemorrhagic fever outbreaks in Gabon, from October 2001 to April 2002. *Bull Soc Pathol Exot* 2005;98(3):224–9.

the laboratory diagnosis. Furthermore, it had been confirmed at the National Institute for Communicable Diseases by my old friend and internationally renowned virologist and zoologist Bob Swanepoel, who simply ran the best and most reliable laboratory in the world. If Bob said that it was Ebola, it was Ebola.

Unlike many other types of outbreaks, by the time outbreak investigations and control efforts for the filoviruses (Ebola and Marburg) are initiated, laboratory confirmation of the pathogen has almost always already occurred.[1] In fact, the unclenching of the entire outbreak response process usually depends on it. Recognizing the severe consequences of both false positives and negatives, a battery of diagnostic tests is usually performed, including the enzyme-linked immunosorbent assay (ELISA), polymerase chain reaction (PCR), and virus isolation; however, there are only a few laboratories in the world where these tests are performed and, paradoxi-

THE INITIAL ASSESSMENT   **329**

cally, very few in sub-Saharan Africa where Ebola is endemic. In contrast to popular belief, this is much less related to the danger of performing the assays (ELISA and PCR can be safely performed using inactivated antigens and samples) than to the unavailability of reagents. There are no commercially available assays for the filoviruses, and existing "in-house" tests rely on the production of antigen derived through the culture of live virus in a high-containment laboratory followed by inactivation, safety testing, and optimization of the assay—a laborious and expensive process that few countries and laboratories have the will and the means to undertake.

The benefit of having a laboratory-confirmed diagnosis before you go has obvious advantages; the considerable resources, both human and financial, required to mount an outbreak response in remote areas of sub-Saharan Africa are not wasted. The wheels are set in motion only when we know that something bad is truly going on; however, the price of this approach is that the response is delayed. In most filovirus outbreaks, transmission smolders at a low level for weeks or even months until a blood sample from a suspected case finally gets drawn and sent, often with the aid of an international NGO working in the area, to one of the few laboratories in the world where filovirus diagnostics are performed. The need to build public health and diagnostic capacity in the endemic area for diseases such as Ebola would later become a major factor in the direction of my career, but that is another story (discussed later here).

In a strange sense, having laboratory confirmation of one of the most lethal pathogens in the world makes things, well . . . more comforting. When you know what you are dealing with, you know the drill—the mode of transmission, the precautions to take in the field and laboratory. I appreciated this a few years later when SARS cropped up and I headed off to Vietnam with just a description of a syndrome, but no pathogen, no mode of transmission, and no concrete guidelines for what safety and control measures were effective. How do you protect yourself with that uncertainty? What advice do you give to others in your role as a public health expert and consultant?

THE INITIAL ASSESSMENT

Getting back to Gabon—okay, it's Ebola. I'll go. I'll do my thing. Anyway, the word from the ground, perhaps reflecting wishful thinking as much as any scientific evidence, was that this was a small outbreak, likely to be rapidly controlled, so maybe I'd even be in Switzerland for New Year's.

The beginning is always easy. You show up in some capitol city in the tropics, in this case, Libreville. Somebody meets you at the airport (in this case, Ray Arthur, who was secunded from the CDC to the WHO and who was often my contact for these outbreaks), takes you to a hotel that is well above the means of 99% of the African population, and then you go to dinner on the same scale. Over lobster and the Gabonese *Regab* beer, Ray and I discussed the situation. It's interesting, almost fun. You feel important. The next day you meet with the national and local authorities and the WHO country office. Still interesting. Still feeling important.

Next day. Time to hit the field! A small plane was chartered for us. We would fly first to Makokou, site of previous Ebola outbreaks and where a suspected case had been recently reported (Figure 17-2). It was only supposed to be a quick evaluation stop before heading on to Mekembo, epicenter for the outbreak. Ray and I showed up at the small hospital in Makokou in the mid afternoon, the peak of the dry season heat, when most sane people are lying as low and still as possible in the shadiest spot that they can find. The place looked deserted, but we managed to drum up a nurse in charge and introduced ourselves. We inquired about the suspected case of Ebola and were informed that the patient, herself a nurse at Makokou, was holding her own and seemed to be responding to anti-malarials. Good news, but I nevertheless thought it was worth taking a quick look at her.

The nurse led us to the patient, being cared for in one of the hospital's small three-bed wards. This being sub-Saharan Africa, I did not expect the patient to be in a negative-pressure room, of which there are precious few on the continent. Furthermore, even if you had one, it would be an extra precaution; although we'd certainly use this with a suspected case of Ebola in the United States, it isn't technically required, given the lack of evidence of natural airborne transmission of the filoviruses.

Of more concern was the absence of personal protective equipment (i.e. gloves, gowns, and masks) necessary to maintain barrier nursing precautions. I was not worried for my own safety during the brief visit with the patient. I knew that Ebola virus was spread by direct contact with blood and bodily fluids.[2,3] I could therefore safely see and speak with, but not examine, the patient as long as I kept out of respiratory droplet range (that is, where droplets the patient might cough up could reach me—about a meter), keeping my arms folded across my chest to not inadvertently touch anything; however, as daily patient management could not be conducted in this way, there were worrying implications for possible exposure to the hospital staff.

The patient, a woman in her early 20s, was quite sick, but there was nothing particularly remarkable from a medical standpoint—fever, headache, malaise, nausea, and vomiting. No bleeding. It could have been a million things, but there was one more unusual and identifying sign— that subtle rash on her face. I'd seen a lot of cases of Ebola during an outbreak in Uganda a few years back[4] and knew that making the diagnosis on clinical grounds was extremely difficult, especially in the early phases of the disease. In contrast to much of the popular press, the infected person's eyeballs don't melt, and the liver does not turn to mush. In reality, even if you're the best doctor in the world, distinguishing a case of Ebola from all the malaria, typhoid fever, and host of other febrile illnesses in the region (which don't take a vacation just because there might be an Ebola outbreak) is usually difficult, if not impossible; however, I knew that a measles-like skin rash is sometimes seen on the face and trunk. The rash doesn't occur in everybody (maybe only approximately 20%) and is usually very fleeting. Its absence doesn't exclude Ebola, but if you see it, the patient probably has the disease. In other words, it is a specific but not very sensitive sign.

Thus, despite the nurse's diagnosis of malaria, her rash made me suspicious of Ebola. Then there was the other clue—the patient was a health care worker. Tragically, the major clue to almost every outbreak of viral hemorrhagic fever I've investigated has been the death of one or more health care workers. Death of a health care worker should always raise the red flag of possible nosocomial, or health care-associated, transmission, especially if there are clusters. Nosocomial transmission lies behind virtually all large filovirus outbreaks. Health care workers in resource-poor settings without consistent supplies of personal protective equipment, clean syringes, and disinfectant (materials usually taken for granted in the United States) are particularly vulnerable. This really hits home when almost every scientific paper you publish is dedicated to someone "who died investigating the outbreak and disease reported in this manuscript."

When you see health care worker involvement, you have to go back to the hospital records and talk with the doctors and nurses. If a hemorrhagic fever virus is circulating, you'll very often find that the health care worker treated a patient with a similar syndrome just a week or so ago. The important point is to make sure that the exposure was within the 3-week maximum incubation period for Ebola, in which case, again, nosocomial transmission should be considered, if not assumed. Indeed, the sick nurse in Makokou had cared for a sick child about 10 days ago—a child brought in from Mekembo.

While Ray and I and the nurse were seeing the patient, another barely noticeable event occurred that was a harbinger of things to come. Although to maintain strict infection control we should not lay a hand on anything, doctors and nurses often can't help themselves from somewhat haphazardly touching things when they're at the patient's bedside. Even if not indicated at that particular moment, we have to check something—the chart, the IV site, the patient's conjunctiva, the turgor of the skin. I suppose that it's the professional equivalent of caring mothers fluffing the pillows when a child is home sick—it doesn't do anything, but it makes her feel better. While seeing the patient, I noticed that the nurse raised his ungloved hand to adjust the patient's IV drip. There was no visible blood anywhere, and the nurse considered the patient to have malaria (which is not generally directly communicable); however, this would prove tragically prophetic for subsequent events in Makokou.

I stayed on in Makokou for a few days, mostly working with local physicians, Julien Mayoun, chief of the Medical Service at Makokou Regional Hospital, and Prosper Abessolo Mengue, regional health director for Ogooué Ivindo, as well as members of the MSF-Belgian team, Catherine Bachy and Christian Katzer, to assist Makokou hospital in setting up an isolation ward. There was considerable debate, mostly out of fear and politics, as to where the ward should be placed. Sadly, the sick nurse I saw the first day died; however, there were no new cases, and I was starting to think that the stateside predictions of a small outbreak with rapid resolution might be true (Switzerland, here I come?), although I knew that things were still more active around Mekembo.

In fact, Makokou being quiet, the plan was for me to move over to Mekembo to lend a hand. On the day before my departure, a mother brought her teenage boy to Makokou Hospital. I didn't consider his story to be suggestive of Ebola at all—low grade fever, no systemic symptoms. True, he had unexplained bleeding, but it was mild and localized to an area around his upper right molars, where he also had pain. I suspected that his problem was primarily dental, perhaps a periapical abscess, the bleeding probably brought on by the mother's constant jamming of her bare fingers into the boy's mouth to show us where the problem was.

ISOLATION WARDS AND INFECTION CONTROL

The principles of an isolation ward are relatively simple—a "souped up" version of barrier nursing precautions, including masks, gowns, double gloves, head covering, and foot protection, are employed, designed to protect against direct contact and respiratory droplets. In contrast to what's often portrayed in the popular press, "space suits" or respirators are not necessary, although these may be required for laboratory manipulation of Ebola virus, where virus culture and techniques such as centrifugation have the potential for significant amplification and dissemination.

Even under the best of circumstances, admission to an isolation ward is a harrowing experience. Sick patients, some of whom may never have been admitted to a hospital, suddenly find themselves surrounded by strangely clad and unrecognizable health care workers, often foreign, in a potentially frightening atmosphere of sterility. Access to one's family is, of course, limited (usually to a single patient attendant, who is also required to wear protective material and not allowed to touch their family member). Perhaps the most daunting aspect of the whole affair is the prospect of dying and being buried by the isolation ward staff without the funeral rituals often so integral to African culture. To this highly charged environment must frequently be added the vestiges of colonial era suspicion of foreigners and present-day frictions between ethnic groups.

Furthermore, because the case-fatality rates for the filoviruses are so high (often approaching 90%), it unfortunately stands to reason that most patients admitted to an isolation ward with confirmed filovirus infection die. This often gives an appearance of causality to the local population—that is, *if* you go into the isolation ward you will surely die. No matter what, *avoid this*. Certainly with this fear in mind, the mother was adamant that her son's problem wasn't Ebola but a "normal disease." Given the very atypical clinical presentation, I was inclined to agree with her. The pressure to not isolate patients also comes sometimes from the political sector; in the worst case scenario, establishing isolation wards and isolating patients can be interpreted as the signal to the community that a terrible disease is circulating in the village, with the implicit, if not explicit message, of *don't come here*. This obviously can have catastrophic consequences to the local economy.

With the presentation seeming so inconsistent with Ebola, I discounted the kid as a real case. Nevertheless, because his fever and unexplained bleeding technically met the case definition (discussed later here), I hedged my bets and took blood to send to CIRMF for testing, to receive the results in a week or so. Partly because of the atypical presentation, but also, it must be said, influenced by the family and political pressure to not isolate patients, I did not place the boy in isolation and didn't think much more about it. Believing Makokou to be pretty well tucked in, the next day I moved on to Mekembo, a 3-hour drive during which (and I am not making this up) our Toyota Land Cruiser, traveling at a swift pace through a deep stretch of bamboo forest, suddenly and sadly collided with a big leopard crossing the road, the wild-eyed cat bounding into the forest, likely to die, I surmised. I elected not to get out of the car to test this hypothesis.

In Mekembo, a larger team of expatriates and Gabonese, maybe 25 altogether, was already hard at work, including Mary Reynolds, the CDC Epidemic Intelligence Officer sent to work with me. The number of cases was still small, and there were only one or two in the isolation ward; however, there was nevertheless plenty to do tracing contacts, collecting specimens, and working on coordinating prevention efforts. I reviewed the isolation ward briefly and, finding little to do there, joined the epidemiologists in the field activities.

THE CASE DEFINITION AND DESCRIPTIVE EPIDEMIOLOGY

One of the earliest and most important steps in any outbreak investigation is to make a case definition. In most previous outbreaks of Ebola, previous contact with a suspected or confirmed case was the biggest risk factor.[2,3,5] Nosocomial risk factors (i.e., being a health care worker or recently being admitted to a health care center) were especially pertinent.[6] Consequently, determination of possible previous contact with an infected human constituted a major part of the standard case definitions and reporting forms developed by WHO. These WHO standards were the ones we were using at the beginning of the outbreak in Gabon (Table 17-1) and most of us on the response team had used these case definitions before and felt pretty comfortable with them.

Table 17-1 Definitions for a Suspected Case of Ebola Hemorrhagic Fever Employed in the Outbreak Response in Gabon and the Republic of the Congo, 2001–2002

Original Case Definition
- Fever and contact with a case of Ebola hemorrhagic fever
- Fever and unexplained bleeding of any kind
- Unexplained death in a person having presented with an acute onset of fever
- Fever and three or more of the following symptoms: headache, vomiting, anorexia, diarrhea, weakness or severe fatigue, abdominal pain, body aches or joint pains, difficulty swallowing, difficulty breathing, and hiccups

Revised Case Definition
- Fever and contact with a case of Ebola hemorrhagic fever
- Fever and unexplained bleeding of any kind
- Unexplained death in a person having presented with an acute onset of fever; fever in a hunter having entered into the forest or other person having contact with wild animals, living or dead, in the 3 weeks before onset of illness
- New onset of fever within 3 weeks of having been hospitalized in Ogooué Ivindo Province
- For patients who do *not* meet any of these criteria: acute febrile illness that persists despite at least 48 hours of appropriate antimalarial and/or antibiotic therapy

There was, however, the usual difficulty of sensitivity versus specificity. To not miss a case, you could consider everybody with fever to have Ebola. The rookie usually feels most comfortable with this strategy, which is indeed prudent in outbreak settings where missing a single case can have disastrous consequences; however, the problem with this approach is that you'll soon fill up your isolation ward with a whole bunch of people who indeed do *not* have Ebola and not have enough room for those who *do*. Furthermore, although infection control guidelines are put in place to prevent it,[7,8] there is still a chance that a patient who does not have Ebola might contract it in an isolation ward. Thus, difficult as it is (and it's *very* difficult), you have to find some balance, to give up some sensitivity for specificity. We add on various signs and symptoms commonly seen in Ebola to try to increase the specificity but, because the early clinical presentation is so similar to most other systemic febrile diseases, they don't help much (Table 17-1).

After some weeks into the outbreak in Gabon, we began to realize that there were some twists on the epidemiology compared with previous epidemics.[1,5] There were a few nosocomial cases, but the numbers were not large. Instead, clusters were noticed in families, sometimes with incubation periods between cases too short to be consistent with human-to-human spread. Furthermore, the initial cases were predominantly male and often members of the same hunting party.

Hunting is the major source of food and protein in inland Gabon, and the killing of a broad array of wild game, including nonhuman primates such as gorillas and chimps, is common (although not necessarily always legal). Like their human cousins, nonhuman primates are susceptible to Ebola virus, rapidly developing severe and usually fatal disease (a fact that excludes them from consideration as the natural reservoir). In fact, over the past decade Ebola has posed a major challenge to the survival of great apes in West Africa, even threatening extinction.[9] Nonhuman primates and perhaps other wild animals are also capable of transmitting Ebola virus to humans who come in contact with them during the course of their illness, usually through hunting.[10,11] An epidemiologic pattern distinct from the nosocomially fueled course seen in most previous outbreaks began to emerge in Gabon; small hunting parties of around five males would head into the forest for expeditions of days to weeks. While there, they would get infected with Ebola virus, perhaps through direct contact with the still unknown primary reservoir or, probably more frequently, through hunting Ebola-infected wild animals (and, logically, the gorilla or chimp suffering from Ebola would be the easier one to catch). Members of the hunting party probably most frequently get infected when they butcher the animal shortly after killing it. Although the hunting party may come home with infected meat, Ebola virus is sensitive to heat and unlikely to last very long in the hot tropical environment. Refrigeration is rarely possible in these areas, and the virus will certainly be inactivated on cooking.

The bigger danger to the family members at home is not the meat, but rather the hunters incubating Ebola virus. In fact, hunters were the index cases of all the chains of transmission except one in Gabon. After a few days at home, one or more members of the hunting party fall sick. The females, traditionally the care takers of sick persons in the household, now become the at-risk group, exposed to infected blood or bodily fluids as they care for their male family members, damping away blood from the mouth or cleaning up after and emptying plastic pails of Ebola-contaminated feces or vomit. In turn, the women fall sick. Still another wave of infection occurs when remaining females in the household take care of their sick mother, daughter, or sister. Over a few weeks, a small cluster can be recognized, males early and females later. This distinct epidemiology relative to other Ebola outbreaks was reflected in the gender ratio of cases. Because of the predominance of female caretakers in the home, most Ebola outbreaks are skewed toward females[1,6]; however, in Gabon, the majority (52%) of the cases were males, reflecting the fact that hunting is almost an exclusively male activity.[5] Recognizing the key role played by hunters in the epidemic in Gabon, we added elements of hunting, forest entry, and exposure to wild animals to our case definition, allowing us to increase the specificity (Table 17-1). We also narrowed the case definition for nosocomial cases by adding a geographic restriction—Ogooué Ivindo Province, where, at that point at least, all the cases had been seen.

THE SCREW UP AND NOSOCOMIAL TRANSMISSION

A few days after my arrival in Mekembo, the results of a batch of samples sent to CIRMF for Ebola testing came back. That kid with the periapical abscess had Ebola! How could this be? How could I have missed this diagnosis? I was shocked and devastated, consumed by guilt and self-doubt. Not having placed the patient in isolation, I wondered how many cases of secondary transmission there would be. How many people might die because of my blunder? I and a small team rushed back to Makokou to address this new crisis and, despite the mother's continued vigorous protest, isolate the boy.

As it turned out, the boy got rapidly better and went home. None of his family members, other contacts, or the health care workers that cared for him got sick, but I passed some nervous days waiting to see what would happen. To their credit, rather than finger pointing, the outbreak team supported and encouraged me. Two members of the MSF team, Christian Katzer and Isabelle Delbeke, were especially kind to me during that time, for which I will always be grateful. Two take home points here are these: (1) Avoid equivocation and half-way measures, which just confuse everybody (including yourself). Decide whether the patient fits the case definition that you have set, and if so, implement your full control strategy as planned. (2) Appreciate the potential for diverse clinical pathogenesis and presentation, especially of diseases that have not been extensively studied.

The interaction between virus, innate and adaptive immune responses is complex and can likely result in a spectrum of clinical presentations.

To this day, I think that there was something strange about that case. If this was Ebola, how could the mother, with so much direct exposure to the boy's blood, possibly have escaped infection? Did she carry some gene that rendered her immune, like the gene for Duffy antigen that confers protection from infection with *Plasmodium vivax* malaria? Perhaps, although unrecognized, she had previously had Ebola herself and survived and was now immune? Seroprevalence studies suggest that circulation of Ebola virus in eastern Gabon is not rare,[10,12,13] and mild and asymptomatic Ebola has been described.[14–16] I'll never be able to explain it (and could not get blood from the mother to test for evidence of previous infection) and still wonder whether maybe the laboratory result was a false positive (although subsequent tests confirmed it). This is, of course, irrelevant now—probably just still hoping to cover for my mistake.

Events such as this boy's case should be a signal to us, stimulating the scientific side of our brains to develop and test hypotheses to understand better the disease and how to control it. Especially with diseases such as the viral hemorrhagic fevers, where the remote and sporadic nature of the diseases usually make prospective study difficult,[17] outbreaks need to be looked at as not only public health responses, but our chance to learn about what is going on. Public health comes first, but scientifically and ethically sound research, with the appropriate safeguards and approvals from the patients and institutional review boards, is an essential part of most outbreak response efforts and indeed is in the best interest of public health. There have been organizations and persons who have opposed this, sometimes with a "damn it—we're trying to save lives here while you're just interested in your data and publishing papers" attitude. I notice that these are often the same people that call to ask you questions such as "how long does the virus last in the blood?" and are disappointed if there is no definitive answer. No blood collected—no research, no answer.

Although the boy, his mother, and those treating him dodged the bullet, it was becoming clear that others exposed at the hospital in Makokou were not so fortunate and that the lack of barrier nursing and infection control practices that I'd noticed the first day was, unfortunately, having an effect after all; the two other patients that shared a room with the nurse I had seen the first day, considered at the time to have malaria, had fallen ill with febrile illnesses, eventually fatal, after returning home from the hospital. Both were subsequently confirmed as cases of Ebola. There were numerous other nosocomial infections of Ebola in Makokou Regional Hospital. The only thing that perhaps prevented a major nosocomial outbreak was that, as word slipped out into the community of a dangerous disease contracted at the hospital, visits and admissions to the hospital drastically tailed off.

FRICTION IN THE COMMUNITY

Meanwhile, the outbreak response efforts in Mekembo were not going well. Power struggles, politics, and infighting among the team members, both expatriate and Gabonese, were deteriorating morale and reducing the team's effectiveness. Furthermore, the outbreak team and their public health prevention messages were generally not being welcomed by the local population. A history of suspicion of white foreigners dating back to colonial times, intertribal frictions, and distrust of the government in Libreville (who had met the outbreak with measures such as cancelling scheduled elections, presumably intended to prevent virus transmission facilitated by the gathering of large groups of people, and imposing a quarantine on the implicated provinces) were among the factors that led to significant resistance by the community. The cancelling of elections seemed proof that political forces were at work. Rumors circulated that Ebola virus was intentionally planted in the nonhuman primates as a diabolical plan to introduce it into and wipe out the local population through hunting. Furthermore, the fact that the malady seemed to concentrate only in certain families was taken as evidence that witchcraft might be at the heart of it, rather than viruses which "should affect everybody equally." To date, virtually all of the patients who had gone into the isolation ward, run in part by the Gabonese military, had died, again arousing suspicion, fueled still more by rumors, that patients were simply being left in their beds to die.

Persons thought to have Ebola increasingly refused to be admitted to the isolation ward. Families refused to cooperate with the outreach teams. Contacts could not be traced. At one point, villagers felled trees along major routes to prevent the outreach team vehicles from reaching the villages. A key meeting of the response team was held in late January. With control efforts ground to a halt and increasing risk of violence, it was decided to suspend operations.[18] Experts in communications and social mobilization were brought in to try to diffuse the tense situation with the community. Operations eventually resumed, but the control of the outbreak definitely suffered a setback. We learned a hard lesson about the dangers of underestimating the importance of building trust and a solid relationship with the local community before delving into outbreak response measures.

THE END OF THE OUTBREAK AND HUNT FOR THE EBOLA VIRUS RESERVOIR

After the convention in filovirus outbreaks of declaring them over when a period of two times the longest incubation period (i.e., 2 × 21 days = 42 days) has past, the outbreak in Gabon was declared over in May 2002, with a total of 65 cases and 53 deaths (case fatality of 82%). Another 59 cases and 44 deaths occurred across the border in the adjacent Cuvette Ouest region of the Congo.[5] The international team was involved in field activities for nearly 5 months in the two countries and included over 70 representatives from 17 institutions. The first human case, retrospectively identified, was a hunter reported on October 25, 2001, 47 days before the outbreak was officially declared on December 11.[1,5] Four distinct primary foci were identified together with an isolated case noted in Franceville in the southeast of Gabon, 580 km away from the epicenter, who subsequently traveled by airplane to Libreville (Figure 17-2). No secondary transmission occurred in Libreville. In addition to the human toll, Ebola was likely responsible for a great number of animal deaths, especially great apes and duikers (small- to medium-size antelopes) in the surrounding forest[5,9,19–21] with animal deaths reported as far back as August 2001. Samples taken from their carcasses confirmed a concomitant animal epizootic (i.e., an epidemic in animals).[22]

Because the reservoir for the filoviruses is unknown, environmental investigations, usually entailing the trapping of a wide range of animals for future laboratory analysis, is usually a component of the outbreak response (Figure 17-3). These usually occur toward the end of the outbreak, even after it has concluded, because of the obvious priority of first combating the spread of disease in humans. Field collections in Gabon in the wake of the outbreak resulted in the identification of Ebola virus sequences by PCR and antibodies to Ebola in fruit bats.[23] Because a virus itself was not isolated (PCR identifies a portion of the virus' nucleic acid, but does not always indicate the presence of viable virus capable of replicating), these

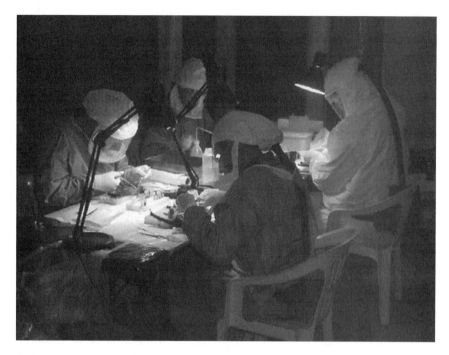

FIGURE 17-3 An ecological investigation team harvests tissues from bats in the Democratic Republic of the Congo in 1999 to test for the presence of Marburg virus. Courtesy of Pierre Rollin.

findings should be considered suggestive, but not definitive, of fruit bats being the reservoir for Ebola. Notably, Ebola's cousin, Marburg virus, has recently been isolated from bats trapped in Uganda (J. Towner, manuscript in preparation).

SOME LESSONS LEARNED

The outbreak in Gabon was one point on the continuum of piecing together the natural history of Ebola virus transmission, both from the natural reservoir to humans and subsequent person-to-person transmission. Major lessons that this outbreak taught us include a greater appreciation of the risk and role of nonhuman primates in the transmission of Ebola to humans. That nonhuman primates could be infected with Ebola and that humans could catch it from them were already known, but these had been isolated incidences. The experience in Gabon and Congo in

2001–2002 helped us understand the much broader scope of human–animal interactions in the context of Ebola, and the danger it poses to both.

Harder lessons were also learned, with issues that remain to be solved. The years of cultural clashes, tension of the populations under pressure, and lack of clinical management options came to a violent head in Gabon. Violence has been seen in subsequent filovirus outbreaks, at times again threatening to derail control efforts. Although these events have engendered a greater appreciation of the need to specifically address issues of communication and cross-cultural understanding, progress must still be made in this regard, perhaps with a renewed focus on the well-being of the individual patient, as opposed to viewing the patient as mainly a source of infection to be isolated for reasons of outbreak control.[24] Although there have been significant research advances on the treatment and vaccine prevention of the filoviruses, no products are yet licensed for use in humans, which continues to pose a major obstacle to the management of outbreaks.[17]

As far me, I still have vivid and surreal memories of spending New Year's Eve 2001 transferring patients to the newly opened isolation ward in Makokou, gowned, gloved, and masked and riding in the back of a pickup truck that served as a make-shift ambulance. I suspect that villagers in Makokou who witnessed this strange and probably terrifying spectacle also call the occasion. I also remember, much later that night, Dr. Abessolo Mengue, a good man doing his best with a difficult situation who also tried to make us feel at home, inviting the outbreak team over to his house for drinks. I couldn't tell you where I was at the stroke of midnight—might have been still hanging on to a beer at his house or maybe already given into exhaustion and sleep.

I eventually did make it back to Switzerland and London, a couple months late for the Christmas celebration or to help my fiancé move. I stuck around the CDC for another year or two after the outbreak in Gabon, continuing to participate in response to outbreaks of hemorrhagic fevers and other virulent viruses, including hantavirus in Bolivia in 2002 and SARS in Vietnam in 2003, as well as work in the laboratory in Atlanta. Although I learned an immense amount from these experiences, I began to feel frustrated by their short-term nature, the feeling that I and the other members of these large international teams, while effective in what we were doing, were inevitably only offering a quick fix for a chronic problem. Without taking more concerted steps to improve the every day capacity on the ground in Africa to respond to outbreaks of all etiologies, we would still be doing the same thing decades from now.

I decided that academia gave me more freedom to pursue some of the goals that I felt important in the field of hemorrhagic fevers, as well to work in aspects of my career that were important to me but largely lacking in my government job, including teaching and interacting with students, more clinical medicine and patient care, expanding the domain of my research to other pathogens, and being able to address more broadly related issues of development, health, and human rights. In 2003, I moved back to New Orleans to rejoin the faculty at the Tulane School of Public Health and Tropical Medicine. At Tulane, one of my major activities is to direct, in contract with the WHO, the Mano River Union Lassa Fever Network (http://www.sph.tulane.edu/ManoRiverLassa), a project to build laboratory and public health infrastructure for the research and control of Lassa fever, a viral hemorrhagic fever prominent in West Africa.[25] I remain interested in the filoviruses, especially directing my attention to how patient care can be improved[24] and how capacity can be built to conduct clinical research in the field on Ebola and Marburg and to translate the laboratory research advances on these viruses through to improved treatment and control in sub-Saharan Africa.[17]

DEDICATION

This chapter is dedicated to my wife, Dr. Frederique Jacquerioz, who admirably weathers the unenviable position of being married to someone interested in field work in the viral hemorrhagic fevers.

ACKNOWLEDGMENTS

The author thanks Katie McCarthy and Catherine Pruszynski for careful review of the manuscript.

REFERENCES

1. Bausch D, Rollin P. Responding to epidemics of Ebola hemorrhagic fever: progress and lessons learned from recent outbreaks in Uganda, Gabon, and Congo. *Emerg Infect* 2004;6:35–57.

2. Bausch DG, Towner JS, Dowell SF, et al. Assessment of the risk of Ebola virus transmission from bodily fluids and fomites. *J Infect Dis* 2007;196(Suppl 2): S142–S147.

3. Dowell SF, Mukunu R, Ksiazek TG, Khan AS, Rollin PE, Peters CJ. Transmission of Ebola hemorrhagic fever: a study of risk factors in family members, Kikwit, Democratic Republic of the Congo, 1995. Commission de Lutte contre les Epidemies a Kikwit. *J Infect Dis* 1999;179(Suppl 1):S87–S91.

4. Bausch D. Of sickness unknown: death, and health, in Africa. *United Nations Chronicle* 2001;38:5–13.

5. Nkoghe D, Formenty P, Leroy EM, et al. Multiple Ebola virus haemorrhagic fever outbreaks in Gabon, from October 2001 to April 2002. *Bull Soc Pathol Exot* 2005;98:224–229.

6. Khan AS, Tshioko FK, Heymann DL, et al. The reemergence of Ebola hemorrhagic fever, Democratic Republic of the Congo, 1995: Commission de Lutte contre les Epidemies a Kikwit. *J Infect Dis* 1999;179(Suppl 1):S76–S86.

7. CDC and WHO. *Infection Control for Viral Haemorrhagic Fevers in the African Health Care Setting.* Atlanta: Centers for Disease Control and Prevention, 1998.

8. Bausch DG. Ebola and Marburg Viruses. In *PIER: The Physicians' Information and Education Resource.* Philadelphia: American College of Physicians, 2008 (http://pier.acponline.org/physicians/diseases/d891/d891.html).

9. Walsh PD, Abernethy KA, Bermejo M, et al. Catastrophic ape decline in western equatorial Africa. *Nature* 2003;422:611–614.

10. Georges AJ, Leroy EM, Renaut AA, et al. Ebola hemorrhagic fever outbreaks in Gabon, 1994–1997: epidemiologic and health control issues. *J Infect Dis* 1999; 179(Suppl 1):S65–S75.

11. Formenty P, Hatz C, Le Guenno B, Stoll A, Rogenmoser P, Widmer A. Human infection due to Ebola virus, subtype Cote d'Ivoire: clinical and biologic presentation. *J Infect Dis* 1999;179(Suppl 1):S48–S53.

12. Monath TP. Ecology of Marburg and Ebola viruses: speculations and directions for future research. *J Infect Dis* 1999;179(Suppl 1):S127–S38.

13. Johnson ED, Gonzalez JP, Georges A. Filovirus activity among selected ethnic groups inhabiting the tropical forest of equatorial Africa. *Trans R Soc Trop Med Hyg* 1993;87:536–538.

14. Leroy EM, Baize S, Debre P, Lansoud-Soukate J, Mavoungou E. Early immune responses accompanying human asymptomatic Ebola infections. *Clin Exp Immunol* 2001;124:453–460.

15. Leroy EM, Baize S, Volchkov VE, et al. Human asymptomatic Ebola infection and strong inflammatory response. *Lancet* 2000;355:2210–2215.

16. Baize S, Leroy EM, Georges-Courbot MC, et al. Defective humoral responses and extensive intravascular apoptosis are associated with fatal outcome in Ebola virus-infected patients. *Nat Med* 1999;5:423–426.

17. Bausch D, Sprecher AG, Jeffs B, Boumandouki P. Treatment of Marburg and Ebola hemorrhagic fevers: a strategy for testing new drugs and vaccines under outbreak conditions. *Antiviral Res* 2008;78:150–161.

18. Larkin M. Ebola outbreak in the news. *Lancet Infect Dis* 2002;3:255.
19. Lahm SA, Kombila M, Swanepoel R, Barnes RF. Morbidity and mortality of wild animals in relation to outbreaks of Ebola haemorrhagic fever in Gabon, 1994–2003. *Trans R Soc Trop Med Hyg* 2007;101:64–78.
20. Rouquet P, Froment JM, Bermejo M, et al. Wild animal mortality monitoring and human Ebola outbreaks, Gabon and Republic of Congo, 2001–2003. *Emerg Infect Dis* 2005;11:283–290.
21. Leroy EM, Rouquet P, Formenty P, et al. Multiple Ebola virus transmission events and rapid decline of central African wildlife. *Science* 2004;303:387–390.
22. Leroy EM, Souquiere S, Rouquet P, Drevet D. Re-emergence of Ebola haemorrhagic fever in Gabon. *Lancet* 2002;359:712.
23. Leroy EM, Kumulungui B, Pourrut X, et al. Fruit bats as reservoirs of Ebola virus. *Nature* 2005;438:575–576.
24. Bausch D, Feldmann H, Geisbert T, et al. Outbreaks of filovirus hemorrhagic fever: time to refocus on the patient. *J Infect Dis* 2007;196(Suppl 2):S136–S41.
25. Khan S, Goba A, Chu M, et al. New opportunities for field research on the pathogenesis and treatment of Lassa fever. *Antiviral Res* 2008;78:103–115.

CHAPTER 18

Whipping Whooping Cough in Rock Island County, Illinois

Mark S. Dworkin, MD, MPH&TM

INTRODUCTION

In 2003, I was the state epidemiologist for the Illinois Department of Public Health (IDPH). One of the many interesting and challenging parts of my job was leading the state health department's rapid response team (RRT). This team was created as a response to several highly publicized infectious disease outbreaks that had occurred in the late 1990s. When Illinois was dealing with those events, I was in Atlanta working at the Centers for Disease Control and Prevention (CDC) as a medical epidemiologist in the Division of HIV/AIDS Prevention in the Surveillance Branch. Working at the CDC was my first job after the long but interesting training of medical school, internal medicine residency, infectious diseases fellowship, and the CDC's Epidemic Intelligence Service (EIS) (where I was stationed in Seattle at the Washington State Department of Health).

Among the Illinois outbreaks that preceded my arrival was a large outbreak of gastroenteritis from *Escherichia coli* O157:H7 among attendees of a big outdoor rural event in which a lot of meat was cooked and served in a cow pasture. Consumption of inadequately cooked ground beef that had been contaminated with cow feces was a well-recognized mode of transmission of this foodborne disease, partly because of the highly publicized Jack in the Box hamburger outbreak in the early 1990s. In the case of the

Illinois rural outbreak, the mystery of what precisely caused the outbreak was summarized by one epidemiologist as "hamburger patty or cow patty?" because it wasn't perfectly clear whether the burgers or the unwashed hands that were holding them were contaminated. Another newsworthy Illinois outbreak involved participants in a triathlon who swam in Lake Springfield and then became ill with leptospirosis.[1] There is something humbling about the ability of one of the tiniest life forms (the bacteria) to bring the strongest athletes down with complaints of feeling weak. There was also a Chicago area outbreak of streptococcal disease that included cases of necrotizing fasciitis (the bacterial disease inaccurately named by the media as the "flesh-eating virus"). I was told that this latter outbreak received a lot of newspaper and television coverage. These and other publicized outbreaks served to increase recognition of the importance of infectious diseases and the state health department's need to respond. Legislation was passed that provided funding to IDPH to create a RRT to help fight these emerging threats to public health and to assist local health departments during these events.

The initial RRT was hired before my arrival. The intention was that a physician hired as the state epidemiologist would be the team leader. The RRT was created as a multidisciplinary group of public health personnel. In addition to being led by a medical epidemiologist, it included a regional communicable disease representative, a veterinarian knowledgeable in animal slaughter and meat processing, a sanitarian with environmental health and restaurant and food establishment inspection expertise, a microbiologist with a PhD and experience working with pathogens that may be used in bioterrorism, an infection control nurse, and someone experienced in data systems and data analysis. With the exception of myself and an infection control nurse, the individuals that were hired were not trained in epidemiology; therefore, an important part of the meetings that I led every 1 to 2 months included epidemiology training and review of published outbreak investigations. What this team may have lacked in not being a team of polished epidemiologists, it made up for with terrific enthusiasm to do what needed to be done and an eagerness to learn and apply that learning. Later, the team gained CDC EIS officers and public health fellows that I recruited to train at IDPH. The team also benefited from its collaboration with enthusiastic members of various sections within the health department who volunteered on outbreaks on an as-needed basis and the program staff who had experience managing outbreaks before their was the RRT. Many of these health department volunteers had experience working on outbreak investigations before the RRT was created, although their job duties did not allow them to focus on such work. The RRT helped to augment the work of experienced program staff members who were spread thin. Most program staff couldn't spare the time to get out into the field as often as would benefit the local health departments of the state, and thus, the RRT helped to fill this gap.

By September 2003, the team had already gained experience working on many outbreak investigations. Our first experience with pertussis (whooping cough) occurred in 2001 when Coles County in rural eastern central Illinois requested assistance with a rise in pertussis. We provided onsite assistance with the outbreak and observed that a large proportion of the cases that were reported were in adults. Because many people, including in the health care profession, had written pertussis off as a childhood disease that was largely controlled in the United States, the finding of many adult cases attracted my attention. I will not soon forget one man who came to the health department after he learned of the local rise in pertussis. A photograph was taken of him because of the impressive sequelae of the chronic cough that he was manifesting. When he walked into the health department, I was told the first impression was that he had been in an automobile accident because both of his eyes looked purplish red as if he had been struck on the back of the head; however, he met the case definition for pertussis, and had no other condition that would explain his facial change. The man had bilateral subconjunctival hemorrhages (Figure 18-1). This

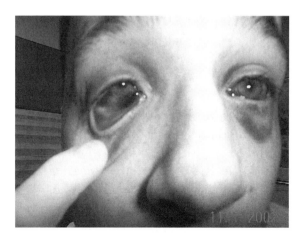

FIGURE 18-1 Man with subconjunctival hemorrhage secondary to paroxysms of coughing.

ocular finding is not specific to pertussis but is one of its possible complications. Other diseases that cause spasmodic coughing for prolonged periods of time are also capable of doing this.

Pertussis is caused by infection with the bacterium *Bordetella pertussis* and is notorious for causing prolonged coughing fits that can occur on and off for weeks or months, vomiting after one or more of these fits, and an inspiratory gasping sound that is known as the whoop. If someone has been previously exposed to pertussis either from a history of having whooping cough or being immunized, they might have a milder illness less likely to be recognized as pertussis but no less deadly to a susceptible infant. Infants are the most likely to be hospitalized or killed by this disease; therefore, control of an outbreak could interfere with transmission to infants and thus prevent hospitalization and death.

In 2002, an outbreak of pertussis occurred in an oil refinery in another downstate rural location, Crawford County. Our CDC EIS officer (Greg Huhn) and others published that outbreak as an MMWR,[2] and it served as another nail in the coffin of the myth that pertussis is just a disease of childhood. No children were working at an oil refinery! My experience with an outbreak among office workers when I was an EIS Officer in Washington State during 1994 to 1996,[3] the Coles County outbreak, and this additional work place outbreak, and reviewing the published literature on pertussis in adults had convinced me that pertussis was not just a disease of childhood. It was a disease of all ages despite widespread immunization with pertussis vaccine for decades. The incidence of pertussis had been gradually rising for 2 decades (Figure 18-2).[4] In 2003, pertussis was the only disease with a rising incidence among the diseases for which there was a recommendation for universal childhood immunization.

In late September 2003, I was called by the administrator of the Rock Island County Health Department, Wendy Trute. Rock Island County is in western Illinois on the Mississippi river and had a population of approximately 148,000 at this time. This region is mostly rural but also is known for its "Quad Cities" (Rock Island and Moline in Illinois, Bettendorf and Davenport in Iowa). The IDPH regional immunization and central office staff were aware of a rise in the number of cases reported from there through their recent communication with the Rock Island County Health Department. As for verifying there was indeed an outbreak, a review of surveillance data revealed that only 15 cases of pertussis had cumulatively been reported in Rock Island County in the past 8 years; however, between July 1

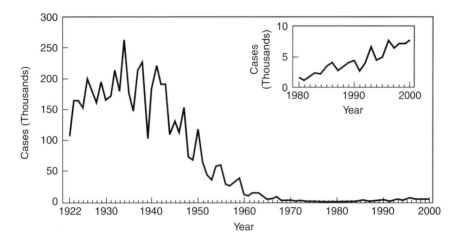

FIGURE 18-2 Number of reported pertussis cases by year—United States 1922–2000.

Adapted from Zanardi L, Pascual FB, Bisgard K, Murphy T, Wharton M, Maurice E. Pertussis—United States, 1997–2000. *Morb Mortal Wkly Rep* 2002;51:73–6.

and September 26 (just a 3-month period), 11 cases had been reported to the health department. It was definitely a situation worthy of additional investigation.

My partner in crime for this outbreak was a seasoned member of the immunization section of IDPH, Chuck Jennings. When he wasn't in his office, he rode around the state in a well-worn Ford van with a personalized license plate that said "CNTAGN 1." At first, I struggled to figure out how to read it until Chuck pronounced it for me, "Contagion 1." He was soft spoken and balding but with a pony tail. Idealistic, passionate about his work, and schooled in the 60s, Chuck began working with immunization preventable disease in the 70s during the "swine flu" vaccine campaign. Only someone who had spent their career excited about the field of immunizations could reveal with great pleasure that he knew where the long since retired jet injectors from the swine flu campaign were stashed.

Chuck recognized the power that our response team could bring to an outbreak. He was eager to apply the enthusiastic personnel resources to fighting the good fight of beating back a disease such as pertussis, and he was a perfect match for the RRT. He knew his way around the state and the subject matter. Despite his experience with pertussis investigation, he very much welcomed having a partner with a different background but equal enthusiasm and at times complimentary knowledge about the pathogen and its manifestations. How we related to each other was a critical feature of the outbreak investigation's ability to succeed.

As the state epidemiologist and a physician, I was an unusual member of a field work team. Many local health department investigations are handled without a physician. Although I knew of several physicians that were warmly regarded years after their assistance, more than once I had been told by local and state health department and hospital staff in Illinois and other states about medical epidemiologists who came in to assist and were condescending, competitive, or left behind a feeling that they were out of touch in some way. I suspect that these ill-remembered medical epidemiologists may have meant well but were ignorant about how they were perceived and the missteps they were taking. The relatively academic culture of medical institutions where physicians are schooled and trained is unlike what one often finds in many state and local health departments and in many community hospitals.

As an example, I recall when I was an EIS officer, a microbiologist in Spokane, Washington told me of his experience with a CDC investigation some years earlier. He had been working with others at his hospital on an investigation of an outbreak of *Pseudomonas cepacia*. The CDC was called to discuss it, and although a breach of good practices related to a medical device was already identified, a CDC investigator requested sending out an EIS officer, as it would be a good training experience. The officer arrived along with his supervisor and additional epidemiologic work was performed without problems.

The point of the story as it was related to me, however, was that another more senior epidemiologist at the CDC had hoped that the Spokane microbiologist would authorize the CDC team to take the investigation data, and then they could publish it themselves. The CDC field supervisor had shared this unsavory plan with the microbiologist, as she had no interest in helping make this happen and was uncomfortable with her requested role. Having not been a part of this investigation or personally knowing the senior epidemiologist, I can't say what was his true intention. In this case, however, it doesn't matter his true intention because the perception of what he was doing was that he was going to publish someone else's data without giving them credit for it. In a phone call that apparently had become an oft-told tale, the senior epidemiologist back at the CDC was on the phone with the field supervisor in Spokane (and the microbiologist was listening in on another line as invited to by the field supervisor so the microbiologist could hear for himself if the issue of taking over control of the outbreak data came up). When the senior epidemiologist asked whether the field supervisor had gotten a release for them to have the data, the field supervisor said that he should ask him himself because he was on the line. This led to an uncomfortable pause and a kind of "gotcha" moment. This story underscores the importance of good communication and the ability for perception (or misperception) to undermine current and future public health work. Needless to say, the microbiologist was hesitant about inviting staff coming from the CDC to assist in an investigation in the future and perhaps others that he may have told the story to retained the same concern.

It is important for anyone, medical or nonmedical, who becomes a guest in a community where they will provide assistance, to be clear and focused on the mission of their work but to maintain an attitude that it is a team effort and not just an opportunity to publish a scientific article as a lead author. Even if one is in the lead of the team, one is also a member of the team. With that thought in mind, Chuck Jennings and the local health department administrator were co-team leaders in this pertussis outbreak investigation. I made it clear very early on that I was not swooping in to take control. I was there to assist them with their efforts. In this and other outbreak investigations at local health departments, this approach was consistently successful.

The conversation with the health department administrator centered primarily on my gathering the facts as known at that time, determining whether onsite assistance was desired (which it was), and outlining what might be done upon arrival of the RRT. The primary work would be (1) to enhance surveillance in order to better determine the extent of the outbreak through case ascertainment and descriptive epidemiology and (2) to control the outbreak through the established public health actions that accompany the identification of a case including antibiotic prophylaxis of close contacts of cases. For my first visit to Rock Island County, to save time, I arranged to fly rather than drive. I was met at the small airport by Chuck Jennings who had a smile on his face like a kid in a candy shop. He really loved the work.

Chuck drove me to the Rock Island County Health Department in his well worn van, and on arriving, we held a meeting of the participating RRT members supplemented by regional immunization section staff, recently hired IDPH bioterrorism preparedness staff (including Judy Conway, an excellent nurse, and Pat Welch, an experienced former environmental health worker from another Illinois county), and local health department staff. This was a crucial meeting because it established what work we would do, allowed for staff to question and then better understand the rationale for the work, and set the tone for organization in the days to come. A "to-do" list was essential, as it laid out what was in front of us and allowed us to see where we were at in the investigation at any given time. A list of everyone relevant to the investigation was also created with contact information including telephone numbers (cell and land lines), pager numbers, and e-mail and text-pager addresses. This was copied and distributed to all of us at the end of the meeting without delay because soon many of us would be going in different directions, including my returning to Chicago where communication would typically be with the staff by phone. Such basic organizational tools as a list of our names and how to reach each other should not be overlooked within the design of a successful outbreak investigation. There was a palpable feeling of relief and excitement by the staff that we had a clear direction to what we each needed to do and where it fell into the big picture.

SURVEILLANCE

Case ascertainment was at the top of our "to-do" list. Passive reporting had allowed for recognition of the pertussis outbreak. Active case finding would benefit our attempt to describe the epidemiology of the outbreak and to control it. The RRT including our communicable disease staff member, Dorian Robinson, and our veterinarian, Karnail Mudahar, helped the local health department to respond to the rise in case reports that followed by performing telephone case investigations on the suspect cases.

Surveillance is information for action. I had emphasized this to the RRT so many times by this point that one day, as we were assembling the team to meet with the Rock Island County staff, Judy walked into the room and stood at attention while saluting, "Judy Conway reporting for duty. Surveillance is information for action!" That action includes respiratory precautions to prevent droplet spread from cases, treatment of cases, and prophylactic treatment of close contacts of the cases. These are the primary methods used to interrupt transmission. It is also important to ensure that the antibiotic used is appropriate for treatment of *B. pertussis* because not just any antibiotic that might get prescribed for a cough illness will reliably kill this organism.

The first way to increase reporting was to enhance the passive reporting system by increasing awareness and encouraging reporting of suspect and confirmed cases. The main reporters of pertussis were physicians and laboratories; therefore, a memorandum was drafted and sent to the local laboratories and to the hospitals for distribution to the physicians. Memorandums were also sent to local day care centers (including one for directors and a separate one for parents), schools, urgent care centers, and chiropractors. There was also communication with neighboring county health departments, including across the river in Iowa (Scott County), to make them aware of the situation and to encourage sharing of information when appropriate. A rise in pertussis was occurring in this part of Iowa which was not a surprise because in this Quad City area some people lived in one state but worked, recreated, or received medical care in the other. After the administrator of the Rock Island County Health Department and the Scott County Health Department spoke, it was agreed that they meet monthly in the future.

In addition to paper communication, I paid a personal visit to several health care facilities to underscore the importance of reporting cases and to provide an opportunity for answering questions that physicians or laboratory personnel might have. I gave a brief lecture on pertussis (including our initial outbreak data) in a doctor's dining room at the Trinity Regional Health System's east campus; met privately with the head of the emergency department, the laboratory director, and then later the adult and pediatric infectious disease physicians at Illini hospital; visited another emergency department at Trinity West; and also visited a community health practice. I made sure that for every visit, I traveled with a health department staff member. I wanted to be certain that the state health department was not given sole credit for the outbreak investigation work. Such a misperception could have undermined the credibility of the local health department. I would come and go, but they would remain in the community. It was therefore very important to boost their credibility and not appear like a "white knight" that came in to save the day. The health department and I both recognized that having a physician knowledgeable in the clinical and epidemiologic side of the pertussis outbreak going out, and personally speaking to other health care staff (especially other physicians) was a rare opportunity to bolster the health department surveillance and investigation efforts. Many health departments outside the largest urban areas of a state lack such a resource, although they may have a community physician who they call on from time to time to assist with medical-related public health decisions. I have had local health department staff confide in me that doctors in their community may dismiss the local health department recommendations because they are coming from a nonphysician.

Another activity was to make the IDPH Division of Laboratories aware of the situation in an effort to increase the speed of communication between the laboratory and the county health department. One of our team members was tasked with being in phone contact with the laboratory regularly. At first, it was daily communication. It was possible to learn of unreported suspect cases by reviewing the state laboratory's list of pertussis tests and comparing the names with the county's list of cases under investigation. When testing was being performed on Rock Island County residents that had not been reported to the Rock Island County Health Department, an investigation was launched to gather information and verify that those persons met the case definition. We used the case definition that was recommended by the Council of State and Territorial Epidemiologists (Exhibit 18-1).

The concepts of sensitivity and specificity come to life within the pertussis case definition because this definition provides for a very sensitive and nonspecific alternative for use during an outbreak. This alternative case definition requires that the case only have cough illness for at least 2 weeks and be reported by a health care provider. It is a great way to catch a lot of cases. The question at this point was whether this case definition is intended for a community outbreak. With a population of approximately 148,000 people, the application of this very sensitive definition could lead to a substantial and even dramatic rise in case reporting with the potential to include large numbers of persons who have other cough illnesses; therefore, a case definition such as this is most useful in a community setting when used for identifying possible cases in order to investigate further whether they satisfy the probable or confirmed case definition and for selective use in outbreaks in special settings such as among a well-defined population rather than the entire county.

We also performed active case finding by sending some of our team members to review the medical records of the emergency department at Trinity West. We picked a limited time period of records to review based

---

Exhibit 18-1   Council of State and Territorial Epidemiologists' 1997 Case Definition for Pertussis

---

Clinical Case Definition

A cough illness lasting at least 2 weeks with one of the following: paroxysms of coughing, inspiratory "whoop," or posttussive vomiting, without other apparent cause (as reported by a health professional)

Laboratory Criteria for Diagnosis

Isolation of *Bordetella pertussis* from clinical specimen

Positive polymerase chain reaction (PCR) for *B. pertussis*

Case Classification

Probable: meets the clinical case definition, is not laboratory confirmed, and is not epidemiologically linked to a laboratory confirmed case

Confirmed: a case that is culture positive and in which an acute cough illness of any duration is present; or a case that meets the clinical case definition and is confirmed by positive PCR; or a case that meets the clinical case definition and is epidemiologically linked directly to a case confirmed by either culture or PCR

Comment

The clinical case definition above is appropriate for endemic or sporadic cases. In outbreak settings, a case may be defined as a cough illness lasting at least 2 weeks (as reported by a health professional). Because direct fluorescent antibody testing of nasopharyngeal secretions has been demonstrated in some studies to have low sensitivity and variable specificity, such testing should not be relied on as a criterion for laboratory confirmation. Serologic testing for pertussis is available in some areas but is not standardized and, therefore, should not be relied on as a criterion for laboratory confirmation.

Both probable and confirmed cases should be reported nationally.

---

on two factors. The first was personnel. Judy Conway and Pat Welch who were primarily assigned to this task were available to realistically perform it for approximately 3 or 4 days at the most. The second factor was the likelihood that we could perform useful actions after identifying cases retrospectively. Perhaps we could have examined records going several months back in time, and in theory, we might have identified additional persons who met our case definition and populated an epidemic curve of the outbreak; however, for every medical record that we screened where their symptoms lasted at least 7 days and were consistent with the possibility of pertussis (such as cough illness but without an obvious explanation), we contacted the patient to interview them with questions to determine whether they met the pertussis case definition. If we had gone back 3 or perhaps 4 months, not only would we have created a huge mound of records to review and had a problem with recall, we would also have identified cases that were no longer contagious and whose close contacts were also unlikely to be contagious because of how long ago their infections had started; therefore, we reviewed emergency department records of patients presenting with cough illness during the previous 2 months starting with the most recent cases.

A spreadsheet of possible cases was generated from this review and health department staff performed the follow-up telephone calls after they cross-referenced with the spreadsheet with cases already reported (to avoid duplication of effort). A similar medical record review was also performed at a local urgent care clinic. Seven suspect cases were identified among the emergency department records reviewed (although the denominator is not available to determine what fraction that was of all reviewed records); however, among 250 urgent care records reviewed, five were suspect cases (2%). Given that our goal was to control a disease that could be passed from person to person to person to infant (who it could hospitalize or kill) and because we had adequate personnel resources at the beginning of the outbreak investigation, we believed that this was an acceptable, although low, yield for this record review.

To help us determine the scope and the impact of the outbreak, we also surveyed local pharmacies. We had an interest in exploring syndromic methods of surveillance to gain experience with these issues. There were no electronic methods in place that obtained data representative of the region so Pat Welch gathered the information directly from pharmacies. She contacted nine large pharmacies to identify what was their experience with sales of over the counter cough medicine and antibiotics that would likely be used to treat pertussis (specifically, erythromycin, clarithromycin, and azithromycin). This identified a modest increase in over-the-counter sales and the antibiotics, but nothing dramatic. We were satisfied to have gone through this exercise to demonstrate what we were capable of doing, but we did not find it very useful as the outbreak was already established; however, if we had identified a marked increase in the sales of these pharmaceuticals, we would have hypothesized that the outbreak might be impacting the community to a greater degree than we currently had recognized, and we would have questioned the sensitivity of our surveillance system efforts. Additional investigation would then have been performed.

The county's outbreak data was maintained using an Epi Info database that RRT member Roland Lucht helped to set up and maintain. Chuck made sure that the data were reported to the Immunization Section at IDPH. As we examined the data regularly throughout our surveillance efforts, there were several factors we had to consider that could influence the case count. The first was heightened awareness. Our efforts led to an increased likelihood that physicians would think of pertussis when a compatible case presented to them. Of course this was an intended result that we hoped would increase reporting so that we could ensure control measures were undertaken for each case; therefore, a rising case count early on would not indicate an outbreak that we were failing to control but more likely an outbreak that we were more accurately capturing through surveillance. There was media coverage as well, and thus, the community was learning about pertussis from their local newspaper and other media outlets. As a result, persons with a cough illness might bring up the possibility that they had pertussis to their health care provider and even could request testing. Given that pertussis was recognized to be circulating among the U.S. population before the outbreak, we had to consider that some of the rise in cases was actually an uncovering of the endemic disease secondary to heightened recognition and increased testing practices. We did not have a way to quantify this issue because we did not have data that defined the true background rate of pertussis in this community. We only had historic passive pertussis surveillance data that are known to underrepresent markedly the true incidence of disease.

Another important factor that impacted on our data was diagnostic testing. Culture of *B. pertussis* is considered the gold standard, but the organism can easily die, which may lead to false negatives. The organism requires a special transport medium that is not as widely available as a rapid test for strep throat or a transport medium used to swab an ordinary wound for culture. Thus, a special effort was made to supply and resupply the local laboratories with plenty of this transport medium and to educate the local physicians that it was needed for accurate diagnosis. A nasopharyngeal swab is performed to collect the specimen; however, not all physicians are aware of this, and therefore, a throat swab can be incorrectly submitted. In addition, the choice of swab used to obtain a nasopharyngeal specimen could also impact on the yield of culture and the more sensitive molecular-based PCR. Dacron and calcium alginate swabs are preferred for culture because cotton swabs can inhibit the growth of *B. pertussis*. Calcium alginate swabs inhibit PCR. When culture and PCR are planned, Dacron and rayon swabs are the best choice.[5] Thus, there were many factors competing to undermine our confirmation of cases, including trying to get physicians, including many unfamiliar with pertussis, to perform the nasopharyngeal swab using the right kind of swab and sending it with the special transport medium.

The timing of the nasopharyngeal swab is also important. The yield is highest in the first 2 weeks after the onset of illness.[6] It may not be worthwhile testing several weeks into the cough illness, although that is when pertussis is most likely to be considered in sporadically occurring cases. Age also impacts on yield. Adults and immunized persons mount an immune response that suppresses the number of organisms more quickly after onset of illness so that diagnostic yield is less with increasing age. What this meant to our outbreak was that we were likely to have a lot of negative specimens because we were observing a large proportion of cases in adolescents and adults and who had been coughing for weeks before being recognized as cases.

Laboratory confirmation is a subclassification of the case definition but is not required for case reporting if the patient met the clinical case definition; however, reporting is affected by the factors that can increase the likelihood of a negative laboratory result in a true case because physicians commonly view negative test results for a pathogen as a rule-out procedure for that diagnosis. Therefore, a patient could meet the clinical case definition and their physician could think of pertussis and even decide that it was worth the extra effort to submit a specimen for culture or PCR; however, if the swab chosen was not the optimal swab for the test being ordered or they swabbed the throat, if the transport medium was not correct, if the patient was several weeks out since onset of illness or was an adolescent or adult, if the specimen was mishandled in transport, or if laboratory difficulties with the specimen were to occur, a negative result would later be received by the health care provider, and no report would follow. As if these were not enough issues with laboratory diagnosis, serology is also another point for confusion. A reliable and Food and Drug Administration (FDA)-approved serologic test for pertussis was not available for use during this outbreak investigation; however, serologic tests (not FDA approved) were available to health care providers and were being obtained.

As a result, serologic test results could not guide definitive conclusions about whether a person had been infected with pertussis, but lack of awareness of this could have caused some physicians to use them as a definitive answer. For this reason, it is important during pertussis outbreaks to stress to health care providers that reporting should not be dependent on the laboratory results. If their patient meets the clinical case definition (or the outbreak case definition in the setting of an outbreak), then the case should be reported. It should also be recognized that there are situations where local or state health departments may decide to limit reporting of cases to only those meeting the confirmed case classification because of the department's inability to handle the volume of probable cases that would result.

THE CONTROVERSY OF DEFINING A CLOSE CONTACT

In the midst of all the surveillance activities, we were made aware of an adult football coach who was positive by PCR for *B. pertussis*. An investigation was begun, and it was learned that the coach had extensive face-to-face contact with others (which, of course, was not unexpected). Interviewing of approximately 110 students and other contacts of the coach at the high school one evening identified 26 persons with an active cough illness. The team physician elected to give chemoprophylaxis to the entire team. Practices continued, and they planned to postpone their next game by 3 days; however, the competing team, apparently driven by fear, would not play their perceived to be contagious competitor, and a forfeit was arranged. The rationale for providing prophylaxis to the team was explained by the Rock Island County Health Department administrator in a local newspaper article entitled "Whipping whooping cough": ". . . If you think about a football team, being in a locker room together, on a bus together, three or four hours everyday together in practice, the coach being positive, there's a lot of reasons why the players would be more susceptible." The finding of this cluster of potential cases within the community illustrates another example of the value of heightened surveillance within an outbreak. It allows for recognition of situations in which additional investigation may be needed such as this football coach or a health care provider or hospital employee who might have routine close contact with patients.

In this and other pertussis outbreaks I have been involved in, how to define a close contact has been controversial. Often there has been a general rule applied but judgment has been allowed on a case-by-case basis. I have seen it defined as prolonged face-to-face contact versus being within 3 feet some period of time such as at least 10 minutes versus much longer. The questions will come up: "What about the child who sits directly behind the case in the classroom? Does that child need prophylaxis?" "What about the other children in the classroom for whom we don't know exactly how much contact they might have had with the child during the day?" "How do we handle the situation where a student does not stay in one room most of the day (such as the high school student) but sits in multiple class-rooms of different students throughout the day, leading to a huge number of potential close contacts?" "How about those who ride on the bus with the child?" The more questions asked and answered liberally to try to inter-rupt transmission completely, the more prophylaxis might be dispensed to the point where it seems excessive. As a result, some health departments have changed their recommendation for close contacts to be only those at highest risk for morbidity or mortality or contributing to the morbidity and mortality of others (such as reserving it for pregnant women and oth-ers who are likely to expose infants).[7]

THE IMPORTANCE OF AGE

By October, a preliminary look at the epidemiology demonstrated some interesting findings that illustrated the importance of this disease in the adolescent and adult population. Recalling that the case definition in-cluded two classic features of the disease that were typically thought to occur mainly in children and the unimmunized (posttussive vomiting and whooping), we examined the data collected from the cases by age group to understand better the distribution of these symptoms in adolescents and adults. The hypothesis was that these symptoms would be uncommon but present; therefore, I was surprised to observe that posttussive vomiting occurred as frequently as 20% to 60% in those older than 21 years of age. Even more surprising was that whooping occurred in 33% to 88% of those older than 21 years of age (Figure 18-3).

When we later examined nearly all of the cases, it was clear that the majority (70%) were in adolescents and adults (Figure 18-4). This was yet another example of the important role of the older population as a reser-voir of pertussis for infants who were most vulnerable to its more severe complications. Our active case finding had identified many persons in the

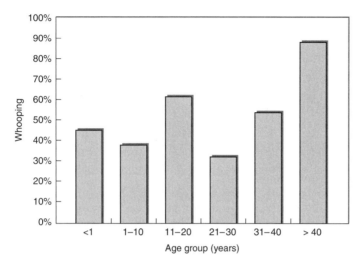

FIGURE 18-3 Preliminary analysis of whooping by age among the first 66 cases reported, Rock Island County, Illinois, 2003.

community that met the case definition who otherwise would have gone unrecognized.

Given that these cases were occurring in persons basically with a history of pertussis immunization as children or old enough to have likely had pertussis in the prevaccine era, the lesson learned here was that the vaccine does not provide lifelong immunity. This was not new information, but given that many vaccines do appear to provide long lasting immunity (such

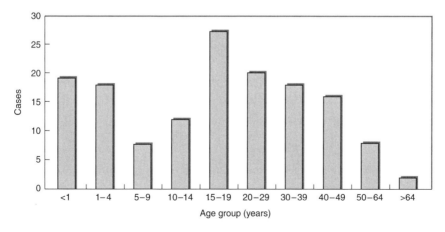

FIGURE 18-4 Distribution by age of 148 cases of pertussis, Rock Island County, Illinois, 2003.

as measles vaccine), it can be overlooked that pertussis vaccine-induced immunity begins to decline relatively soon after completion of the pertussis immunization series of vaccines. The duration of immunity after vaccination ranges from approximately 4 to 12 years and for infection-acquired immunity ranges from 7 to 20 years[8]; therefore, a vaccinated child can be fully susceptible as early as 9 or 10 or during their adolescent years. What was nicely illustrated here was that adults with surprising frequency could get the more classic symptoms such as whooping rather than only very mild illness, as had been the common anecdote when I interacted with a variety of physicians in various settings over the years. Certainly, adults can and do get mild illness, but I had not before seen documented such a relatively high frequency of these more severe symptoms. I recall one of the investigation staff commenting that an adult patient was having a coughing fit and whooping during their telephone interview with them.

COMMUNICATION

Finally, a variety of communications issues had to be dealt with during this outbreak investigation. Communication targets included the media (and through them to the public), other public health jurisdictions, and others who can be viewed as stakeholders of the investigation and pertussis surveillance system, including health care providers, laboratories, and the local college, schools, and day care facilities. In addition, internal communications were vital, including among the investigation staff and with personnel off site within the state health department, including program staff and those higher up the chain of command.

Communication with the media should be handled with forethought and ideally is performed by someone with experience. Although health departments in jurisdictions with large populations may have a public information officer whose role can be critical during outbreaks, emergencies, and day-to-day communication with the media, most health departments do not have this luxury and the Rock Island County Health Department fell into this category of serving a moderate sized population; however, we were able to consult with IDPH on these issues and also found that once we had our overriding communications objectives decided on, the anxiety of communicating with the media decreased.

A concern with communicating with the media about an outbreak is primarily that although you can control what you write in a press release or speak in an interview, what the journalist does with the information after that is completely out of your control. As a result, they could choose to write an article about how the health department is incompetent, or they can make heroes out of the staff, or something in between. In one outbreak investigation, the local newspaper referred to our investigation team as a "crack team" of experts who "descended" on the local jail where the outbreak was occurring. They made us sound like a bunch of superheroes. I have been fortunate not to have the other extreme, but I have seen news that put health departments in an unfavorable light.

The media can play a vital role within the response to the outbreak. They can help disseminate prevention information and calm fears about the emerging problem. You won't usually see public health prevention as front-page news, but if it is going to occur, an outbreak is a likely time for it; therefore, we made how to prevent disease transmission and advocacy for disease reporting among our major communications objectives in interviews with local newspapers and other journalists who contacted the health department. We were pleased to see information about the disease symptoms, who was susceptible, and how to prevent it on the front page of the Quad City Times (Exhibit 18-2). Wendy, the local health department administrator, had not been on the job very long when this outbreak occurred, but she and her staff did a great job with handling it, as well as with communicating with the media. I made myself available for some interviews, especially when it would lend credibility to the dissemination of medical information; however, as mentioned earlier, it was important to have the local health department speak for themselves to the media with assistance from the state as needed rather than giving the unhelpful impression that the state deserved all the credit for the control of the outbreak.

Another of the important messages to impart through the media was that the case count was expected to rise. Communicating this properly was of great importance because as we performed case ascertainment successfully, the number of cases reported would rise sharply. If not forewarned that this was a planned outcome, the media could issue news reports that the outbreak was worsening despite health department efforts. The last thing we wanted to see was a headline such as "Cases of Whooping Cough Soar Despite Health Department's Attempts at Control." This would undermine credibility and be inaccurate; therefore, we made it clear during early interviews that our efforts would likely lead to a rise in case counts and that this was our intended result.

Exhibit 18-2   Newspaper Article in the Quad City Times, Including Information on Transmission and Prevention of Pertussis as Front-Page News

---

Friday, September 26, 2003

WHOOPING COUGH STRIKES Q-C

LOCAL AUTHORITIES CONFIRM 22 CASES OF DEADLY DISEASE

By Cherie Black
QUAD-CITY TIMES

An outbreak of a disease many thought was no longer a threat has invaded the Quad-City area.

Pertussis, more commonly known as whooping cough, has appeared in a cluster of cases throughout Rock Island and Scott counties in recent months, prompting local health departments to begin investigating the extent of the outbreak and educating physicians and residents of the possible dangers.

Since July 1, there have been 11 confirmed cases among Rock Island County residents between the ages of two months and 37 years old with more than a dozen other cases being investigated. This compares with just 15 cases reported between 1995 and 2002.

In Scott County, 11 cases have been diagnosed since Aug. 1, including one confirmed Thursday. Nine of the cases came from the same day care facility. Last year, 25 cases were diagnosed; there were six in 2000 and 2001.

"Even though pertussis is an old disease, it is considered to be making a comeback," said Chuck Jennings, a member of the Illinois Department of Health Rapid Response Team, which has teamed with the Rock Island County Health Department to investigate the outbreak. "We now see that adults serve as a reservoir for this bacteria. Ten to 12 years ago, we didn't think adults could get this."

Whooping cough is a highly contagious bacterial infection that causes coughing and gagging with little or no fever. An infected person has cold-like symptoms and prolonged cough episodes that may end in vomiting or cause a "whoop" sound when the person tries to breathe in. Once diagnosed by a nasal swab or a DNA-type test, whooping cough can be treated with a 14-day dose of antibiotics. Household contacts who may have also been exposed are also asked to be tested. Although it is a disease most people have been vaccinated against, it is more dangerous in infants 12 months and younger and can be fatal.

"Because it's a vaccine-preventable disease, we don't expect to see it as much as we have in our population," said Roma Taylor, a clinical services counselor with the Scott County Health Department. "But the effectiveness of the vaccine tends to wane in teenagers and adults."

Because of this, health officials are encouraging residents and especially physicians [to be aware] of the symptoms to avoid the spread of the disease.

"We're into allergy season and also going into flu season, and we want physicians to be thinking of whooping cough as a possibility and not just think patients just have allergies or bronchitis," Taylor said.

Rock Island County Health Department administrator Wendy Trute and state epidemiologists have been visiting hospitals, schools, day care facilities and health care clinics to make sure staff is aware of symptoms.

"I think a lot of them were surprised this wasn't even on their radar," Trute said. "This spreads from person to person to person and is highly contagious. We want to try and stop the spread and break that chain of development."

BY THE NUMBERS

Pertussis is a highly contagious bacterial infection that causes coughing and gagging with little or no fever. An infected person has cough episodes that may end in vomiting or cause a "whoop" sound when the person tries to breathe in.

THE SYMPTOMS: Symptoms appear between 6 to 21 days after exposure to the bacteria. The disease starts with cold symptoms like a runny nose and a cough. Sometime in the first two weeks, episodes of severe cough develop that can last one to two months. The infected person may look and feel fairly healthy between these episodes. During bouts of coughing the lips and nails may turn blue for lack of air. Vomiting may occur after severe coughing spells. During the severe coughing stage, seizures or even death can occur, particularly in an infant.

WHO GETS IT: Anyone who is exposed can get pertussis. Unimmunized or inadequately immunized people are at higher risk for severe disease. Many cases occur in adults because protection from the vaccine lasts only 5 to 10 years.

TREATMENTS: The vaccination against pertussis is included in the DTP and DTaP vaccines. Before age 7, children should receive 5 doses of the DTP or DTaP vaccine. These usually are given at 2, 4, 6, and 15–18 months of age and 4–6 years of age. Persons with pertussis should avoid contact with others until no longer contagious. If you live with someone who has pertussis or are exposed in any way, antibiotics are necessary.

Reprinted with permission of the Quad City Times.

As mentioned earlier, the Rock Island County Health Department maintained regular contact with their colleagues across the river in Iowa. They also shared information with other health departments in their region of Illinois. Within Illinois, these activities were facilitated by a regional IDPH employee who also shared information with the central office at IDPH. This kind of communication with other jurisdictions was especially important to minimize the chance of inconsistent information being released. The media could go to other jurisdictions and to the state health department for information on this outbreak because it was not exclusively involving Rock Island County. With so many potential voices, it would be easy for inconsistent messages to be released.

Appropriate prescription of antibiotics for prophylaxis of all close contacts was another important communications issue. Prophylaxis has been a routine part of pertussis control for many years (although recently its efficacy as a control measure has been called into question). In outbreaks of limited size, it may be feasible to treat all close contacts with an antibiotic that is effective at killing *B. pertussis*. Some health care providers enthusiastically attempted to comply with this recommendation, and we even heard from one physician that there was a shortage of erythromycin at one or more of the local pharmacies; however, in conflict with this kind of recommendation was the recent public and health care provider targeted campaign by authoritative organizations such as the American College of Physicians and the CDC aimed at minimizing inappropriate prescription of antibiotics.[9,10] This campaign was an effort to respond to the rising rates of antibiotic resistance among bacterial pathogens. As a result, there was a lot of pushback on the recommendation to treat asymptomatic children and adults with the drug of choice at that time (erythromycin). It didn't help that the drug needed to be given for 14 days and was known to cause an upset stomach; therefore, our communication needed to stress the rationale for the recommendation and to explain that prophylaxis was indicated for close contacts regardless of age and even if they had a history of pertussis immunization.

Although I am now less convinced that every single "close contact" of a pertussis case needs to receive prophylaxis as part of the control of a pertussis outbreak, during this outbreak I spent a great deal of time talking to individuals and groups of physicians explaining the rationale for this policy. It was intended to aggressively interfere with the spread of pertussis; however, as a policy, it was difficult to enforce and ensuring that close contacts took the antibiotic for the full 14 days was not even a part of the activities of the outbreak response. Although there is biologic plausibility to a policy like this and I assumed it must have been derived from some carefully performed population studies of pertussis, I have not seen such studies and am not certain there are any. I now endorse the more prioritized policy of focusing on those most likely to spread the disease to infants and those who are more likely to have severe disease,[11] as well as a case-by-case judgment call for other situations.

Communications with the local laboratories was another important activity. They were highly impacted by the outbreak. Testing for pertussis increased substantially as we advocated for increased awareness of the disease as a means of increasing case ascertainment and the media further increased awareness among health care providers and the public. Testing was occurring in persons who had the classic clinical presentation, persons who had some overlapping clinical presentation but were not highly likely to be true cases, and even some who were asymptomatic (apparently the worried well); therefore, there was an influx of inappropriate testing going on and the local laboratories (as well as the more distant reference laboratories) observed a large increase in their workload including acquiring the appropriate test kits with the transport media, processing the samples, notification of laboratory test results, sending samples to the state laboratory, and reporting results to the county health department. It was clear in one of my meetings with a local hospital laboratory manager that they were upset about the situation, and it was my impression from them that they felt as if I and the health department had been overreacting leading to their having to deal with the consequences. This was understandable given that their staff had not previously dealt with a pertussis outbreak like this one, that they had not been forewarned of what to expect nor explained the rationale for the activities, and that they were witnessing a large number of negative results (as so many of the specimens submitted were from low likelihood clinical scenarios combined with the relatively low yield for pertussis culture and PCR in the setting of advanced illness and older age). They were processing lots of samples from patients who did not have pertussis and from patients who probably had it but it was too late into their illness to identify it. All in all, it was an unsatisfying experience for the laboratory. Our state laboratory was also unenthused with the situation; therefore, communication with the laboratory was important throughout the outbreak. The investigation team needed to be aware of the laboratories' concerns and to respond to them by encouraging appropriate testing by the affected health care community (which we did).

FINAL THOUGHTS

It should be emphasized that during the first 2 weeks of our assistance with this outbreak, it felt like there was nonstop activity. Serving as the lead consultant to the health department, there were numerous questions and issues that needed to be settled. One moment someone interviewing a possible case needed clarification, and then there might be an interview with the media, then a visit to a hospital, then review of some data, again more questions. At one point, to lighten things up a bit, I asked that some of the health department personnel and RRT members hold one of our daily update meetings at a local old famous ice cream parlor in Moline. One of the things I enjoyed about being state epidemiologist was visiting the many small towns and finding little pearls of history or local culture. I drove thousands of miles of Illinois highway during my approximately 5.5 years in this job and loved the big skies, migrating birds, and the variety of small towns and their characteristics. A few months before this outbreak I had received a magazine in the mail that mentioned that in Moline, Illinois was an ice cream parlor in business for 100 years named Lagomarcinos. I had clipped the little story of this place and saved it. When I realized I was working nearby, I decided it would be a great place for our meeting. We sat in a cramped mahogany booth with a Tiffany-style lamp overhead. From the unique floor to the metal ceiling, it was a great place to go over data and enjoy each others company. The hot fudge sundaes were fantastic, and who knows, maybe the "sugar rush" enhanced our epidemiologic minds.

The number of cases with onset of illness had declined by early November. The state health department needed to have its staff members resume their routine duties. The local health department that experienced three retirements around this time needed to stop performing active surveillance work. The outbreak response was then largely completed in November with ongoing passive surveillance demonstrating relatively low level continued community transmission in December (Figure 18-5).

This outbreak investigation illustrates some of the many issues that are relevant to the response to a community outbreak of a respiratory illness. Unlike some outbreaks where the expected final outcome is an eradication

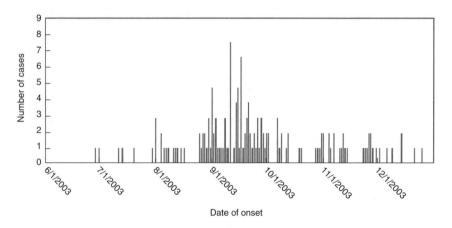

FIGURE 18-5 Epidemic curve of 151 pertussis cases by date of onset, Rock Island County, Illinois, 2003.

of the disease in the impacted population, for a community-wide outbreak where endemic low level disease is the norm, a more modest outcome is acceptable. Pertussis continues to be a problem nationwide; however, I am optimistic that since the approval of licensure by the FDA in 2005 of two booster vaccines (one initially licensed for use in adolescents and the other for adolescents and adults) the burden of pertussis in the United States will fall to hopefully historically low levels in the coming decades, and pertussis outbreaks will be less frequent.

REFERENCES

1. Morgan J, Bornstein SL, Karpati AM, et al. Outbreak of leptospirosis among triathlon participants and community residents in Springfield, Illinois, 1998. *Clin Infect Dis* 2002;34:1593–1599.
2. Skaggs P, Jennings C, Hunt K, et al. Pertussis outbreak among adults at an oil refinery—Illinois, August–October 2002. *Morb Mortal Wkly Rep* 2003;52:1–4.
3. Dworkin MS, Spitters C, Kobayashi JM. Pertussis in adults. *Ann Intern Med* 1998;128:1047.
4. Zanardi L, Pascual FB, Bisgard K, Murphy T, Wharton M, Maurice E. Pertussis—United States, 1997–2000. *Morb Mortal Wkly Rep* 2002;51:73–76.
5. Cloud JL, Hymas W, Caroll KC. Impact of nasopharyngeal swab types on detection of Bordetella pertussis by PCR and culture. *J Clin Microbiol* 2002;40: 3838–3840.
6. Sotir MJ, Cappozzo DL, Warshauer, et al. Evaluation of polymerase chain reaction and culture for diagnosis of pertussis in the control of a county-wide outbreak focused among adolescents and adults. *Clin Infect Dis* 2007;44:1216–1219.
7. Pertussis prophylaxis passé? CD Summary. Retrieved September 18, 2008, from www.oregon.gov/dhs/ph/cdsummary/2005/ohd5409.pdf.
8. Wendelboe AM, Van Rie A, Salmaso S, Englund JA. Duration of immunity against pertussis after natural infection or vaccination. *Pediatr Infect Dis J* 2005; 24:S58–S61.
9. Centers for Disease Control and Prevention. Get smart. Know when antibiotics work. Available June 4, 2008, from http://www.cdc.gov/drugresistance/community/faqs.htm.
10. Maguire P. Your patients are sick but do they need antibiotics? *ACP-ASIM Observer* November 2001. Retrieved June 4, 2008, from http://www.acponline.org/clinical_information/journals_publications/acp_internist/nov01/antibiotics.htm.
11. Pertussis. Oregon Public Health Division. Oregon Department of Human Services. 2007:1–10 (see page 5). Retrieved June 4, 2008, from http://www.oregon.gov/DHS/ph/acd/reporting/guideln/pertussis.pdf.

CHAPTER 19

Emergency Yellow Fever Mass Vaccination in Post-Civil War Liberia

Gregory Huhn, MD, MPH&TM

INTRODUCTION

The Call

The last few months of the Epidemic Intelligence Service (EIS) are usually set aside as wrap-up time for the officer. Their supervisors usually divert new assignments to others as we double check analysis of surveillance projects, write and edit manuscripts (if not already plunged in the dreadful purgatory of the Centers for Disease Control and Prevention [CDC] clearance process), and perhaps most importantly cobble together enough annual leave to catch a sunset or two while sipping caipirinhas on a Brazilian white sand beach; nevertheless, as commissioned officers with our own public health service march,* we know that any expectation of a reserved sabbatical at the end of our tour of duty is a sucker's bet. We can get "the call" at any time. On March 8, 2004, with less than 4 months remaining in my EIS fellowship, I didn't get the call. I made a call, and suddenly I was cashing in my chips on a new outbreak.

I was stationed with the state branch at the Illinois Department of Public Health, revising a manuscript describing the first human outbreak of

---

*"In the silent war against disease no truce is ever seen; We serve on the land and sea for humanity." Available at: http://coa.spsp.net/phsmusic.html.

West Nile virus in Illinois in 2002 when I needed clarification of a new term that the CDC had developed, "neuroinvasive disease," for surveillance purposes in categorizing West Nile virus meningitis or encephalitis cases. I called the guy who I knew would give me a straight answer, Dr. Tony Marfin, deputy director of the Division of Vector-Borne Infectious Diseases in Ft. Collins, Colorado. Both Tony and I have San Diego roots, so, not only did I trust his acumen in all things arboviral, but I also enjoyed just catching up with him. "So what's new, Tony?" "We just got a report this week from a UNICEF representative that there may be a yellow fever outbreak in Liberia." Yellow fever, how fascinating. Liberia, how sublime. A country under United Nations security protectorship with a transitional government 5 months removed from the end of a macabre 14-year civil war, this small nation of 3 million people was awakening from the devastating rule of warlord president Charles Taylor that witnessed 250,000 killed, millions uprooted as refugees or internally displaced persons (IDPs), and nearly all institutions ruinous. Most physicians are asked at some point when or why they first wanted to become doctors. For me, the answer was Liberia.

In 1990, 25 years old and seeking some sort of muse beyond the borders of my job as a research assistant at the Research Institute at Scripps Clinic, I volunteered as a clinical lab technician with a Spanish order of Brothers who operated St. Joseph's Catholic Hospital in the capital of Monrovia. By my fifth month, we were the only hospital functioning in the city, as the genesis of the civil war rapidly spilled into Monrovia. Two factions of rebel forces led by Charles Taylor and Prince Johnson battled the government soldiers of President Samuel K. Doe. By this time, Medicins Sans Frontieres (MSF) had established a field surgical unit within our compound, and I had redirected my job description to start a blood bank for which I exchanged 5 cups of rice, valuable currency in this time of desperation and starvation, plus iron and folate tablets, for a unit of blood from community donors. By mid-August, my nascent apprenticeship in Liberia was vanquished when our hospital was bombed behind two battle lines by government soldiers. We were forced to evacuate within a matter of hours. Mortars blasts had damaged much of our transportation vehicles; however, we quickly repaired a cadre of cars and rolled out in the Charles Taylor rebel-controlled streets. After a 2-day journey through the bush, the last I saw of Liberia was the shores of a rebel training ground lined with young fighters lying prone on the sand, with their AK-47s aimed toward the helicopters of the unarmed U.S. Marines who had been hastily deployed to pick us up and fly us off into safe waters.[1–3]

From this experience, I decided to enter medical school and study tropical medicine. I did not elaborate all of this to Tony; I simply told him that I had worked previously in Liberia and was familiar with the people and political situation. To investigate this yellow fever outbreak would be an opportunity of a peaceful homecoming, I thought. Tony said, "You know, it might be useful to have an EIS officer who knows the lay of the land over there." UNICEF was initiating an emergency yellow fever immunization program and requested assistance from the CDC. A year beforehand, the UNICEF representative in Liberia had been supervising UNICEF's aid program in Afghanistan. An EIS team had established a surveillance system for unexploded ordinance throughout the country after the U.S. military involvement. Pleased with the performance of the EIS, the representative felt confident that the CDC could provide expertise in controlling this yellow fever outbreak. Before acting on the invitation, however, we still needed to invoke the first rule of outbreak investigations—verify that there is an outbreak.

THE OUTBREAK

On January 1, 2004, a 26-year-old male living in an IDP camp in Totota, Salala District, Bong Country, Liberia (Figure 19-1), one of roughly 531,600 Liberians[4], or one-sixth of the nation's estimated population living in such camps throughout the country, returned from his work as a day laborer in a nearby rural farm complaining of fevers, chills, headache, and muscle aches. Over the next week, he had transient fever and chills with a persistent headache and abdominal pain. He continued to work in the fields. By day 8 of his illness, he was unable to work, as the fevers, chills, and headache continued, the abdominal pain worsened, and he developed nausea and back pain over the next 3 days. From days 11 to 13, he noted an onset of epistaxis (bleeding from the nose), emesis, and weakness, with ongoing constitutional symptoms. On day 14, he was seen by Dr. Hansel Otero of MSF at the camp clinic. Vital signs recorded a temperature of 39°C, hypotension with a blood pressure of 90/50 mm Hg, a heart rate of 80 beats per minute, and noticeable jaundice. The patient was confused and was vomiting blood. The patient was admitted to the field hospital on site, which consisted of a large tent with rows of beds separated by white

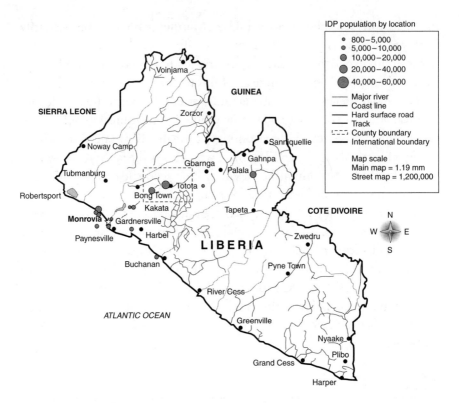

FIGURE 19-1 Salala District, Bong County, Liberia.

From Humanitarian Information Centre of Liberia. Available at
http://www.humanitarianinfo.org/liberia/mapcentre/catalogue/index.asp. Accessed
November 4, 2008.

cloth curtains. Blood was drawn for laboratory testing. Intravenous fluids
were administered, and the patient was treated empirically for malaria.
By the next day, the patient developed progressive confusion with seizures,
had profuse bloody vomiting, and his fevers were unrelenting. He died
within 24 hours of admission.

Dr. Otero was a relatively recent graduate of the Universidad Central de
Venezuela medical school, class of 2002. After graduation, he worked for
1 year in a small town on the Caribbean coast in Venezuela, and then he
joined forces with MSF France. His first assignment was delivering basic
health care to the IDPs of Bong County in the interior of Liberia. On the
job for approximately 6 weeks, he suspected that the young rural farm
laborer he encountered with fevers, jaundice, and apparent hemorrhage

might be suffering from a disease that he had never seen before but that he had read about in his medical texts. Nearly everyone in West Africa presenting with fever and headache is treated for malaria. Dr. Otero made this perfunctory step in his treatment plan; however, he knew that his diagnostic plan demanded a more critical exercise. Dr. William Osler once said, "The value of experience is not in seeing much, but in seeing wisely." As an astute clinician (and most all outbreaks, before they are realized as outbreaks, start with the "astute clinician" type, ranging from medical professionals to even concerned parents), processing the constellation of signs, symptoms, and setting—the nosebleed, the bloody vomit, the fever and jaundice—this he insisted appeared to go beyond the commonplace malaria that he was already accustomed to seeing in a healthy young man. In medicine, "zebras" are the rare diagnoses. Clinicians are cautioned not to seek them out without due cause. So, Dr. Otero went zebra chasing, as he began to piece together these tropical hoof beats while perhaps hearing echoes of Dr. Osler's edict. He ordered a blood test that he knew would take several weeks to finalize a result and probably would not save his patient's life.

In 2003, during the scare of SARS, the New York Times published "The Epidemic Scorecard" (Figure 19-2). Ensconced in the bottom right-hand corner among 10 other deadly diseases sat yellow fever, with 30,000 deaths and 200,000 new cases per year worldwide. Although viral diseases such as Ebola and Marburg may grab more headlines, yellow fever is the "original" viral hemorrhagic fever, untreatable in its clinical course and responsible for over 1,000 times the number of infections and death than these more recent emerging diseases. Yellow fever has been described for centuries, dating back to the 17th century Mayans, who inscribed a manuscript detailing an epidemic of *xekik*, the black vomit. The virus likely evolved from other mosquito-borne viruses approximately 3,000 years ago, probably from Africa from which it was transported to the New World through the slave trade. Despite an effective vaccine, first introduced in the 1930s as derived the 17D strain from a patient from Ghana, with over 400 million immunized hence worldwide, yellow fever continues to inflict endemic and epidemic disease in sub-Saharan Africa and South America, where vaccination programs are lacking. This is the case in countries such as Liberia. Within the yellow fever belt in Africa (latitude 15° north to 10° south), these developing countries have been targeted by the World Health Organization (WHO) Expanded Program on Immunization (EPI) for

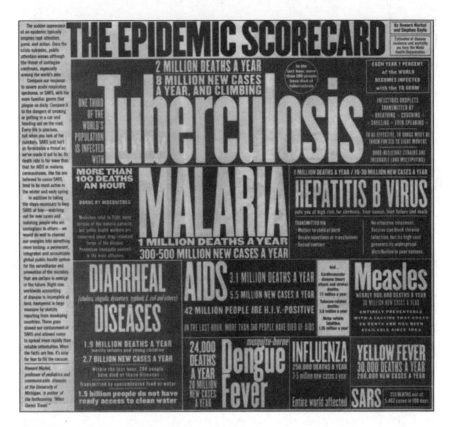

FIGURE 19-2 "The Epidemic Scorecard."
New York Times, Op-Ed Section, April 30, 2008.

decades to support sustainable efforts against a wide range of vaccine-preventable diseases, including yellow fever. Analytic models since the 1990s have advocated for inclusion of yellow fever vaccination in EPI in endemic areas.[5] In Liberia, however, 14 years of civil war through 2003 devastated much of the country's health care infrastructure and severely disrupted public health disease surveillance and immunization programs. Since 1999, Liberia has had a surveillance system sanctioned by the Liberia Ministry of Health (MOH) for eight diseases: acute flaccid paralysis, neonatal tetanus, meningitis, bloody diarrhea, cholera, Lassa fever, measles, and yellow fever. Weekly reports from county health centers filter into Monrovia, comprising an early warning system to monitor incidence patterns of these diseases. Because of ongoing civil conflict, the system had never been fully operational. Laboratory support for the system was minimal, with yellow fever diagnostic capacity first initiated in 2001 through grants from WHO and the Global Alliance for Vaccine Initiatives. Crippled by lack of reagents, however, testing had never been performed in the country. A resurgence of vaccine-preventable diseases would not be surprising and in reality likely expected.

During the last couple of weeks in January, initial reports of suspected yellow fever in Dr. Otero's patient began to filter back to MOH and aid agencies such as UNICEF and WHO in Monrovia, prompting the MOH to alert all IDP camp medical personnel, government-run clinics, and nongovernmental organization (NGO) health care systems throughout the country to report all suspected cases with appropriate serum testing to the MOH. By February 13, 2004, the WHO declared an outbreak of yellow fever in Liberia following laboratory confirmation of four cases, three fatal, all with onset of illness between January 1 to 9, 2004, in Bong County and Nimba County, near the Cote d'Ivoire border. The first case as cared for by Dr. Otero had a blood specimen shipped to the nearest diagnostic laboratory for yellow fever at the Institut Pasteur de Cote d'Ivoire in the capital Abidjan. The preliminary serology was negative for IgM anti-yellow fever antibody. A positive anti-yellow fever IgM enzyme-linked immunosorbent assay result in late acute or early convalescent phase, which peaks by the end of the second week of illness and was the time point for which Dr. Otero's patient had his blood drawn for testing, provides a presumptive diagnosis. Demonstration of a rising antibody response from two blood samples collected several weeks apart from each other beginning after onset of illness is confirmatory. This was not an option for Dr. Otero's patient. IgM antibody testing for yellow fever requires exquisite laboratory technique, and the sensitivity of IgM enzyme-linked immunosorbent assay serology is approximately 70%; thus, Dr. Otero's patient's blood was then sent to the Institut Pasteur in Dakar, Senegal for more advanced polymerase chain reaction (PCR) testing. In early February, the PCR test for yellow fever was positive, and by the second week in February, all four cases were likewise confirmed. WHO considers even one case of confirmed yellow fever worthy of outbreak investigation because of the concern for human-to-human transmission, particularly in urban areas. Two of the four cases occurred in men aged 19 years and Dr. Otero's 26 year old patient living in densely populated IDP camps in Bong County. The WHO announcement of a yellow fever outbreak set in motion an international response to control the epidemic quickly to prevent potential rapid spread to surrounding areas and urban settings.

In the early stages of the outbreak, it was uncertain just where the mosquito-borne sources for yellow fever truly lied. In West Africa, the virus is transmitted in three cycles—a sylvatic or "jungle" cycle, in which transmission occurs between forest-dwelling mosquitoes and nonhuman primates; an intermediate cycle, in which transmission occurs between mosquitoes and both nonhuman primates and humans in moist savanna areas referred to as "emergent zones"; and an urban cycle where it causes large epidemics (Figure 19-3). Urban cycle epidemics develop from anthroponotic, also known as human-to-human, transmission in which humans serve as the sole host reservoir of the peridomestic *Aedes aegypti* mosquito vector. Urban epidemics occur when persons who do not have the tell-tale sign of jaundice but do have virus circulating in their blood (and are not yet severely ill) travel from emergent zones of transmission in jungles and savannas to cities where they infect local *A. aegypti* mosquitoes. This species of mosquito is abundant in urban areas and in areas where humans store water. It was well known that thousands of men in the IDP camps would travel routinely to Monrovia in search of work. Low background

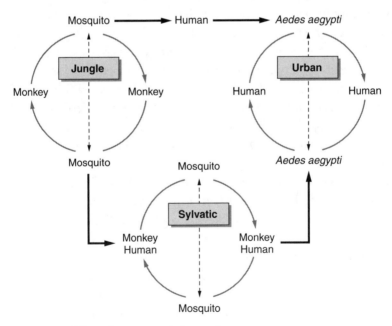

FIGURE 19-3 Yellow fever transmission cycles.
Adapted from Monath TP. *Lancet Inf Dis* 2001 (1):11–20.

prevalence of neutralizing antibody to yellow fever virus in the population because of lack of previous vaccination or naturally acquired infection and poor disease surveillance systems are also contributing factors to epidemics in West Africa. Human-to-human transmission to an urban area such as Monrovia could be ominous. The last urban yellow fever outbreak to hit West Africa occurred in neighboring Abidjan, Cote d'Ivoire just 3 years before in 2001, claiming 14 lives and requiring an emergency immunization campaign to vaccinate 2.6 million people over a 4-week period. Dr. Muireann Brennan, a veteran CDC epidemiologist dispatched to Liberia in late 2003 to supervise EIS officers during a mass immunization campaign of children against measles after the fall and exodus of the Charles Taylor regime, recognized the urgency of this threat. In a February 9 e-mail to Dr. Barry Miller, a director of the arbovirus diseases branch of the CDC in Ft. Collins, CO, Dr. Brennan wrote,

> "Greetings from Liberia. I have a vector question that I hope you can help with. We have suspected yellow fever in Monrovia. We are concerned about 200,000 IDPs living in camps in very crowded conditions with poor sanitation. We also have the population of greater Monrovia. Less crowded but still poor sanitation. We are wondering what would be the most effective vector control measures. We have eight trained sprayers and spraying equipment. What is the best use of these people? How many gallons of 'stuff' do we need and what is the best chemical? Should we save spraying for the IDP camps, near drains and water outlets? Do you have a number I could call you at? My number is *** 47 525 *** thanks, Muireann." Dr. Miller replied one hour later, "Dear Dr. Brennan. I assume you are worried about *Aedes aegypti*. The only effective means of controlling this mosquito is to cover water storage containers and to dump all containers on property that hold water. Spraying is a last ditch effort and it only helps if every residence is sprayed inside. Outdoor spraying is not very effective. Although covering containers that hold water seems simple, getting the population to implement it is not. Mass vaccination with 17D is your best bet in my opinion."

This dialogue is instructive to our understanding of outbreak investigation. Dr. Brennan, in the final throes of the measles mass vaccination campaign, has been watching another soon-to-be-confirmed outbreak unfold and believes identifying, controlling, and eliminating the source of the outbreak should be a top priority. In most classic settings, controlling the source of the epidemic is generally a critical component in outbreak investigations. Dr. Miller, a wisened entomologist, counters though that the source, the ubiquitous *A. aegypti* mosquito, is an entrenched menacing force that will not back down even if a gazillion gallons of "stuff" were carpet-bombed on every field, house, spare tire, and tin can in the area. He essentially tells Dr. Brennan that if you want to best protect the people, do what you do best and start mass immunization with yellow fever 17D vaccine.

CONTROL THE OUTBREAK— YELLOW FEVER MASS VACCINATION

After the worldwide announcement of a yellow fever outbreak on February 13, UNICEF, WHO, and MSF convened with the Liberian MOH on February 18 to draft an emergency vaccination proposal to immunize the approximately 722,000 Liberians aged 6 months or older at risk for yellow fever in Bong and Nimba counties. WHO and UNICEF would fund and supervise the effort, whereas MOH, MSF, county public health departments, and other NGOs would implement the campaigns. The plan was split into two phases. Phase I was termed outbreak intervention and divided into two steps. Step 1 encompassed mass vaccination in Salala District IDP camps and their host communities in Bong County, and step 2 outlined mass vaccination for two districts from which two of the confirmed and fatal cases originated in Nimba County. Phase II was designated outbreak prevention to later canvass remaining areas within Bong and Nimba counties for mass immunization not covered during phase I. Though there were many obstacles, two issues predominated before the vaccination campaign launched into action. Where was Liberia going to get the money, and did the country have enough vaccine for such an undertaking? The country was nearly completely dependent on outside aid for most aspects of civil services, including health care, and the Liberia MOH only had 80,000 doses of yellow fever vaccine in stock. As the number of suspect cases climbed to nine (symptoms compatible with yellow fever, but not yet laboratory confirmed), UNICEF and WHO released a joint statement on February 25 through the WHO Disease Outbreak News network on ProMED mail (a global electronic reporting system for outbreaks of emerging infectious diseases and toxins, http://www.promedmail.org/pls/otn/f?p=2400:1000). They appealed for $1.3 million to cover costs for vaccine and injection materials, operational logistics, and the strengthening of epidemiological surveillance and public awareness.[6] The situation was described as "urgent" with a potential for "exploding to larger populations in displaced persons camps and urban areas" and "even more favourable (conditions) for the disease with the onset of the rainy season in April." The governments of Ireland and Norway pledged financial commitments and the WHO set aside 400,000 doses, approximately one tenth of its entire worldwide supply, for the campaign. The next day, MSF France received 72,000 vaccine and syringe doses with official Liberia Yellow Fever vaccination verification cards from WHO. UNICEF provided 2 refrigerators, 4 deep freezers, 15 cold ice-pack containers, 32 cool boxes, 991 ice packs, and syringe safety disposal boxes for the initial phase of the campaign at MSF IDP camp clinic facilities and surrounding villages to implement the first phase of the campaign in Bong County, the epicenter of the outbreak. Essential elements to emergency mass vaccination quickly took form.

Operations and Organization

Nine vaccination teams each with six members and one supervisor, comprising public health officials from MSF France, the district hospital, Save the Children, and the Bong County Health Department, were formed and trained in appropriate techniques in yellow fever immunization. Vaccination centers within the four IDP camps where two of the confirmed cases originated, Totota and Maimu I, II, and III, were set up with a registration table, vaccine administration area, and an exit station where vaccine verification cards were documented and distributed. There were two vaccinators per team, with a goal of 300 immunizations delivered per vaccinator. Each member of the team was paid 5 U.S. dollars per day.

Cold Chain System

The yellow fever vaccine is manufactured from live-attenuated virus and unstable at room temperature; maintaining a functional cold chain for vaccine storage between 2°C and 8°C is vital to ensuring potency of the vaccine. Cold chain systems are a series of storage and transport links through a network of refrigerators, freezers, and cold boxes that keep vaccines at a safe temperature throughout their journey (Figure 19-4).

A generator was secured to provide electricity from 5 a.m. to 11p.m. to maintain temperatures in the refrigerators between 0°C and 8°C and < 0°C for the freezers. Supervisors delivered ice packs from the freezers to the field vaccination teams at 2-hour intervals to maintain the cold chain.

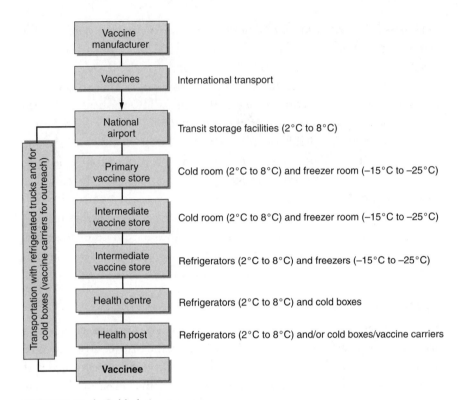

FIGURE 19-4 Cold chain system.

Each cold box was affixed with a 3M MonitorMark card that served as an in-field alarm system in case the cold box reached temperatures beyond the range recommended for usable vaccine. A cold chain coordinator recorded the temperature of each cold box daily each morning and evening (Figure 19-5).

Social Mobilization

Social moblilization is a process that is used to increase awareness of a program and stimulate community participation. Social mobilization brings a marketing atmosphere to generate community interest in mass vaccination campaigns. This enterprise began one week before the immunization kick-off date and continuing throughout the campaign. Messengers with megaphones delivered announcements throughout the camps, villages, and even by shelter-to-shelter visits describing the symptoms of yellow fever, modes of spread of the disease, methods to eliminate household

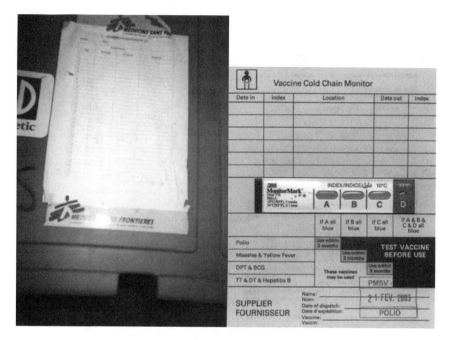

FIGURE 19-5 Cold chain cold boxes and temperature monitoring card.

mosquito breeding sites, and the need for vaccination. The vaccines were advertised as free of charge. These messages were translated in English and five different local languages (Kpelle, Mende, Loma, Vai, and Southern Kisi). In the town of Totota, a local radio station transmitted details of the disease and campaign. The social mobilization efforts were reinforced midway through the campaign with testimonials by church elders, heads of schools, and other leaders of local institutions. Signs were posted as guideposts to the vaccination sites (Figure 19-6).

Adverse Events Following Immunization

The day before the campaign launch date, vaccination team supervisors were briefed on recognition and reporting of adverse events following immunization (AEFI) by MSF campaign managers. AEFI surveillance is important to preserve the integrity of the campaign and cultivate public confidence overall in immunization programs. Monitoring events related temporally to immunization enable campaign managers to reduce risks even further as AEFI are investigated in search of idiopathic reactions versus potential program-related discrepancies in storage and handling of the

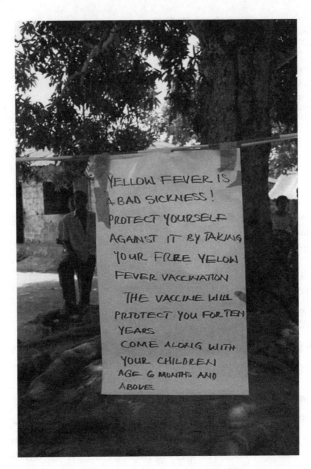

FIGURE 19-6   Social mobilization. Yellow Fever mass vaccination campaign, Liberia, February–March 2004.

vaccine, or inconsistencies in vaccine administration technique. Supervisors were instructed to be vigilant for all injection site abscesses, severe reactions such as anaphylaxis, toxic shock, sepsis, encephalitis, febrile jaundice illnesses, and deaths potentially related to immunization within 4 weeks of vaccine receipt. Although rare, viscerotropic and neurotropic reactions, or a fulminant yellow fever infection from the reactivated live attenuated 17D vaccine strain, have resulted in death following yellow fever immunization, primarily in immunocompromised or elderly persons receiving vaccine.[7–16] Given the urgency of the campaign and because screening every vaccine recipient for HIV was not feasible, AEFI surveillance was important to ensure safety and public acceptance of the campaign.

The campaign lasted 10 days, from February 26 to March 6. An extension of the campaign occurred from March 16 to March 20 in two additional Bong County IDP camps, Salala and Tumutu, as well as the town of Salala. Outreach vaccination teams also immunized persons living in outlying villages in Bong County. Two vaccinees developed mild self-limited facial rashes after immunization, and there were no serious AEFI reported. Among the estimated 87,000 population living in the IDP camps, only 47,763 (56.8%) were vaccinated. The vaccination coverage fell far short of the 80% goal, which is believed to be a threshold level for immunoprotection within a community to limit person-to-person transmission of yellow fever.

What happened? The MSF coordinators had several theories. Insecurity in the area with unconfirmed rumblings of rebel activity contributed to lower campaign turnout. Some outlying communities could not be accessed. The rainy season perhaps had restricted movement of some people, and some IDPs and villagers may have been absent from the area as itinerant farmers. The overriding suspicion, however, was that the original target population estimate was too high. Julie Gerberding, director of the CDC, once said in a lecture of the principles of epidemiology, "Anyone can count numbers for the numerator, but the real skill of what makes an epidemiologist a scientist is determining the correct denominator." If the denominator is wrong, then the most well-designed plans, as apparently engineered during this first phase of the emergency yellow fever vaccination campaign, can appear fruitless in the end. Meanwhile, in the middle of the vaccination campaign, before all the final tallies were in, another missive was posted from the WHO Disease Outbreak News network on ProMED Mail on March 11: "A total of 39 suspected cases including 8 deaths are reported to WHO from 5 counties."[17] The outbreak was not yet over and appeared to be claiming more victims.

THE CDC RESPONSE

On February 25, the day before the first phase of the mass vaccination campaign, Angela Kearney, the UNICEF representative to Liberia e-mailed Tony Marfin at the CDC requesting "urgent technical assistance from CDC and specifically the Division of Vector Borne Diseases in controlling a yellow fever outbreak in Liberia, in particular, support in planning and implementing a mass vaccination campaign." Ms. Kearney had already conferred with WHO and the Liberia MOH, agreeing to a 6-week time period for CDC involvement "as soon as possible."

Tony replied that day after reading the WHO/UNICEF joint proposal that Ms. Kearney had attached to her e-mail:

> I think that you have done a very good job to cover all the aspects of the mass campaign and certainly have addressed the more pressing needs in terms of operational research issues such as AEFI. I see that MOH, WHO, and UNICEF have covered the majority of the work tasks and that the plan enlists the assistance of multiple groups, such as MSF, Africare, and the International Red Cross. With all of this expert assistance already in place, I am a little confused as to what you see as the function of CDC personnel that may participate. I suspect that we are not being asked to partake as another independent partner (too many partners can be as big a problem as too few). It seems that you may be asking us to participate as a UNICEF resource that is being contributed to this effort and that we would be working more directly with UNICEF. That would be a fine paradigm, but I just want to more fully understand if that is correct and what you see as the scope of work. If you would, please clarify for me to whom a senior yellow fever subject matter expert would be reporting. Please pardon my caution. We are always ready to pitch in; it is just when there are so many organizations that we must be sure that we actually have a function when we arrive. One thing that Dr. Brennan may not have mentioned to you was that most of the people in our division work on the surveillance, epidemiology, laboratory, and ecology aspects of yellow fever—more research aspects of the disease and vector control than operational aspects of running a mass yellow fever vaccination campaign. Still, we have some people (including me) that have also overseen the operation of such campaigns and set up surveillance for adverse events. Because we do not have anyone that has regularly performed the logistical activities, our division may be able to provide the senior staff subject matter expert and possibly an experienced EIS officer as team leaders. Then we would work closely with other CDC groups to find people that are much more experienced in the logistical aspects of these campaigns. I will work to get you an answer as quickly as possible.

As a seasoned CDC epidemiologist, Tony exhibits a prescient assessment of UNICEF's request for CDC assistance. One of the CDC's unspoken ground rules for accepting invitations from outside organizations to help investigate outbreaks is that unless otherwise explicitly stated, the locals are in charge. Local officials are central stakeholders in outbreak settings, and the CDC is exquisitely mindful of avoiding any perceptions of commandeering an investigation and undermining the authority of on-the-ground forces and institutions. In seeking clarification of CDC's proposed role, Tony wanted to ensure that he lined up the right people for the right reason. EIS officers, with burgeoning epidemiologic skills and energy, are usually the right answer. Indeed, Ms. Kearney wanted to bolster UNICEF's support system with EIS officers, a blueprint that had worked so effectively for her in Afghanistan 1 year prior and most recently with measles mass vaccination in Liberia. Tony identified two EIS officer veterinarians from the CDC arboviral branch in Ft. Collins, Colorado, Drs. Susan Montgomery and Jennifer Brown, for the assignment. Both had worked tirelessly in the United States on surveillance for West Nile virus that was sweeping the country during 2002 to 2003 and were ready for an international field experience. Sue was in my EIS class, and I knew her well from shared experiences with West Nile virus. I had not yet worked with Jen. Both were scheduled to arrive in the capital Monrovia on Monday, March 15. As the senior EIS officer, Sue would assist in the interpretation of the yellow fever surveillance data, review appropriateness of the response, coordinate activities among Liberia MOH, UNICEF, WHO, and any other partners, and assess laboratory capacity for in-country diagnosis of acute yellow fever—all in 8 days. Conversely, Jen had a 33-day itinerary to more intensely participate in yellow fever disease surveillance activities and enhance AEFI surveillance, as well as assist in any possible vaccine coverage surveys. Once travel documents and security clearance were obtained for Sue and Jen, Tony replied to Ms. Kearney on Friday, March 12, "We have had some difficulty identifying someone with campaign experience who could help in performance of the vaccination campaign for 4–6 weeks, but we will keep working on this part this weekend." Tony had told me to keep my bags packed later that week after our serendipitous phone conversation on May 8. The shoe-leather epidemiology that the EIS prides itself often allows officers to assert themselves in unfamiliar situations. Tony assured me, "I know you can handle it. You know the place." Apparently I was the guy with mass vaccination campaign experience. I had never seen, let alone helped organize, a mass vaccination campaign as far as I was aware.

The duo from Ft. Collins had 3 weeks to prepare for the deployment. I had 1 week, tentatively scheduled to depart March 15. The day after my initial phone conversation with Tony, I drove up to the Great Lakes Naval Training Base, about 30 miles north of Chicago, which was considered the commissioned corps' local health center. Along with malaria prophylaxis, I received three catchup vaccines, quadrivalent meningococcal, typhoid, and of course, yellow fever. I needed emergency visas and country clearance from the respective embassies of Cote d'Ivoire and Liberia (there were limited commercial flights into Liberia and local air carriers usually routed through Cote d'Ivoire or Ghana), government travel orders from the United States (granted only after country clearances were obtained), and a seat on a flight. For a tour of duty slated for 30 days, I packed rather light—some clothes, cash (no traveler's checks, Liberia was a cash economy, with the U.S. dollar as the hard currency), bug spray and a mosquito net, 90 energy bars (three a day, just in case), my laptop with the season 1 DVD collection of "Curb Your Enthusiasm," and my old St. Joseph's Catholic Hospital ID card for those unforeseen instances when I might need a little "street cred" (Figure 19-7). By the morning of March 15, I had no Liberian country clearance and therefore no travel orders. A cable from Monrovia was sent to CDC at 11:54 a.m. for my country clearance. At 12:20 p.m., my travel orders were secured. On a freezing day in Chicago at 2:00 p.m., I was out the door and on a 5:45 p.m. flight to Paris and then on to Abidjan for an overnight stay until touching down in Monrovia 2 days behind Sue and Jen on March 17. As I looked down from my window seat on the plane flying over the tropical savanna into Liberia, I felt a sense of hopefulness.

UNICEF had arranged rooms at the Mamba Point Hotel, in the heart of the diplomatic district in Monrovia. Bungalow style, it was nice and clean, with air conditioning, satellite television, and a full-service restaurant. The spread probably ranked between 2 to 3 stars by U.S. standards. It was touted as one of the premier hotels in Liberia. At $120 U.S. a night, it was outlandishly expensive. Despite the breezy beaches across the street, this stretch of real estate, or really anywhere else in Liberia, could not be considered a tourist destination. Most guests were foreign aid workers, journalists, or diplomats, with governments or NGOs footing the bill. A good proportion of the room rate was in fact for shadow security, imperative in this still volatile country. Romeo, an engaging Liberian in his 30s, was the desk manager and chief broker agent for the folk art street hawkers outside the lobby. His easy smile and animated graciousness brought back my recollections of an otherwise friendly people who were pulled and

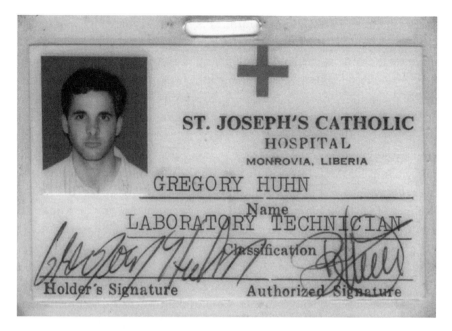

FIGURE 19-7 St. Joseph's Catholic Hospital identification card, 1990.

mangled by tribal-based conflicts, ultimately manipulated into brutality by ruthless and greedy warlords.

I checked in, took a quick shower, and headed to the UNICEF compound down the street to start digging into our roles in the yellow fever outbreak. I first met with Dr. Bjorn Forssen, the UNICEF emergency medical officer from Sweden, and Ms. Carmen Michielin, the UNICEF staff security officer from South Africa, for a security briefing. An international peacekeeper force, with the characteristic blue helmets, patrolled most all major cities in Liberia, including Monrovia, as authorized by the United Nations Mission in Liberia (UNMIL). UNMIL was established by the U.N. Security Council resolution 1509 in late September 2003 to support the ceasefire agreement and peace process; protect United Nations staff, facilities, and civilians; support humanitarian and human rights activities; as well as assist in national security reform, including national police training and formation of a new, restructured military.[18] In Monrovia, the national police force had disintegrated, replaced by an international civilian police contingent called CIVPOL.[19] There were reports of kidnappings and even cannibalism of both Liberians and expatriates, so, Carmen encouraged us to always use a UNICEF security escort when walking or traveling at night in Monrovia. Eleven thousand peacekeepers were in place by the time we arrived, but 15,000 were needed to secure the borders. There were still active rebel incursions from the Cote d'Ivoire border in Nimba County in the eastern part of the country, where the other two confirmed yellow fever cases were detected. To implement the next step of the mass vaccination campaign, targeting the population of Nimba County, we would need an UNMIL military escort while in the field. The Bangladeshi UNMIL unit stationed in the Nimba County capital of Sanniquellie was alerted of our intention to start the campaign imminently. Radio call-ins every hour to UNICEF offices in Monrovia would be required to provide updated security situation reports (known as SitReps) during our field operations. I left the meeting with a UNICEF symbol embossed certificate stating, "Gregory Huhn has successfully completed Basic Security in the Field—Staff Safety, Health, and Welfare" and quickly realized why we received an extra few hundred bucks in commissioned corps hazardous incentive pay for "hostile fire/imminent danger" during our assignment here in Liberia.

During the first couple of days before I arrived, Sue and Jen had been reviewing the line list of suspected yellow fever cases reported since January. A suspect case was defined as acute onset of fever followed by jaundice within 2 weeks of onset of first symptoms. Several were already IgM antibody negative for yellow fever, yet were still counted as suspect cases. The chief WHO surveillance medical officer, Dr. Mekonnen Admassu from Ethiopia, maintained that these may have been true yellow fever infections with IgM antibodies that had waned. The IgM antibodies usually persist for 30 to 60 days after acute illness and then decline over several months.[20] The case definition for confirmed cases used by WHO in Liberia also included an "epidemiologically linked" category. To EIS officers disciplined in precision in tracking West Nile virus cases, this extension of the case definition appeared unsound in the arboviral world and prone to over inflation of the true case rate. Tony was in daily e-mail communication with our team for the first week and put this practice into context:

> This is exactly what many countries do. They use a syndromic case definition for surveillance to add cases, but do not use serology or PCR results to remove cases. This is the way you end up with a lot of P. *falciparum* malaria on the list. Epi-linked is exactly as you state. . . . There is a geographic and temporal relationship between a person who meets

the surveillance case definition and a person with a serologically confirmed case of yellow fever. . . . This is the part that is often left out. What happens is you have someone with fever and jaundice and they get added to the case list. Then the sister or some other family relative gets ill (not always fever and jaundice) a week later and they get added to the list because of the relationship to a case that was never confirmed. It is not wrong to continue to emphasize the importance of lab confirmation. If there were many hundreds of cases and the first 25–50 cases were serologically confirmed as the "real deal," then no one would have a problem doing syndromic surveillance beyond that point. But, what happened in Cote d'Ivoire and it sounds like it may be happening here is there are 'some' cases and only some of those are serologically or PCR confirmed. Then syndromic surveillance with a highly sensitive and unspecified specificity starts to run the program . . . even though many of them turn out to be negative on serology.

By the time I arrived to meet Sue and Jen at the UNICEF offices, the two of them had pressed the WHO and UNICEF surveillance leadership, which also included Dr. Nuhu Maksa from Nigeria, UNICEF Project Officer for Nutrition and Health, on tightening up to a more specific case definition, to delete at least the IgM-negative cases. Our overtures we could sense hovered among this multinational team with mild skepticism (change can sometimes move as slow as a goat roast in this equatorial land). We were nonetheless ready to then concentrate our efforts on the second step of immunization campaign targeting high-risk populations in Nimba County. Two days into my time in Liberia, Jen and I had finished a new case investigation form emphasizing duration and onset of symptoms and dates for yellow fever acute and convalescent serology submission for public health officials in Nimba County. I had the opportunity to pilot this form as I was called to investigate a case of a 2-year-old boy from Monrovia hospitalized at an MSF clinic down the road from the UNICEF office. Five days after onset of symptoms, primarily dyspnea, the boy developed fevers and then 7 days later jaundice and hematemesis. He died 1 day later. Yellow fever serology was submitted to MOH on the day of death. I spoke with his parents just after he died. The boy did not spend any recent time outside Monrovia. The working diagnosis was pneumonia. We learned later that the yellow fever serology was negative.

Within the first couple of days in Liberia, I bought a cell phone. Minutes could be bought freely from calling cards on sale at many outposts throughout the city without a contract. Although much of the country was physically in decay, Liberia was as wireless as any developed nation. Advances in communications technology, from our Internet hookups at our UNICEF office to our slick cell phones, were quite a revelation for me when looking back to my past experience in the country 14 years prior. We were without any communications except for a fuzzy ham radio for my last 6 weeks during the battles around our hospital in 1990. Now I was able to call my wife daily from most anywhere (except the deepest parts of the bush), preferably from across the street of the Mamba Point Hotel, on the beach next to a lobster shack. With our reliable Ethernet connection, I also downloaded and printed a chapter from a WHO website on how to organize a mass vaccination campaign. Acquiring on-the-fly expert-level knowledge by sometimes unconventional means becomes almost instinctual for EIS officers in the field. I read it on the 6-hour jeep ride out to Nimba County to commence our roles as supervisors in phase I, step 2 of the campaign.

As Sue wrapped up her reports on yellow fever surveillance and a summary of diagnostic laboratory capacity she had researched in Monrovia (there essentially was none so Dr. Juliet Bryant, an arboviral biochemist from Ft. Collins, was summoned later in April to revive the yellow fever lab), Jen and I set out for Sanniquellie on Sunday, March 20 after receiving UNICEF security travel clearance. We went shopping the day before at a Monrovia market as if we were provisioning for a Yosemite hiking trip. We bought a camping stove, canned and dried foods, peanut butter, cheese sticks, crackers, bottled water, and toilet paper. I also brought along a good bulk of my energy bars. We stayed at a hostel across the street from the Bangladeshi UNMIL compound. The place was fairly sparse, outfitted with a few single bedrooms with plug-in fans, clean sheets, and a shared hallway bathroom. Electricity ran during the day, but not at night. A patio out front served as our commissary where we sparked up our stove for bean or soup dinners. Our hostel hosts provided a cooler of cold beers, which actually creates a relaxing tonic as you snooze away under the mosquito net in the humid hot nighttime air. The buzz also probably took the edge off those vivid dreams that usually accompanied my weekly dose of mefloquine malaria prophylaxis.

On Monday, March 22, we met up with the Bangladeshi UNMIL team and traveled out with our WHO and UNICEF colleagues to supervise the mass vaccination activities just underway as coordinated by MSF Holland and Swiss, Liberia MOH, and the Nimba County public health department. As compared with the recent mass immunization in Bong County, there were no IDP camps in Nimba County. Rather, vaccination sites were decentralized throughout towns and villages in the two high-risk districts of Zoegeh and Gbehleygeh. The Zoegeh district was demarcated into two zones based on security factor; a western zone comprised an estimated population of 35,000, and an eastern zone was bordering Cote d'Ivoire with an estimated 15,000 target population. The eastern zone was essentially off-limits to foreign NGOs and international aid groups such as UNICEF and WHO because of ongoing cross-border armed skirmishes; therefore, the MOH conducted the immunization campaign in this area. The target population for the Gbelaygeh district was 75,000 for a planned 10-day campaign. WHO provided vaccines, and the same mass vaccination organization structure employed in Bong County was instituted in the Nimba County campaign; however, the nature of village life provided obstacles not encountered in the Bong County IDP camps. Terrain was rugged and there were no paved roads village to village (Figure 19-8). The largest towns along the perimeter of the district zones were selected as vaccination sites to create accessibility to the villages' populations. Still, many villagers had to walk 2 hours to get to a vaccination center, particularly taxing on older people. Satellite vaccination sites were then created by mobile vaccination

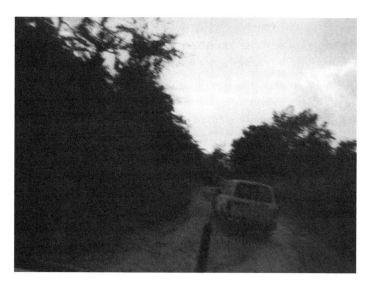

FIGURE 19-8 UNMIL Bangladeshi unit escort in Zoehch District, Nimba County, Liberia.

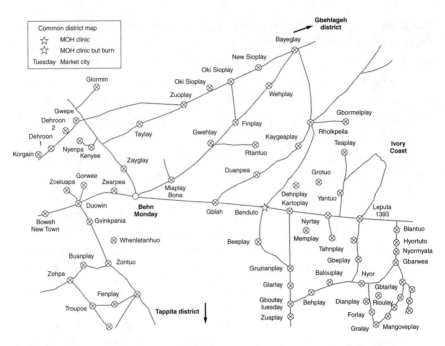

FIGURE 19-9 Map of towns and villages, Zoegeh District, Nimba County, Liberia.

teams to reach out to some of these outlying villages (Figure 19-9). There were disagreements over money transfers between UNICEF and WHO to the MSF, MOH, and local public health department teams that did the actual implementation of the mass vaccination in the western Zoegeh district. Rumors stirred that some county public health vaccinator teams "boycotted" the campaign over these financial disputes, resulting in poor social mobilization and low campaign turnout rates in some areas.

Inconsistencies in vaccine delivery systems were uncovered. Standard multidose vials for WHO 17D yellow fever vaccines are reconstituted with 10 cc of diluent and administered as 0.5-cc subcutaneous injections. Vaccinators in the Gbelaygeh district campaign disclosed to supervisors 3 days into the campaign that the diluent vials contained 12 cc of solution, allowing 24 injections per vial. After consultation, we recommended that vaccinators first draw up 2 cc from the diluent vial, waste it, and then proceed with resuspension with 10 cc for proper dilution concentration. Vaccinators in the Zoegeh western district were already 6 days into the campaign, and 49% of target population had been immunized by this time, when this correction was applied in that campaign as well. Minimal potency require-ments established by WHO for standard yellow fever vaccine exceed the 90% immunizing dose by fivefold; therefore, it was unlikely that the excess dilution affected vaccine immunogenicity.[21]

The cold chain system in Gbehlaygeh campaign was particularly imper-iled. "Running on the limits of what was acceptable," according to Steven de Bock, chief logistician for MSF Holland. Approximately one third of the large cold boxes supplied by the public health department for vaccine storage in the field vaccination sites were defective and could not close and lock properly. Six different sizes of ice packs, rather than a uniformly sized ice pack, made loading of the cold boxes awkward, leading to "unnecessary delays, confusion, and inefficient use of the cold chain equipment," by De Bock's account. Perhaps most distressing was the mystery surrounding the whereabouts of essential heavy equipment. UNICEF apparently promised MSF Holland a freezer and generator to be stationed in the district capi-tal town of Karnplay, population 11,000, as the central ice pack and vac-cine storage center. They never showed up. (We were later informed that the equipment had been destroyed in heavy fighting in the rebel strong-hold town of Ganta in 2003). MSF Holland improvised, renting two freez-ers and a generator at a local bar, but they were in need of renovation. De Bock rehabbed the equipment, but the generator broke down after the first day of the campaign. The head MSF office in Monrovia quickly sent a new generator up to Karnplay the next day; however, the largest refrig-erator on site gave out by the third day of the campaign. De Bock simply stated, "There was no room for error." As supervisors, we observed watery ice packs shuttled from Sanniquellie every 2 hours by car to Karnplay and then onto to vaccination sites in villages by car or bicycle. There were no temperature-monitoring cards on the cold boxes, and only a few ther-mometers were spotted to accurately record cold box temperatures. Even our jeep limped into one of the villages with a flat tire, burning fumes on a near empty tank of gas. Pulling up to a lean-to gas station, a jack and a patch, along with petrol poured from recycled beer bottles that were sit-ting on a rickety table, got us back on our way (Figure 19-10). Through improvisation and grit, the logisticians displayed the resiliency and resourcefulness vital to public health emergency operations.

In regards to AEFI, surveillance was erratic, and some public health department vaccination teams believed that an emphasis on AEFI report-ing actually undermined their credibility as protectors of public health and

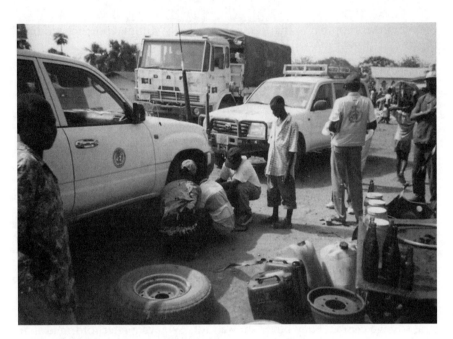

FIGURE 19-10 Gas station in Gbehlaygeh District, Nimba County, Liberia.

deterred villagers from participating in the immunization campaign. We attempted to reinforce the importance of AEFI surveillance with tutorials on proper case form completion during our daily supervisory visits to vaccination centers. Ultimately, there were no AEFIs reported nor any other suspect yellow fever cases identified during the western district Zoegeh and Gbehlaygeh campaigns. We were not in communication with the MOH campaign in the eastern district of Zoegeh. We felt that no news was probably good news. If there happened to be an unfortunate breach in safety, we thought we would have heard about it.

Despite setbacks, there was success. Vaccinations started promptly at 6:30 a.m. at most sites. With four vaccinators per site, people sped through waiting lines and could make it back off into the farms for their usual daily routine (Figure 19-11). Among the target population of 75,000, 66,469 (87%) people were immunized.

By March 25 in the western Zoegeh district, 23,680 among the 35,000 target population (67.5%) had been immunized. There had been efforts to mobilize the population to get vaccinated (social mobilization). We were uncertain how adequate those efforts had been. Jen and I developed a rapid

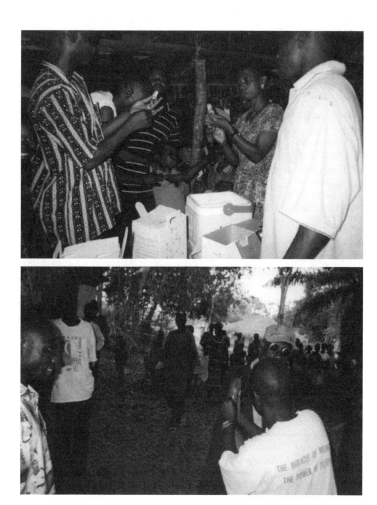

FIGURE 19-11 Young boy and elderly man immunized with 17D Yellow Fever Vaccine in Gbehlaygeh District, Nimba County, Liberia, in March 2004.

coverage survey to determine whether lapses in social mobilization efforts may have given rise to disproportionate vaccination rates among various communities. A survey such as the one we performed here is useful to better understand the initial tally data collected at the vaccination site registration tables because it is important to ensure that resources have adequately been dedicated to all at-risk populations. We selected three villages within a 45-minute to 2-hour walking distance from one of the five main vaccination sites as a convenience sample (Figure 19-9). Holding true to our principle that the locals always need to be engaged and sign off on our activities, we met with village elders in roundtable sessions to explain our intentions and reinforce the importance of controlling yellow fever in their communities. We visited 10 houses in each village. We asked the head of the household how many people lived in the house 6 months of age or more, if they heard about the yellow fever vaccination campaign, whether they did get vaccinated, and if not vaccinated, what were the reasons. Two villages ranked 86.8% and 99.2% vaccination coverage, respectively. A mobile vaccination had been deployed to each of these communities for at least one day. A third village, Gweley, showed a dismal vaccination rate, 2.4%, primarily because of lack of awareness of the campaign, inaccessibility to a vaccination center, and the expectation that vaccination teams would come to their community as had previously occurred during polio eradication campaigns year ago (Table 19-1). Our suspicions were confirmed. Based on these results, MSF Swiss agreed to provide vaccine and cold chain supplies to the MOH to extend the campaign during March 27 to 29 for these uncovered communities, resulting

Table 19-1 Yellow Fever Convenience Coverage Survey, Zoegeh District, Western Zone, Nimba County, Liberia

			GWELEY VILLAGE		
Number	Number of Family Members Older than 6 Months	Is the Family Aware About the Ongoing Yellow Fever Campaign?	Number of Family Members Vaccinated with Card	Number of Family Members Unvaccinated	Core Reason for Nonvaccination
1	15	Y	0	15	Access
2	7	Y	1	6	Waiting for vaccinators
3	8	Y	1	7	Access
4	20	N	0	20	Don't know about it
5	8	N	0	8	Access
6	10	N	0	10	Access
7	15	N	1	14	Access
8	29	N	0	29	Access
9	5	N	0	5	Access
10	7	N	0	7	Access
Total	124	3	3	121	Access
Percentage	100	30.00	2.42	97.58	Access

Table 19-1 (Continued)

ZAYGLAY VILLAGE

Number	Number of Family Members Older than 6 Months	Is the Family Aware About the Ongoing Yellow Fever Campaign?	Number of Family Members Vaccinated with Card	Number of Family Members Unvaccinated	Core Reason for Nonvaccination
1	12	Y	12	0	N/A
2	8	Y	7	1	Was absent
3	9	Y	9	0	N/A
4	10	Y	10	0	N/A
5	15	Y	15	0	N/A
6	8	Y	8	0	N/A
7	10	Y	10	0	N/A
8	20	Y	20	0	N/A
9	20	Y	20	0	N/A
10	12	Y	12	0	N/A
Total	124	10	123	1	N/A
Percentage	100	100.00	99.19	0.81	N/A

GBLAH VILLAGE

Number	Number of Family Members Older than 6 Months	Is the Family Aware About the Ongoing Yellow Fever Campaign?	Number of Family Members Vaccinated with Card	Number of Family Members Unvaccinated	Core Reason for Nonvaccination
1	14	Y	14	0	N/A
2	7	Y	6	1	Was absent
3	7	Y	7	0	N/A
4	6	Y	6	0	N/A
5	6	Y	6	0	Was absent
6	12	Y	10	2	N/A
7	10	Y	6	4	Were absent
8	15	Y	15	0	Access
9	25	Y	25	0	Access
10	27	Y	17	10	Were absent
Total	129	10	112	17	Were absent
Percentage	100.00	100.00	86.82	13.18	

in 32,318 persons (92.3%) overall receiving immunization. For me, a truly astonishing figure emerged from our study—the absolute value of our coveted denominator. As epidemiologists, we treasure the denominator, but sometimes lose sight of the intimate witness that it may bear. Through our treks into rather sparse and withered two to three room homes, the median household size was about 12 people. Households numbering 20 or more residents were not uncommon. Village life, the poverty, and the family commitments that solidify a community in times of strife, peace, and disease can be breathtaking.

REASSESSMENT—BACK TO BONG COUNTY

After 8 days supervising the campaign in Nimba County, Jen and I returned to our UNICEF base in Monrovia to update ourselves on case surveillance and review options for a catchup campaign in Bong County, where coverage rates fell far below threshold goals. Sue had flown back to the United States during our sojourn in Sanniquellie, and as she regrouped with the CDC powers in Ft. Collins, an understanding of where our Liberia work fit into a bigger picture, with global political implications, began to emerge.

Liberia was still smoldering with guns and disillusionment. Young uneducated fighters had spent most of their formative years simmering in a cesspool of violence, without a moral playbook that formal schooling can often provide. Quickly after Charles Taylor's exile in late 2003, the United Nations Development Programme established a multidisciplinary international mandate, DDRR (Disarmament, Demobilization, Reintegration, Rehabilitation), to disarm the approximately 80,000 combatants throughout the country to reeducate and reintroduce these factions into society. Launched in December 2003, DDRR's credibility had been challenged by the time we showed up in mid March with a high number of ex-fighters registered, exceeding preparatory estimates, although with a sub par number of weapons confiscated.[22] With few weapons confiscated, the term "disarmament" became a worrisome misnomer within the international donor community.

Sue was now preparing to testify with Muireann Brennan and Tony in Washington, DC to a USAID Office of Foreign Disaster Assistance (OFDA) panel on the success of yellow fever control in Liberia and need for long-term support of vaccine-preventable disease programs. OFDA had also been keeping close tabs on DDRR and was concerned that DDRR had thus far failed. UNICEF, United Nations Development Programme's subsidiary, was largely responsible for executing many of DDRR's objectives. Thus, funding of our work depended on perception from those far away. There was concern that DDRR was not getting its job done. Therefore, reassurance was needed that we were getting our job done. Sue wrote in a March 29 e-mail to us, "My impression was that OFDA was reluctant to fund UNICEF since they seemed to be dropping the ball on that program so why would the vaccine program be a success?" As UNICEF received extensive funding from USAID for their overall activities in Liberia, offering a compelling narrative from U.S. commissioned corps officers on the scene could prove persuasive. Yet could we really call our efforts a success with the wimpy Bong County numerators dangling like stale cassava in a dry harvest line? Recall that among the estimated 87,000 population living in the IDP camps of Bong County, only 47,763 (56.8%) were vaccinated and that the vaccination coverage goal was at least 80%.

Dr. William Perea, from the communicable diseases emergency operations division of WHO, had just arrived in Monrovia from Geneva, Switzerland to provide further expertise on control of the epidemic. The question now was if there was still an outbreak? This was an issue because by March 30 the WHO reported 46 suspect cases from eight counties; however, 31 cases were IgM negative, and the initial four confirmed cases from the first 2 weeks in January were the only confirmed cases. The outbreak may have been over; therefore, a shift toward absorbing yellow fever immunization resources into routine EPI throughout the country began to germinate among the WHO and UNICEF leadership. Jen compiled a summary presentation of the mass vaccination campaigns, and I was designated to create a strategic plan with a budget for yellow fever immunization EPI integration. I had some bystander experience at the Illinois Department of Public Health in pandemic influenza planning, which accelerated during 2003 with the SARS experience, although now potentially millions of dollars in funding appeared riding on my rudimentary bookkeeping aptitude. Yet, being epidemiologists, we were still hung up on the less than satisfying numbers calculated out of the Bong County campaign. We needed some rational consensus before we could sensibly close the book on Bong County and declare victory.

Toward the end of the perceived finish line in outbreak investigations, fatigue often sets in among the pertinent players. You just want to move on to the next outbreak, those unfinished manuscripts lingering on your desk, or that cold caipirinha your wife poured up that's tantalizingly within reach back home. Dr. Perea reenergized our focus to examine the attributes of the campaigns and take one of the last steps in an outbreak investigation, the outcome assessment. He encouraged formulating a strategy to formally survey vaccination coverage in Bong County. On April 1, Jen and I met for the first time with Dr. Otero, who too was troubled with the low calculated vaccination rate. He spent 3 days after the campaign going shelter-to-shelter looking for yellow vaccination cards and found most occupants had one. The IDP camps were built in 2002 and administered by the Liberian government through the Liberia Refugee Repatriation and Resettlement Commission. Food was supplied by the World Food Programme (WFP). The last government census in Liberia occurred in 1984.[23,24] MSF France wanted to perform a census of the Bong County IDP camps, but was not granted permission by the Liberia Refugee Repatriation and Resettlement Commission or WFP. A WFP formula of five persons per shelter was used to estimate the camp population. But how was this formula derived?

As a denominator detective, I finally learned of its rather imprecise origins about 6 weeks after we left Liberia in an e-mail reply to my inquiry with the WFP. "There seems to be a general agreement that the average family size in Liberia is 5 to 6," and "on average, the shelters in Liberia IDP camps are 4×5 meters, well below recommended area per person," according to Alfred Nabeta, a representative for the WFP director in Liberia (Figure 19-12). Mr. Nabeta added this:

> In the camp environment, there are some cases of families that are compelled to occupy more than one shelter because they cannot fit in one single shelter. In addition to the prevalence of large nuclear families, perhaps the other thing that tends to have a bearing on the family sizes in reality is the very strong bond between the nuclear family and the extended family.

Long ago I realized that if you want the real dirt on a new town, ask a cab driver what's really going down in the place. Jefferson Cooper, our trusted driver from UNICEF, took an interest in what we were doing in these IDP camps. When we told him we wanted to survey people in their shelters, he said, "If you want to really know how many IDPs actually

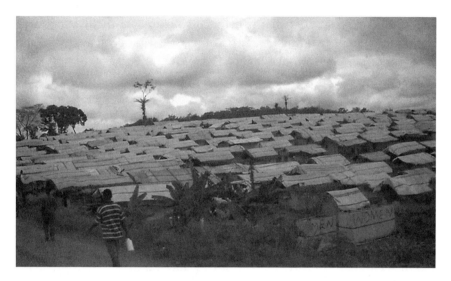

FIGURE 19-12 Physical design and spatial location of shelters in IDP camps, Salala District, Bong County, Liberia.

occupy a shelter, ask them how many people sleep there overnight. Otherwise, if you ask them how many people just live there, they're used to getting that question from the WFP and will always give a higher number because more people means more food rations." In developing countries, a reliable driver can be more valuable to your well-being than potable water, vaccines, or the "tourista" antibiotics you pack along. Road accidents kill more expatriates than exotic diseases. Thus, Mr. Cooper was doing double duty for us as both our eyes on the road and epidemiologic mole. I felt like deputizing him as an honorary EIS officer for his inscrutable insight.

Jen and I devised a two-prong attack to determine vaccination coverage in IDP camps and outlying host communities. For the IDP camps, I designed a two-stage cluster sampling survey with the assistance of local maps and registration logs of habitable shelters in each of the six camps.[25] Each camp was partitioned into alphabetical blocks, and each shelter within each block was given a sequential integer number. Each of the 17,384 total shelters in these six camps had a unique identification that included the camp name, a block letter, and a shelter number. Sample size was calculated based on 5% allowable margin of error. The design effect was equal to one because one person per shelter cluster was to be randomly selected for the survey. We chose the conjectured vaccination coverage rate to be 80%, the threshold that is believed to eliminate the likelihood of human-to-human transmission.[26,27] Sample size was calculated by a standard random cluster formula[28]:

$$(t^2)(\text{design effect})(\text{coverage rate})(1 - \text{coverage rate})/(\text{margin of error})^2 = 248 \text{ persons } [t = 1.96 \text{ for } 95\% \text{ level of confidence}]$$

As a contingency for missing persons in selected shelter households, an additional 5% (12 persons) were added for a total sample size of 260.

The sum total of all shelters (n = 17,384) served as the overall denominator for the population. At the first stage, we constructed a single sampling frame (x) among all six camps by using an alphabetical and numerical hierarchy of shelter addresses to create a linear list of all shelters. Thus, the first cluster on the list was shelter A1 from Totota camp and the 17,384th and final cluster was shelter D361 from Tumutu camp (Figure 19-13). We divided the total number of shelters by the sample size (17,384/260 = 67) to determine an interval-sampling instrument (r) to select shelter clusters systematically. A two-digit number x, between 01 and r, from a random number table was chosen as the first sampling point on the frame, with subsequent points provided by $x + r$, $x + 2r$, $x + 3r$, etc., until $x + 259r$.

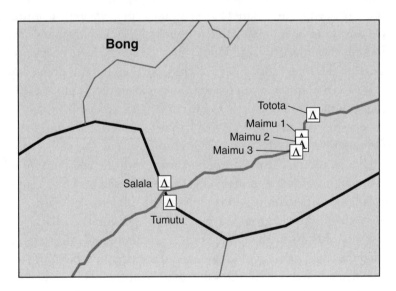

FIGURE 19-13 IDP (internally displaced person) camps, Salala District, Bong County, Liberia.

Wherever a point fell on the cumulative shelter population list, that shelter was assigned as a cluster. The number of clusters chosen per camp was proportional to camp size.

The second stage sampling was performed on site. Persons aged 6 months or more living in the shelter were assigned a number based on their height, from the shortest person in the shelter to the tallest. We invoked the newly minted "Jefferson Cooper" definition of a person considered to be a household member if he or she routinely slept overnight in the shelter during the vaccination campaign. Household members present during the survey supplied height estimates for absent persons who lived in the shelter. One person per shelter cluster was randomly chosen for the survey using a random number table. No replacement of shelters or persons in shelters occurred during the survey.

Approval for the survey was granted by local authorities in the Liberia Refugee Repatriation and Resettlement Commission. A standardized questionnaire in English eliciting demographic information, household size, awareness of the yellow fever vaccination campaign, yellow fever vaccination status, and reports of AEFI was distributed to 12 teams of interviewers. In addition, a signed and dated yellow fever vaccination card was requested from each person who was interviewed. Each team consisted of three to four interviewers proficient in English and at least five of the other local languages spoken by a substantial majority of IDPs in the camps. We formed one team from each camp among local MSF and county public health department workers and trained them in the use of the questionnaire by role playing on April 4. Our UNICEF and WHO colleagues joined us as supervisors on the teams. On my team, I had two local MSF workers who were also IDPs in one of the Maimu camps. Both were college educated, yet their career paths had been derailed by the civil war. They told me that the IDPs were issued tarpaulins, and then each had to build their own shelters to reside in the camps (Figure 19-14).

During April 5 to 7, teams conducted face-to-face interviews with randomly selected survey participants. Questionnaires were translated as needed. If an absent adult was selected, the survey team queried present household members to schedule a return appointment based on the availability of the selected adult. If after 3 consecutive days the selected adult remained unavailable, a present household member was surveyed as a proxy regarding the adult's information. If a young child was selected, a present adult household member was surveyed as a proxy about the young

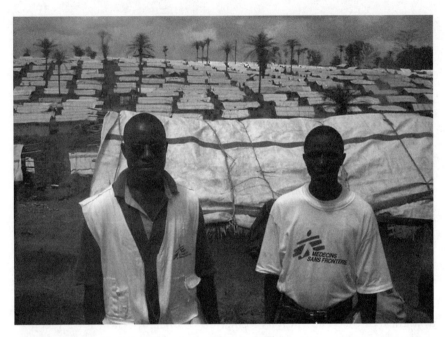

FIGURE 19-14 Medecins Sans Frontieres survey team, Maimu IDP camp, Salala District, Bong County, Liberia.

child's information. Oral, informed consent was obtained from all respondents before interviews. To minimize response bias of overreporting household size, respondents were clearly informed that the survey was not linked to a registration or food-distribution process.

Of the 260 shelters we visited, one of the 260 shelters did not exist. Among the 259 existing shelters, 22 were either unoccupied for 3 successive days during the survey (15 shelters) or were incomplete shelters that were not yet inhabited (seven shelters). Data were analyzed for 237 survey respondents (one person per shelter). There were no missing data from IDPs surveyed and no AEFI reported.

We drove in and out from Monrovia daily for about a 2.5-hour trip each way, and thus, I was able to enter data from our survey forms and analyze it in real time using Epi Info.[29] The median number of household members living in a shelter was four (range, 1–8). We estimated that 69,536 persons lived in these six camps, or 20% less than the WFP-based estimate of 87,000 used before the campaign. This disparity in the denominator was the greatest factor in the low vaccination rates initially tabulated

Table 19-2 Age and Yellow Fever Vaccination Status Among Internally Displaced Persons Living in Salala District, Bong County, Liberia, 2004

	Age (Years)*		
Population (Number)	Median	Range	Interquartile Range (25th and 75th percentile)
Total sample (237)	20	1–87	10, 36
Vaccinated (215)	20	1–87	10, 37
Unvaccinated (22)	21	1–62	16, 31

* No significant difference between vaccinated and unvaccinated; $p = 0.86$.

through the onsite administrative tally data sheets. The median age of respondents was 20 years (Table 19-2); of the 237 respondents, one half ($n = 119$) were aged 15 to 44 years. Females outnumbered males by an almost 2:1 ratio (Table 19-3).

Of the 237 respondents, 230 (97.6%) were informed of the vaccination campaign; 215 (91.9%) had been vaccinated during the campaign by their self-report, and 196 (83.5%) possessed a signed and dated vaccination card from the recent campaign. Self-reported vaccination rates were highest in the 5- to 14-year age group (94.8%) and lowest in the 15- to 44-year age group (89.7%) (Table 19-4). Gender distribution was similar among vaccinated versus unvaccinated respondents ($P = 0.63$), and no difference existed in the median age among respondents reporting vaccination (aged 20 years) during the campaign compared with unvaccinated respondents (aged 21 years) ($P = 0.86$).

Among 22 unvaccinated respondents, 8 (38%) did not participate in the campaign because of prior yellow fever vaccination within the past 10 years; 5 (24%) stated that they were unaware of the campaign, and 5 (24%) stated that vaccination was "inconvenient." Two respondents were absent from the IDP camps during the campaign, and one respondent had no access to the vaccination site. One respondent provided no explanation. Including respondents reporting prior yellow fever vaccination within the past 10 years with the persons with self-reported recent vaccination, 223 respondents (94.8%) were immunized against yellow fever.

Our study had at least four limitations that may have affected data interpretation. First, some interviews were conducted by proxy; however, proxy

Table 19-3 Yellow Fever Vaccination Coverage Estimates Using Administrative and Survey Methods Among Internally Displaced Persons Living in Bong County, Liberia, 2004

Number

Characteristic	Total	Vaccinated in 2004	Coverage (%)	95% CI
Administrative				
Total	87,000	47,676*	54.8	NA[†]
Age group (%)				
6 months to 4 years	13,920 (16.0%)	9,422	67.7	NA
5–14 years	25,230 (29.0%)	12,238	48.5	NA
15–44 years	34,800 (40.0%)	18,427	53.0	NA
> 44 years	13,050 (15.0%)	7,589	58.2	NA
Gender				
Female	NA	NA	NA	NA
Male	NA	NA	NA	NA
Survey				
Total	237	215	91.9	88.4–95.5
Age group (%)				
6 months to 4 years	28 (11.8%)	26	96.2	90.9–101.6
5–14 years	54 (22.8%)	51	94.8	89.0–100.7
15–44 years	119 (50.2%)	105	89.7	84.1–95.2
> 44 years	36 (15.2%)	33	91.5	81.2–101.9
Gender[‡]				
Female	151 (63.7%)	138	92.7	88.6–96.9
Male	86 (36.3%)	77	90.2	84.2–96.8

*An additional 1,719 IDPs reported YF vaccination within the past 10 years and did not participate in the 2004 campaign. Ages of previously vaccinated IDPs were not collected. The total number of IDPs considered appropriately immunized using the administrative method was 49,395 (56.8%).

[†]NA = not applicable.

[‡]No significant difference between vaccinated females and males; relative risk = 1.0 (95% confidence interval 0.94–1.1, $P = 0.63$).

Table 19-4 Survey Results of Yellow Fever Vaccination Coverage Survey for 237 Internally Displaced Persons, Bong County, Liberia, 2004

Characteristic	Positive Response	Percentage	95% Confidence Interval
Knowledge of campaign	230	97.6	95.5-99.6
Vaccinated, 2004	215	91.9	88.4-95.4
Possessed 2004 vaccination card	196	83.5	78.6-88.5
Vaccinated, 1994–2003	8	2.9	0.9-5.0
Appropriately vaccinated*	223	94.8	92.0-97.7

* Vaccinated either in 2004 or within past 10 years.

interviewees were members of the same shelter and usually very familiar with the demographic and vaccination status of the selected person. Second, proof of vaccination was not obtained from 19 persons (9%) who claimed to have been immunized during the campaign, which may have introduced recall bias. This occurred most commonly when an absent person was selected and their vaccination card was unavailable either because the card was locked with their personal belongings inside the shelter or the absent person had taken the card with them outside the camp for documentation if traveling on main roads, registering for school, or seeking medical treatment. Also, because no other vaccination programs occurred within the IDP camps during the yellow fever immunization campaign, bias by inadvertently attributing yellow fever immunization to another vaccine was likely diminished. For these reasons, self-report or proxy report of vaccination was considered an adequate indicator of immunization status. Third, although we verified the dates and county of vaccination in 2004 for nearly all (> 90%) survey participants because data were not available on the validated vaccination cards specifying the exact vaccination site during the campaign, we could not quantify estimates of IDPs vaccinated outside the camps in 2004. Finally, the reason for the low proportion of males surveyed remains unclear. More men may have moved from IDP camps in search of employment near the capitol city Monrovia since the civil war ceasefire. Of the estimated 200,000 Liberians killed during the civil war, most were male combatants,[30] which may have changed the distribution of gender in the country overall.

As lords of the denominator, we were confident now that the mass vaccination campaign in IDP camps in Bong County did in fact meet its target goal. In addition, we were able to determine that there was near-universal knowledge and broad acceptance of the campaign among IDPs, which highlights the high degree of yellow fever disease awareness in this population generated through effective social mobilization. We were able to avoid a costly and unnecessary mass immunization mop-up campaign in the IDP camps through our rapid assessment coverage study. We then looked to the surrounding villages to fill in the missing pieces of the Bong County coverage data.

LOT QUALITY ASSURANCE SAMPLING

In the host communities surrounding the IDP camps, where 24,866 persons were vaccinated during the Bong County campaign, we did not have the luxury of a documented address system as we had in the camps. We therefore could not perform a similar survey format as conducted in the IDP camps. Because of population upheavals from the civil war, even rough estimates of village populations collected as recently as 2002 were considered inaccurate by local officials. For these host communities, Jen opted for a lot quality assurance sampling (LQAS) survey to assess communities.[31] This technique was originally developed by Westinghouse in the manufacturing industry in the 1950s for quality control purposes. To determine whether a batch, or lot, of light bulbs met desired specifications, a sample of light bulbs from each lot was inspected for defects. If the number of defective items in each sample exceeded a decision value, then the entire lot was rejected. The sample size and decision value are based on user-defined risks of type I and type II errors. The WHO adopted this method in the 1990s to assess vaccination coverage rates. When delivered in the context of an immunization coverage survey, the "lot" is a community and a "defective item" is an unimmunized person. The LQAS method has been used to identify communities with inadequate coverage without the need for precise population denominator verification. It can also estimate the overall immunization coverage in a group of communities by taking a weighted average of the estimated coverage in each community.

The sample size and decision value were calculated using WHO guidelines. The desired level of accuracy for the survey results was ± 8% and the desired level of confidence for the survey results was 95%. Given these levels of accuracy and confidence, the required sample size according to WHO guidelines was 150 households. MSF France and the Bong County public health department supplied us with maps with labeled villages of the surrounding area. All communities were eligible for the survey, but major population centers had a higher probability of being identified. Ten communities were systematically selected and the size of each relative to the others was used to determine the weight of its contribution to the overall target population (Table 19-5). The minimum lot sample size was therefore 15 households per community. The low threshold level, at which immunization coverage was judged "unacceptable," was set at 50%. The high threshold level, at which immunization coverage was judged "acceptable" was set at 80%, as this was the goal set by campaign coordinators. Given these thresholds, the decision value, the number of unimmunized persons necessary to call coverage "unacceptable" in a specific community, was 4.

The same survey teams used in the IDP camps study ventured into the communities on April 7 and 8. Teams first visited the village chief to request permission to conduct the survey, ask for an estimate of the population of the community, and seek guidance on what time was best to start the intervention. The teams walked to the center of each community

Table 19-5 Estimated Weighted Populations, Host Communities LQAS Study, Salala District, Bong Country, Liberia

Community	Estimated Population	Weight
Central Totota	5,000	0.23
New Totota	3,000	0.13
Maimu	4,000	0.18
Salala	4,000	0.18
Frelela	3,000	0.13
A-99	1,000	0.04
Tumutu	1,000	0.04
Wreputa	1,000	0.04
Tokpaipolu	500	0.02
Velengai	250	0.01
Total	22,750	1.00

or at focal points such as schools, places of worship, or health facilities. The teams then determined a vector direction at random by spinning a pencil on the ground and proceeding outward to the first house in the selected direction.

At noon on April 7, we all suddenly stopped and fell silent for one minute. It was the International Day of Reflection on the Genocide in Rwanda, marking the 10th anniversary of beginning of the massacre. U.N. Secretary General Kofi Annan called on people of the world "everywhere, no matter what their station in life, whether in crowded cities or remote rural areas" to observe this somber memorial.[32] To be in Liberia at this moment doing what I was doing struck me with solemn pause that just perhaps as a global community we have grown in solidarity to offer empathy and protection to the world's vulnerable and suffering whether by conflict or disease.

One person from each household in the vector line was asked for the names of all of the residents in the house aged 6 months or more, including anyone not present at the time of the survey. Each name was assigned a number. One number was then selected using a random number table. The person whose number was selected was the person for whom the survey was administered (Figure 19-15). The standardized questionnaire used in the IDP camps study was the same survey tool used for the LQAS study. If the person selected was too young to answer the survey, then the questions were directed to his or her parent. If the person was not present, then a proxy interview was conducted with another member of the household. When the interview was completed, the protocol was repeated at the next house, following in the same vector that was pinpointed by the spin of the pencil.

One person was surveyed in each of a total of 158 households across the 10 communities. The median household size was 10 people (range, 1–32). Eighty seven (55%) of the residents randomly selected were female. Fifteen (9%) were 6 months to 4 years old. Thirty three (21%) were aged 5 to 14 years. Seventy nine (50%) were aged 15 to 44 years, and 31 (20%) were 45 years or older. There were no AEFI reported. An estimated 95% of the population of the 10 communities was aware of the 2004 immunization campaign. If self-report of immunization was used as an indicator of campaign coverage, then an estimated 89% of the population was immunized in the campaign. If proof of immunization by yellow card was used as an indicator of campaign coverage, then an estimated 71% of the population

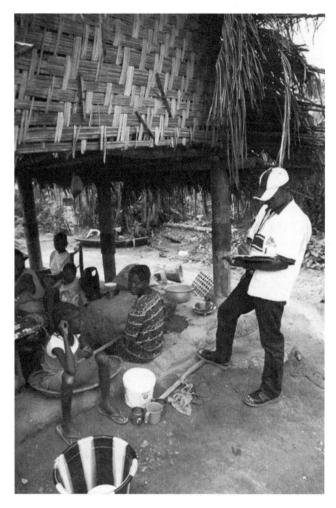

FIGURE 19-15 IDP camp host community LQAS Survey, Salala District, Bong County, Liberia.

was immunized. The self-report figure we believed was a fairly accurate portrayal of the true vaccination rate for the same reasons also illustrated in the IDP camps study. Immunization coverage in the overall target population was estimated by calculation of a weighted average of the proportion of people reporting that they were immunized in each sample. When weighted according to the rough figures provided by town chiefs and public health department personnel of community densities, the overall immunization coverage was 89% (95% confidence interval, 0.84–0.94), similar to the IDP camps survey and again indicating that the target levels of immunization were achieved.

There were differences, however, in vaccination coverage in discrete villages. Using the binary decision value established at four, 4 of the 10 communities were "rejected" as not achieved adequate vaccination coverage (Table 19-6). Two of these communities, Frelala and A-99, were located on the main road between camps but somewhat distant from major immunization sites. The two other communities, Tokpaipolu and Velengai, were less populated and very remotely isolated within the district. Because of their distant locations, social mobilization was challenging, limiting the duration of the campaign in these areas. These neighboring communities also hosted weekly market days attracting many IDPs. Numerous IDPs were reportedly vaccinated at community sites on market days and not in the camps. This would have resulted in extra doses being administered in the villages, but not necessarily to town residents, further deflating the actual coverage rates in some host communities.

One of the disadvantages of the LQAS sampling method is that there is no measure of magnitude in unacceptability of individual lots. Although this survey design did provide information on deficiencies in some communities, the overall vaccination rate revealed in the study enabled us to finally conclude that the Bong County mass vaccination campaign successfully met target goals.

Table 19-6 Level of "Acceptable" Vaccination Rates in Host Communities, LQAS Study, Salala District, Bong Country, Liberia

Community	Number Not Immunized	Sample Size	80% Coverage
Central Totota	1	16	Yes
New Totota	0	15	Yes
Maimu	1	17	Yes
Salala	1	15	Yes
Frelela	5	16	No
A-99	7	17	No
Tumutu	1	17	Yes
Wreputa	1	15	Yes
Tokpaipolu	5	15	No
Velengai	4	15	No

Concerns with the quality of administrative data used to estimate vaccine coverage have prompted several retrospective surveys after National Immunization Days in other settings[33–40]; however, to our knowledge, this was the first reported survey to evaluate yellow fever vaccination coverage in IDP or refugee camps. Worldwide, nearly 35 million refugees (9.7 million) and IDPs (25 million) existed by 2004; more than 7 million of these persons have been warehoused in camps and settlements for at least 10 years.[41–43] Our studies underscored the importance of accurately estimating the population at risk for yellow fever to assist programmatic decisions regarding future vaccination strategies.

FINAL RECOMMENDATIONS

Jen and I returned to our Monrovia office on April 9. With information on phase I activities now fully complete, I finalized a revision of the WHO and UNICEF Response to Yellow Fever Outbreak Control in Liberia, along with a new draft budget. An overall total of 199,729 persons were immunized against yellow fever in Bong and Nimba counties during February 26 to March 31. We reviewed the document with Dr. Forssen, Dr. Maksha, and Ms. Kearney of UNICEF, who were in agreement with its content. We presented our findings to a group meeting among WHO, UNICEF, and MSF, in particular to answer this question: Now should we move on to phase II of the original plan targeting an additional 320,000 persons in Bong and Nimba counties? The group agreed that "catch-up" immunization campaigns are important to boost background immunity in endemic areas where yellow fever immunization is not yet routinely administered as part of EPI; however, the group also agreed with our conclusions that the implementation of phase II should be deferred in favor of investing resources in reinforcing yellow fever immunization integration in EPI in Liberia. The demographic distribution and stagnant number of confirmed cases—no other cases had been confirmed since early January—suggested that the outbreak was over. Mass immunization campaigns would require the reallocation of already limited health care resources and might preclude control of other causes of morbidity and mortality. We identified yellow fever outbreak preparedness as a priority by bolstering the fledgling MOH surveillance system and strongly recommended that provisions for outbreak preparedness be supported to ensure in-country readiness and capacity to respond to future outbreaks immediately. With lessons learned and laid forth from implementation of phase I, this response capacity included a capital and technical network to vaccinate rapidly and efficiently a population of 200,000 persons. Funding requirements within our draft budget to maintain outbreak preparedness were $396,000 and were requested by UNICEF from donor agencies throughout the international community.

BRINGING IT ALL HOME

I had the opportunity to twice visit St. Joseph's Catholic Hospital on the other side of town from the diplomatic district in Monrovia. As I first approached the entrance, the compound looked about the same as I recalled before mortar shells had torn holes in the building and ripped off one of the roofs. They had been firmly repaired, and the adjacent coconut grove, stripped bare for firewood after all the coconuts had been consumed by a starving population during the war, had grown back. I recognized one of the hospital's drivers named Lhame standing out front. He looked at me as if I was a ghost (well, my hair had grayed a little bit over the past 14 years). I flashed my old ID card. He smiled, gave me one of those rhythmic African handshakes, and then took my card and ran into the back administrative offices. Brother Justino Izquierdo, the long-standing chief operating officer, came barreling through the hallway and threw out a big bear hug. We spent the next couple of hours reminiscing of those hospital workers who died during the war, the survivors, and the dedication of the staff throughout the war (after they came back about a month after our evacuation, they never left again). It was the homecoming I had wished for, filled with fondness, regret, and hope. My next and last visit was on the request of Angela Kearney to consult on a French expatriate employee of UNICEF hospitalized with malaria. I assured her that St. Joseph's Catholic Hospital was still regarded as the best medical center in the country.[44] Her care was excellent, and she was recovering.

I am now an assistant professor in the division of infectious diseases at the John H. Stroger Jr. Hospital of Cook County and Rush University Medical Center in Chicago. The last I searched proMED mail as of August 2008 with the words "yellow fever" and "Liberia" I found no other accounts, neither cases nor outbreaks, announced since the 2004 epidemic. A long list of outbreaks in neighboring West African countries in the interim 4 years popped up, so, perhaps our presence in 2004 and recommendations for enhanced surveillance and EPI uptake have paid off. I present this investigation as an example not only of an international public health response to an isolated outbreak of yellow fever in a small tropical country, but as a paradigm to the obstacles both practical and political that need to be addressed if a viable vaccination strategy for HIV were ever to take hold in Africa. I am often reminded of our mission as epidemiologists to protect populations at risk of injury or diseases, whether ancient afflictions such as yellow fever or new threats such as HIV, when I look at a watercolor portrait hanging on my otherwise nondescript office wall in Chicago. As I stepped out of the Mamba Point Hotel on April 11, 2004, to throw my bags into Jefferson Cooper's jeep for a lift to the airport, Romeo was behind the front desk and made sure that I met an artist friend of his named Mitchell before I vanished. I handed over 8 U.S. dollars and rolled up one of his paintings. A traditional Liberian couple is dancing, smiling, celebrating (Figure 19-16).

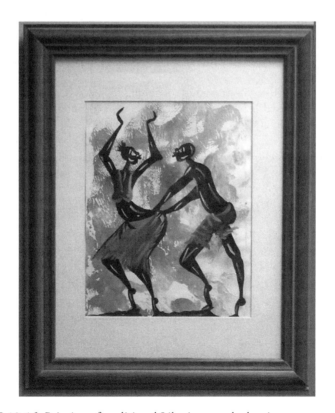

FIGURE 19-16 Painting of traditional Liberian couple dancing.

REFERENCES

1. Evacuees from Liberian capital city describe battles, bodies in streets. *The Washington Post*, August 15, 1990, A18.
2. Liberians' brutality stuns U.S. volunteer. *The Chicago Tribune*, August 15, 1990, 3.
3. San Diego lab tech helped in Liberian evacuation. *Los Angeles Times*, August 21, 1990.
4. United Nations. Office for the Coordination of Humanitarian Affairs. December 18, 2003. Retrieved August 19, 2008, from http://www.humanitarianinfo .org/liberia/.
5. Bryce JW, Cutts FT, Saba S. Mass immunization campaigns and quality of services. *Lancet* 1990;335:739–740.
6. ProMED mail. Retrieved August 19, 2008, from http://www.promedmail.com/ pls/otn/f?p=2400:1202:3246059765909252::NO::F2400_P1202_CHECK_ DISPLAY,F2400_P1202_PUB_MAIL_ID:X,24586.
7. Robertson S. Yellow fever: the immunological basis for immunization. Document WHO/EPI/GEN/93.181993.
8. Merlo C, Steffen R, Landis T, Tsai T, Karabatsos N. Possible association of encephalitis and 17D yellow fever vaccination in a 29-year-old traveler. *Vaccine* 1993;11:691.
9. Kengsakul K, Sathirapongsasuti K, Punyagupta S. Fatal myeloencephalitis following yellow fever vaccination in a case with HIV infection. *J Med Assoc Thai* 2002;85:131–134.
10. Centers for Disease Control and Prevention (CDC). Adverse events associated with 17D-derived yellow fever vaccination—United States, 2001–2002. *Morb Mort Weekly Rep* 2002:51;989–992.
11. Chan RC, Penney DJ, Little D, Carter IW, Roberts JA, Rawlinson WD. Hepatitis and death following vaccination with 17D-204 yellow fever vaccine. *Lancet* 2001;358:121–122.
12. Vasconcelos PF, Luna EJ, Galler R, et al. Serious adverse events associated with yellow fever 17DD vaccine in Brazil: a report of two cases. *Lancet* 2001;358: 91–97.
13. Martin M, Tsai TF, Cropp B, Chang GJ, Holmes DA, Tseng T, et al. Fever and multisystem organ failure associated with 17D-204 yellow fever vaccination: a report of four cases. *Lancet* 2001;358:98–104.
14. Adhiyaman V, Oke A, Cefai C. Effects of yellow fever vaccination. *Lancet* 2001; 358:1907–1908.
15. Troillet N, Laurencet F. Effects of yellow fever vaccination. *Lancet* 2001;358: 1908–1916.
16. Werfel U, Popp W. Effects of yellow fever vaccination. *Lancet* 2001;358:1909.
17. ProMED mail. Retrieved August 19, 2008, from http://www.promedmail.com/ pls/otn/f?p=2400:1202:3246059765909252::NO::F2400_P1202_CHECK_ DISPLAY,F2400_P1202_PUB_MAIL_ID:X,24687.

18. United Nations Mission in Liberia. Retrieved August 19, 2008, from http://www.un.org/depts/dpko/missions/unmil/index.html.

19. International Civilian Police. Retrieved August 19, 2008, from http://www.civpol.org/portal/html/index.php.

20. Monath TP. Yellow fever: An update. *Lancet Infect Dis* 2001;1:11–20.

21. *Prevention and Control of Yellow Fever in Africa*. World Health Organization, Geneva, 1986.

22. Liberia Disarmament Demobilisation and Reintegration Programme (DDRR) Activity Report, United Nations Development Programme Administered Trust Fund—December 2003 to August 2004. Retrieved August 19, 2008, from http://www.lr.undp.org/DEX/DDRR%20Trust%20Fund%20%20Report.pdf.

23. Ministry of Planning and Economic Affairs. *1984 Population and Housing Census of Liberia: Summary Results in Graphic Presentation, PC-1*. Monrovia, Liberia, 1986.

24. Population Reference Bureau, Washington D.C. Retrieved August 19, 2008, from http://www.prb.org/Articles/2008/liberia.aspx.

25. Huhn GD, Brown J, Perea W, et al. Vaccination coverage survey versus administrative in the assessment of a mass yellow fever immunization in internally displaced person camps—Liberia, 2004. *Vaccine* 2006;24:730–737.

26. Brés P. Benefit versus risk factors in immunization against yellow fever. *Dev Biol Stand* 1979;43;297–304.

27. Monath TP, Nasidi N. Should yellow fever vaccine be included in the Expanded Program of Immunization in Africa? A cost-effectiveness analysis for Nigeria. *Am J Trop Med Hyg* 1993;48:274–299.

28. Lemeshow S, Robinson D. Surveys to measure programme coverage and impact: a review of the methodology used by the Expanded Programme on Immunization. *World Health Stat Q* 1985;38:65–75.

29. Dean AG, Dean JA, Coulombier D, et al. Epiinfo Version 6: A Word Processing, Database, and Statistics Program for Public Health on IBM-Compatible Microcomputers. Atlanta, GA: Centers for Disease Control, 1996.

30. United Nations, United States, World Bank. International reconstruction conference on Liberia. June 2–3, 2003. Retrieved June 6, 2005, from http://www.un.org/News/Press/docs/2004?ARF827.p2.doc.htm.

31. Brown J, Huhn G, Perea W, et al. Yellow fever immunization coverage in host communities for internally displaced persons—Liberia, 2004. 53rd Annual Meeting of the American Society of Tropical Medicine and Hygiene (abstract 989), Miami Beach, Florida, USA, November 7 – 12, 2004.

32. United Nations General Assembly resolution A/RES/58/234. International Day of Reflection on 1994 Genocide in Rwanda. Retrieved August 25, 2008, from http://www.un.org/events/rwanda/.

33. Reichler MR, Aslanian R, Lodhi ZH, et al. Evaluation of oral poliovirus vaccine delivery during the 1994 National Immunization Days in Pakistan. *J Infect Dis* 1997;175(Suppl 1):S205–S209.

34. Reichler MR, Darwidh A, Stroh G, et al. Cluster survey evaluation of coverage and risk factors for failure to be immunized during the 1995 National Immunization Days in Egypt. *Int J Epidemiol* 1998;27:1083–1089.

35. Rojas JC, Prieto FE. National immunization day evaluation in Columbia, 2001: an ecological approach. *Rev Salud Publica* 2004;6:44–62.

36. Bhattacharjee J, Gupta RS, Jain DC, Devadethan, Datta KK. Evaluation of pulse polio and routine immunization coverage: Alwar District, Rajasthan. *Indian J Pediatr* 1997;64:65–72.

37. Guyer B, Atangana S. A programme of multiple-antigen childhood immunization in Yaounde, Cameroon: first year evaluation 1975–76. Bull World Health Organ 1977;55:633–642.

38. Borgdorff MW, Walker GJ. Estimating vaccination coverage: routine information or sample survey? *J Trop Med Hyg* 1988;9135–9142.

39. Tawfik Y, Hoque S, Siddiqi M. Using lot quality assurance sampling to improve immunization coverage in Bangladesh. *Bull World Health Organ* 2001;79:501–505.

40. Cutts FT, Othepa O, Vernon AA, et al. Measles control in Kinshasa, Zaire improved with high coverage and use of medium titre Edmonston Zagreb vaccine at age 6 months. *Int J Epidemiol* 1994;23:624–631.

41. United Nations High Commissioner for Refugees. Refugees by numbers, 2004. Geneva, Switzerland. October 14, 2004. Retrieved June 6, 2005, from http://www.unhcr.ch.

42. United States Committee for Refugees. World refugee survey 2004. Washington, DC. May 24, 2004. Retrieved June 6, 2005, from http://www.uscr.org.

43. Global IDP Project. Internal displacement: Global overview of trends and developments in 2004. March 2005. Retrieved June 6, 2005, from http://www.idp-project.org/publications/2005/Global_overview_2004.final.high.pdf.

44. From Liberian war, tales of brutality. *New York Times*, July 9, 1990.

CHAPTER 20

A Mumps Epidemic, Iowa, 2006

Patricia Quinlisk, MD, MPH

INTRODUCTION

Outbreaks often begin with obvious circumstances. For example, you get a call on Friday afternoon reporting that almost everyone who ate at the church supper Wednesday night now has diarrhea, but sometimes these outbreaks, as Carl Sandburg once said about fog, "come on little cat feet," and not until some time has passed do you realize that you are at the beginning of a very large epidemic. This one was like that.

A BRIEF HISTORY OF MUMPS

Hippocrates described mumps in the 5th century BCE, and its correlation with orchitis (testicular inflammation) was noted in the 1700s. Before the vaccine era, mumps was endemic in the United States, with spring and early summer seasonality. The mumps virus is spread by airborne transmission, respiratory droplets, and direct contact with saliva from an infected person. It was one of the most common causes of deafness in the prevaccine era and was associated with sterility in men. Since 1967, after the introduction of a live mumps vaccine, there has been more than a 99% decline in the annual incidence of mumps with seasonal variation no longer occurring. Before this epidemic, the most recent large U.S. outbreak had occurred in Kansas in 1988–1989 in school children, with 269 cases.[1] Because of outbreaks of vaccine-preventable diseases that occurred

in the late 1980s (primarily of measles), in about 1990, the national recommendation changed from one dose of measles containing vaccine to
two doses, most of which was given as the MMR (measles, mumps, and
rubella) vaccine (Figure 20-1). States changed their child care and school
entry laws to reflect this.

During the 15 years after the two-dose vaccine recommendations, no
large outbreaks of mumps were reported in the United States, and by 2005,
only 906 cases of mumps were reported nationally; however, in less vaccinated populations in other parts of the world, outbreaks had continued.
The United Kingdom experienced a very large epidemic of mumps between
2004 and 2007 with over 56,000 cases, primarily occurring in poorly vaccinated young adults (see http://www.cdc.gov/mmwr/preview/mmwrhtml/
mm5507a1.htm). This outbreak was caused by a serotype G mumps virus.
An introduction into the United States of mumps from this outbreak had
occurred in the summer of 2005 at a camp in New York, resulting in a
contained outbreak of 31 cases (see http://www.cdc.gov/mmwr/preview/
mmwrhtml/mm5507a2.htm).

Before this epidemic, Iowa's children were highly vaccinated, with over
97% of children starting school in 2004 having received two doses of
MMR vaccine; however, because the mandatory second dose of vaccine for
school entry didn't start until 1991 in Iowa, many of those in college, particularly juniors and seniors, had only received one dose.

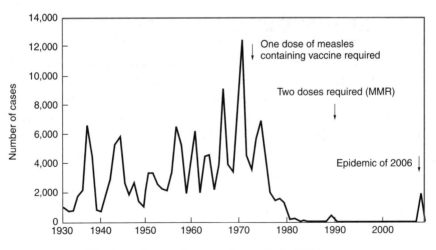

FIGURE 20-1 Number of cases of mumps, Iowa, 1930–2007.

THE IOWA EPIDEMIC

In the early winter of 2005, a cluster of possible mumps cases in eastern Iowa were reported to the health department. Earlier cases may have occurred, but it is difficult for health care workers or public health personnel to identify cases of diseases that only rarely occur and are not expected because of widespread vaccination. Also, health care workers lose experience in diagnosing these diseases as they become so rare. Testing was done for mumps on two people in this cluster, and they had positive mumps IgM tests (but because of the low positive predictive value of tests when disease prevalence is low, these could have been false-positive tests). It was not unusual for a few cases of mumps to be reported. Since the beginning of the 1990s, Iowa had about five cases of mumps reported to the state health department each year, with most of the recent cases having been imported. Thus, at this point, the normal public health follow-up investigation by the local health department was performed, but not much else.

By January of 2006, seven more cases of mumps-like illness had been reported to the public health surveillance system, which were more cases than expected, meeting the definition of a possible outbreak. Because we wanted to confirm that the symptoms of these cases were actually caused by the mumps virus (see Exhibit 20-1), we arranged for clinical specimens (both blood and cheek swabs) to be taken from these patients and sent to Iowa's public health laboratory, the University Hygienic Laboratory (UHL). Mumps viruses were isolated from the cheek swab samples of two patients, and several of the other patients in this cluster had mumps IgM antibodies in their blood. The isolated mumps viruses were sent down to the Centers for Disease Control (CDC) for further identification; the viruses were found to be serotype G (similar to the virus causing the U.K. outbreak). All of these patients were considered to be confirmed cases of mumps using the case definition at the time (see Exhibit 20-2). At this point, we knew we were having an unusual number of mumps cases, so several public health actions were taken:

1. Free laboratory testing began being offered to any Iowan with symptoms consistent with mumps to decrease economic barriers to diagnosis and to assure the identification and reporting of all cases.
2. Messages were sent out to Iowa's health care providers warning them that mumps was spreading in the state and to laboratorians on the

---

Exhibit 20-1   Laboratory Issues

The University Hygienic Laboratory (UHL), Iowa's public health laboratory, provided almost all of the laboratory support during this epidemic. Unlike what might be seen in a clinical trial, the laboratory methods chosen to confirm mumps cases evolved with the outbreak.

The first IgM-positive laboratory tests were thought to be possible false positives because the laboratory reagent used to perform the IgM serology test was not Food and Drug Administration approved (validation had been done with a minimal number of samples). At the UHL, as the outbreak swelled, the large volume of serologic testing for IgM (testing for acute disease) resulted in the decision not to accept specimens for IgG testing (testing for immunity). Thus, when hospitals and clinics began testing their staff for immunity, these specimens had to be sent to reference laboratories. Although all of the mumps tests performed at UHL were done free of charge, those sent to reference labs were not.

Viral cultures were desirable, but the virus is known to be difficult to grow. The cell cultures using primary rhesus monkey kidney (PRMK) cells were used. Because PRMK cells in tubes were in short supply, UHL converted to using PRMK shell vials on April 4. When the outbreak escalated, the demand for any PRMK cells became too great for the suppliers to provide enough; therefore, UHL switched to vero cells (after performing the necessary validation to confirm that vero cells would support the growth of the mumps virus). Vero cells are also of monkey kidney origin.

In the beginning of the outbreak, the patients were asked to provide both urine and buccal swabs specimens, but weeks later, after analysis of the data, it was determined very few positives were being detected from the urine cultures; thus, from then on, only buccal swabs were requested.

At the start of the outbreak, the laboratory questioned whether developing a test using the newer technology of a polymerase chain reaction (PCR) assay for mumps virus should be developed. As the outbreak continued to escalate, it became obvious that the culture method needed to be abandoned because of the amount of labor and time involved; thus, a PCR method was developed. After validation of the test (in collaboration with CDC), proving that this method was as sensitive as a culture, it became the method of choice. The method was then posted on the Association of Public Health Laboratory's website to make it available to other states.

---

process for having laboratory specimens tested (see http://www.idph .state.ia.us/adper/common/pdf/epi_updates/epi_update_060906.pdf for Iowa's weekly EPI update, a newsletter on health events in Iowa).

3. A review of all public health department mumps information material was updated, which included a new case report form (revised to ensure information pertinent to this outbreak was collected).

4. Follow-up investigation of each case was performed.

By late February, with over 20 reported cases via our standard passive disease surveillance system, we were seeing the beginnings of the largest outbreak of mumps to occur in the United States in decades, although we were

---

Exhibit 20-2   Case Definitions

1999 National clinical case definition: An illness with acute onset of unilateral or bilateral tender, self-limited swelling of the parotid or other salivary gland, lasting longer than or equal to 2 days, and without other apparent cause. *Laboratory criteria for diagnosis:* (1) isolation of mumps virus from clinical specimen or (2) a significant rise between acute- and convalescent-phase titers in serum mumps IgM antibody level by any standard serologic assay, or (3) a positive serologic test for mumps immunoglobulin (IgM) antibody. A "case" could be a person with positive laboratory test(s) but no clinical symptoms.

As a consequence of this epidemic, it changed to the following:

Iowa's outbreak case definition in 2006: Because of variation of the symptoms patients with mumps were presenting with and because of limited supplies of mumps laboratory reagent, we modified the 1999 clinical case definition to only include those with symptoms consistent with mumps, which could include no salivary gland involvement but other glandular involvement such as testicular inflammation (orchitis), and the patient had to have a laboratory test positive or be epi-linked to a confirmed case.

2007 National clinical case definition: An illness with acute onset of unilateral or bilateral tender, self-limited swelling of the parotid and/or other salivary gland(s), lasting at least 2 days, and without other apparent cause. *Clinically compatible illness:* Infection with mumps virus may present as aseptic meningitis, encephalitis, hearing loss, orchitis, oophoritis, parotitis or other salivary gland swelling, mastitis or pancreatitis. *Laboratory criteria:* (1) isolation of mumps virus from clinical specimen or (2) detection of mumps nucleic acid (e.g., standard or real time RT-PCR assays), or (3) detection of mumps IgM antibody, or (4) demonstration of specific mumps antibody response in absence of recent vaccination, either a fourfold rise in IgG titer as measured by quantitative assays or a seroconversion from negative to positive using a standard serologic assay of paired acute and convalescent serum specimens. A "case" must have clinically compatible symptoms. This was changed because of experience with the 2006 epidemic.

For more information on case definitions, see http://www.cste.org/Positionstatement.asp.

---

still unaware of that at the time. Because many of Iowa's early cases occurred in college age students (Figure 20-2) and transmission was occurring on several college campuses, we responded by starting active surveillance in five Iowa counties (including those with the three largest universities and the three colleges where transmission was already confirmed) (Exhibit 20-3). To do this, we coordinated with the local health departments to contact local hospitals and clinics, student health services, and similar health care facilities, and asked that anyone with possible mumps be immediately reported. Education of health care workers and college authorities was expanded across the state. On all college campuses, we recommended[1] education of all students on the symptoms of mumps, the importance of isolation for ill persons, and how to seek medical care if symptoms are suspected. We also recommended that all students be assessed for vaccine status and vaccines be given to any student or staff without two documented doses.

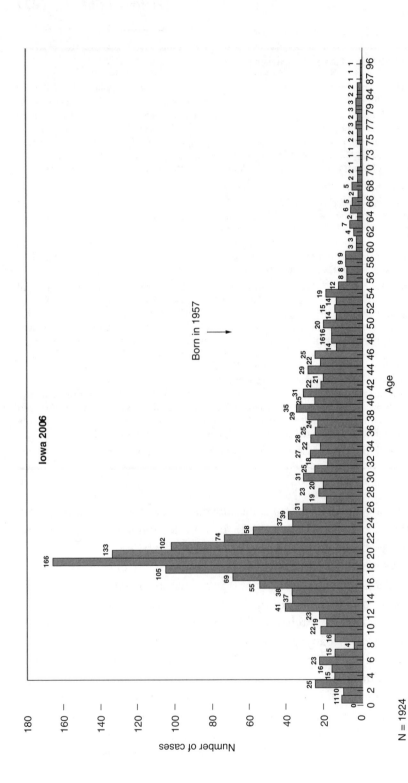

N = 1924

FIGURE 20-2 Age distribution of mumps cases, Iowa 2006.

Exhibit 20-3 Outbreak Data Management

At the beginning of the epidemic, we quickly realized that the mumps investigation form used for routine reports of mumps disease would not be sufficient. We had to assess quickly what questions in a form would answer the many questions surrounding this outbreak.

- Was this due to improper handling of the vaccine causing inactivation? Were there one or a few medical clinics that could be pin-pointed as the source?
- How many doses did our mumps cases receive and when, where, and from whom?
- Were these cases related to travel?
- What mild symptoms and complications were patients experiencing that we did not capture with the old form?
- Were the cases occurring in college students? If so, what types of colleges (e.g., private, public)? What exposures on college campuses would lead to mumps disease?
- What laboratory tests were being done to confirm disease?
- What occupations did our cases have?

Because we initiated active surveillance, we were able to have those sites complete a supplemental form. From that we determined improper handling of the vaccine was not an issue, neither was timing or dosage of the vaccine. We then modified our standard mumps investigation form to include expanded demographics, specific and numerous manifestations of clinical symptoms, several options for laboratory testing, and extensive vaccine and travel history.

Creating the form was the easy part. Entering every form into a database with epidemiology staff already stretched beyond capacity was the next challenge. Approximately 1 month into the epidemic we started prioritizing daily disease reports. Those with the potential to cause outbreaks were processed with mumps (e.g., *Salmonella*, *Shigella*), and those that were not spread person to person (e.g., Lyme disease) were held until everything else was processed. We hired and trained temporary data entry staff. Everyone took turns entering follow-up forms.

On a typical day, we might process 20 reports of all reportable communicable diseases covered by the Iowa Administrative Code. During the mumps epidemic, we handled up to 20 cases of only mumps in addition to the normal number of reports for other diseases. After the outbreak was over, we determined that the number of mumps cases in Iowa nearly doubled the disease reports processed by the Iowa Department of Public Health for 1 year.

With control measures in place, we hoped to interrupt transmission of the virus; however, on college campuses, student's adherence to the isolation recommendations was sporadic and difficult for the student health center staff to enforce. (We had symptomatic students admitting to attending beer parties where they "shared saliva" via glasses of beer and other behaviors: there were three beer parties where spread of mumps virus was confirmed.) Mumps continued to spread on college campuses and into communities around these campuses. Because the spread was occurring and research on mumps had not been feasible for decades because of low numbers, the epidemiologists at the CDC asked whether they could come into Iowa to do a special study on these college campuses looking at transmission of the virus and immunity. We agreed, and by early March, three CDC investigators had arrived, met with IDPH staff, and were conducting their study on a couple of the affected eastern Iowa college campuses.

Quarantine for the public was not used for several reasons, unlike during a measles outbreak in Iowa 2 years earlier. Those reasons included (1) 20% to 30% of cases are asymptomatic, (2) mumps virus can be spread up to 3 days prior to symptoms, (3) some mumps cases are so mildly ill that they do not seek medical attention thus are not reported to public health, and (4) mumps is generally a mild illness. Isolation and work quarantine (i.e., restrictions on patient contact during the incubation period), however, were used for health care workers because of the risk of spread to vulnerable patients. We did recommend at this time that all health care workers in Iowa be assessed for immunity and offered vaccination (two doses of MMR were recommended for anyone without documented immunity; this was defined as laboratory evidence of antibodies, documented receipt of two doses of MMR or physician diagnosed mumps).

In February, we knew that everyone in the state needed to be aware of the situation, and thus, getting information out was of critical importance. When looking at a response to an outbreak, epidemic, or any other biologic emergency, the most challenging aspect is almost always communication. Getting the right information to the right audience at the right time can be difficult. Thus, it was at this point that the communications aspects of this outbreak really began (Exhibit 20-4).

During outbreaks like this, you have exportation of the disease that must be followed up to contain spread. Early in the outbreak, several business travelers from eastern Iowa went to Washington, DC to visit politicians on "the hill." A couple days later, it was determined that one of them was infectious during those visits. IDPH contacted the offices of both of the Senators and Representatives that were visited and the Washington, DC Health Department. The Washington, DC Health Department worked with the Medical Director of Congress and quickly offered vaccine to all the potentially exposed nonimmune persons. No mumps cases were identified as a result of this incident.

Exhibit 20-4   Communications in Iowa

The communication pathways used in this situation included the following:

Face to face: Conferences were held at IDPH each morning to review what had happened the day before and to determine the actions to be taken that day. This was attended by IDPH staff, visiting CDC consultants, and UHL staff (public health laboratorians).

Telephone: Conference calls were held weekly with the local health department officials and as needed with Iowa's Infectious Disease Advisory Committee. Also, regular conference calls were done with CDC, and as the outbreak spread, to involved states, and then to all states.

E-mail: Electronic methods were used to send documents and other information to public health and health care workers, particularly the "Epi Update" a weekly IDPH newsletter. Colleges used their student e-mail systems for getting information to their students on symptoms of mumps, and where vaccine clinics were held.

HAN: The Health Alert Network, and statewide alerting system, was used to both alert public health and health care workers around the state about new events and as a secure, password-protected website for accessing confidential information.

IDPH website: Biweekly updates on numbers of cases, the process for submission of clinical specimens, worksheets for patient assessment, forms for reporting of cases, mumps information sheets in various languages, and other information were placed on the website. This information was used by Iowa's health care workers and newspaper reporters and, as the outbreak spread beyond Iowa, by public health officials in other states as a template for addressing their communication needs. We also posted a running list of the most frequently asked questions and their answers (access this website at http://www.idph.state.ia.us/adper/mumps.asp).

Media: Newspapers, radio, television, and nontraditional media (websites) were used to get information out to the public. Seven official press conferences/news releases occurred during this time with the last one on August 21. IDPH's public information officer worked full time for weeks on this issue alone because the need to get information out and to respond to media inquiries was so critical.

CDC: The *Morbidity and Mortality Weekly Report* (MMWR) published several articles on this situation, the first as it started in Iowa (see http://www.cdc.gov/mmwr/preview/mmwrhtml/mm5513a3.htm), the second as it spread (see http://www.cdc.gov/mmwr/preview/mmwrhtml/mm5520a4.htm), and a third update as the epidemic wound down (see http://www.cdc.gov/mmwr/preview/mmwrhtml/mm5542a3.htm). On this site is also found the Advisory Committee on Immunization Practice's recommendations for use of vaccine to control mumps (see http://www.cdc.gov/mmwr/preview/mmwrhtml/00053391.htm).

In other examples, there was fear of the spread of mumps when a bus load of eastern Iowa college students traveled down to Missouri for an athletic competition. They were not allowed off the bus and were sent back to Iowa by local college officials immediately, even though no one on the bus had mumps. When a wrestling tournament occurred between Nebraska

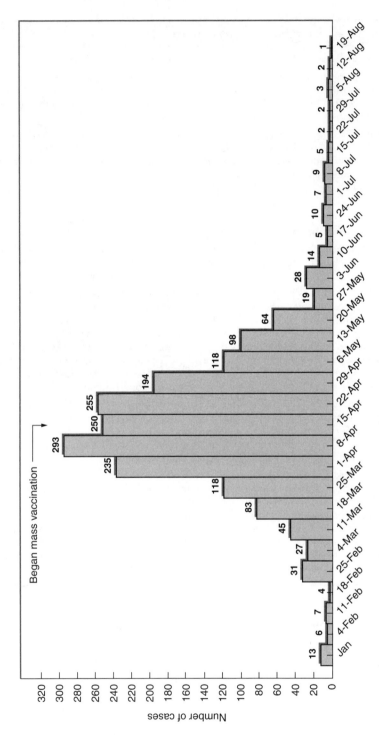

FIGURE 20-3 Number of cases of mumps, by date of onset—Iowa, January 1–August 22, 2006.

and Iowa, mumps was spread not among the athletes, but among specta-
tors and parents in the bleachers, beginning an outbreak in Nebraska
among non–college-aged adults.

In March, the number of cases began skyrocketing; by the end of the
month, over 300 additional cases had been reported, mostly in eastern
Iowa, and another 14 possible cases were being investigated in the bordering states of Illinois, Minnesota, and Nebraska (Figures 20-3 and 20-4).[2]
This compares with an annual average of 265 cases reported in the entire
United States between 2001 and 2005. By March 15, eastern Iowa papers
were printing: "Mumps making comeback." By April 5, the outbreak was
on the front page of the Iowa's largest newspaper, the *Des Moines Register*,
above the fold. (Of course, the *Des Moines Register* headline "Mumps cases
have doctors confounded" would not have been my choice, but at least the
word was getting out to the public.) Other *Des Moines Register* articles
included "Health Officials: Mumps vaccine still effective" (April 7, 2006)
and "Young adults targeted in Mumps fight" (April 21, 2006). We even
made page 3 in *USA Today* on April 3 and page 13 in the *New York Times*
on April 1.

More control measures were instituted in March. They included targeting health care workers with immunity assessments (either check for

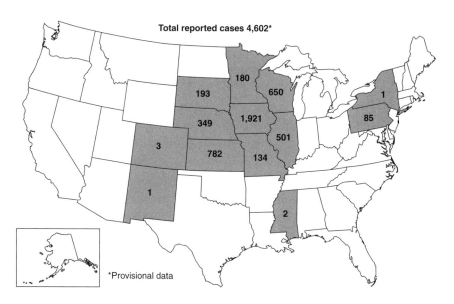

FIGURE 20-4 Mumps outbreak, United States 2006.

documented doses of MMR, or serologic test for immunity—primarily used with the older members of this population because they grew up in a time when mumps was quite common in the community and no vaccines were available). We also changed the recommendations for isolation of case-patients to be reduced from 9 days after onset to 5 days. This was done because of the difficulty of ensuring isolation of college students for 9 days and because the science was showing almost all of the transmission was occurring early in the illness; thus, we felt we would get better compliance with the 5 days, and this could help us slow the transmission of the virus. Our web page on mumps was expanded, and given its own specific site, HAN (health alert network) messages were used as a means to keep public health officials and medical personnel across the state up to date on the epidemic. Questions about vaccine efficacy were common (Exhibit 20-5).

We also began regular conference calls with each of our partner groups: local health departments, infection-control professionals in hospitals, and bordering state health departments/CDC (which very quickly were expanded to all affected states, then to all states). All of these groups were encouraged to copy any of the information/forms/fact sheets that we had produced, to use it however they might need. When you are busy with follow-up investigations and outbreaks, you don't need to reinvent the wheel. Because many similar questions were coming into our hotline system, we began keeping a list of the common questions and how we answered them on our website—a "running Q&A."

By April, the outbreak had reached epidemic levels, and over 50 cases were being reported each working day (Exhibit 20-6). The epidemic was no longer contained in any localized area but had spread across Iowa (Figure 20-5) and to several neighboring states. When situations such as this occur, the importance of good relationships cannot be emphasized enough. Relationships, not only with your public health partners like the local health departments, other state health departments and the CDC, but with other state agencies like emergency management, the governor's office, the legislature, and the media are critical. If you have good relationships, the issues are resolved quickly, and you are able to focus your time and efforts on stopping the epidemic. If your relationships are poor, you may find your time being spent on side issues, stalling your efforts. These relationships are best forged prior to any emergency and are based in understanding each others assets/abilities and roles and responsibilities.

Exhibit 20-5   Vaccine Efficacy

As the public became more aware of the outbreak and the fact that many of those with mumps had been vaccinated, questions arose about whether or not the vaccine was effective at preventing disease. Because we did not want people to falsely use this situation as a reason to not vaccinate their children, we provided information and examples of why this was occurring. (This was created early in the outbreak when vaccine efficacy was still thought to be around 95% after two doses of MMR.)

Examples Explaining Mumps Vaccine Effectiveness

Or Why Are So Many Mumps Cases Occurring in Vaccinated People?

There have been many questions about why people, who have been vaccinated, are getting mumps. As you read through the examples that follow, keep these key points in mind.

- The mumps vaccine (part of the MMR vaccine) is about 95% effective.
- This means out of every 100 people vaccinated, 95 will be protected; however, the vaccine will not "take" in 5 people, and these people will remain susceptible to the disease.
- By comparison, the measles vaccine (also part of the MMR vaccine) is about 98% effective and the annual influenza vaccine is about 70% to 85% effective.

Example 1

In a community of 100 people, 100% have been vaccinated. Everyone is exposed to mumps. What happens?

- Ninety-five people (95%) in the community are protected by the vaccine and do not get mumps.
- Five people (5%) in the community become ill with mumps because the vaccine did not "take."
- Of the 5 people who get mumps, all (100%) have been vaccinated.

Example 2

In a community of 100, 98% have been vaccinated (a similar rate to what is being seen today in Iowa's K-12 schools and some colleges). Thus, 98 people are vaccinated, and 2 people are not. Everyone is exposed to mumps. What happens?

- Ninety-three people (95% of the 98 who are vaccinated) in the community are protected by the vaccine and do not get mumps.
- Five people (5% of the 98 who are vaccinated) become ill with mumps because the vaccine did not "take."
- Two people who have never been vaccinated get ill because they have no immunity to the disease.
- Of the 7 (5 vaccinated + 2 unvaccinated) people who get mumps, 71% (5 of 7) were vaccinated (similar to what is happening now in Iowa)

Thus, a large percentage of the people with mumps have been vaccinated. This is expected in a highly vaccinated population when dealing with a vaccine that is 95% effective and a contagious disease like mumps. This does not mean that the vaccine is not working; in fact the mumps vaccine is working as expected (http://www.idph .state.ia.us/adper/common/pdf/mumps/explaining_effectiveness.pdf).

Exhibit 20-6   What Is an Epidemic

Epidemic definition [from the Greek *epi* (upon), *d_mos* (people)]: the occurrence in a community or region of cases of an illness . . . clearly in excess of normal expectancy. The community or region and the period in which the cases occur are specified precisely. The number of cases indicating the presence of an epidemic varies according to the agent, size, and type of population exposed; previous experience or lack of exposure to the disease; and the time and place of occurrence. Epidemicity is thus relative to usual frequency of the disease in the same area, among the specified population and the same season of the year.

Outbreak definition: An epidemic limited to localized increase of a disease, for example, in a village, town, or closed institution.

At this point, we began using the incident command system (Figure 20-6). I will be honest—a decade ago, when I began to realize that the incident command system was going to be used during outbreaks and epidemics, I was not thrilled. I was concerned that this system would get in the way of the science and epidemiologic response; however, today, after several large outbreaks, including this one, I am a believer. This system was first put into place to deal with forest fires and allows those knowledgeable in emergency response, administration, and intra-agency coordination to deal with those issues, allowing the epidemiologists/scientists to focus on the epidemic and medical aspects of the situation. The result is a better handled situation and more effective epidemiologists. One of the first things completed under this system was the establishment of a phone bank to deal with all of the calls coming into the health department. Most of the calls were from health care providers; very few were from the public. Thus Iowa's phone bank was used only to deal with the medical issues (because we could answer the situation specific questions best), and the public was sent to CDC's answering system where their more general questions could be answered (although the public probably didn't realize this was happening), freeing up our people to deal more directly with the response issues.

Since the beginning of the epidemic, a targeted vaccination strategy had been used; vaccinating college students and health care workers, for example; however, as the disease expanded across the state and showed no signs of slowing, various options were considered. Because there had been no outbreaks of mumps for almost 20 years, I had no experience with outbreaks of mumps and wanted the advice of someone with experience at the state level. It took some effort to find epidemiologists experienced with

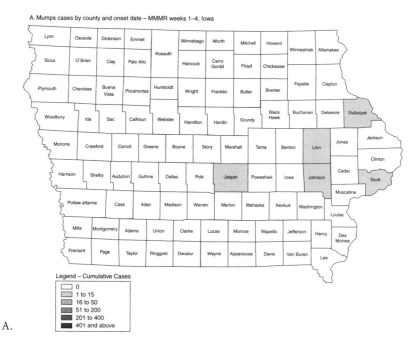

A. Mumps cases by county and onset date – MMMR weeks 1–4, Iowa

B. Mumps cases by county and onset date – MMMR weeks 5–8, Iowa

FIGURE 20-5 A. Mumps cases by county and onset date—MMMR weeks 1–4, Iowa. B. Mumps cases by county and onset date—MMMR weeks 5–8, Iowa.

(continues)

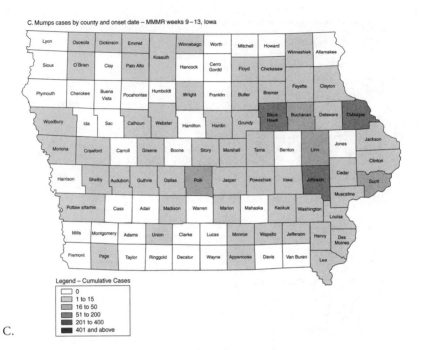

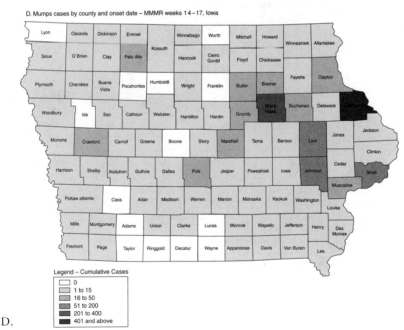

FIGURE 20-5 C. Mumps cases by county and onset date—MMMR weeks 9–13, Iowa. D. Mumps cases by county and onset date—MMMR weeks 14–17, Iowa.

E. Mumps cases by county and onset date – MMMR weeks 18–22, Iowa

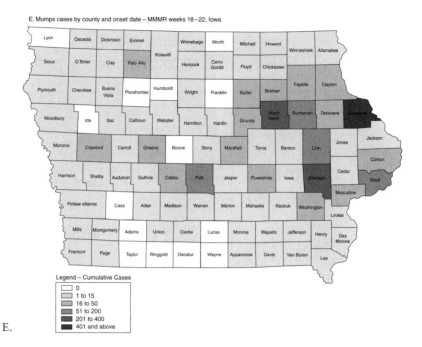

Legend – Cumulative Cases
- 0
- 1 to 15
- 16 to 50
- 51 to 200
- 201 to 400
- 401 and above

E.

F. Mumps cases by county and onset date – MMMR weeks 23–33, Iowa

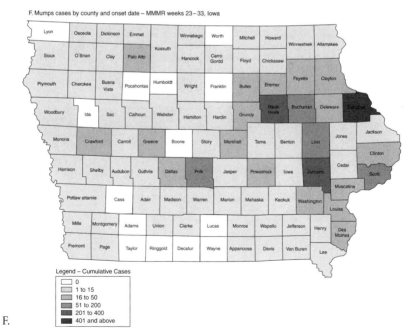

Legend – Cumulative Cases
- 0
- 1 to 15
- 16 to 50
- 51 to 200
- 201 to 400
- 401 and above

F.

FIGURE 20-5 E. Mumps cases by county and onset date—MMMR weeks 18–22, Iowa. F. Mumps cases by county and onset date—MMMR weeks 23–33, Iowa.

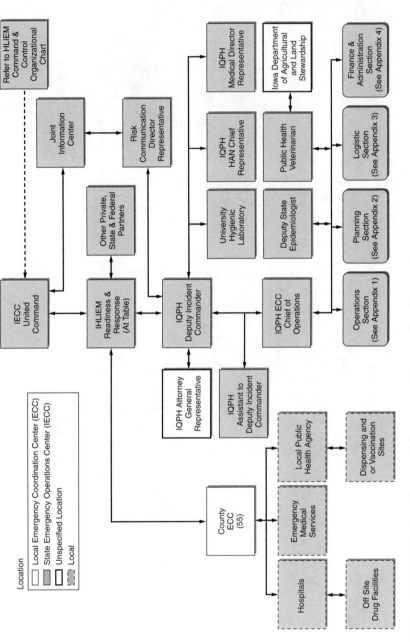

FIGURE 20-6 IDPH Incident Command Structure—Command and Control.

mumps control efforts. I am still grateful to the three state epidemiologists who gave up a Saturday afternoon to have a conference call with me. In the end, with the advice of these epidemiologists and CDC and lots of discussion at the state level, mass vaccination of the whole state was considered (Exhibit 20-7). This is obviously a very difficult strategy; there were issues of vaccine supply, payment of vaccine purchased, distribution of the vaccine to each county, determination of the amount needed by each county, getting the word out about the program, and efforts to have clinics in the midst of the highest risk groups (such as on college campuses). A special committee meeting of legislators with the Director of the Iowa Department of Public Health was needed to release the emergency funds required to buy the vaccine. (For the best uptake of vaccine, it had to be offered free of charge; thus, public funding for the vaccine had to obtained.) This whole process took about 10 days from the decision to do a statewide mass vaccination program, purchase the vaccine, have it shipped to Iowa, distribute it to the local health departments, and have vaccination clinics. In the end, a total of 37,500 doses of MMR vaccine were purchased and made available. This was no small task.

Exhibit 20-7   Policy Issues

Whenever complicated situations such as this occur, there will always be issues that require far-reaching decisions, or "policy decisions." These decisions have to be made carefully because they not only impact on the present situation, but will effect future situations. When these types of decisions needed to be made, usually one person proposed it, and it was discussed over a period of time with the appropriate people, such as the director, our public health lawyer, and other department directors that might be affected by this policy. Invariably, it was modified, and then the director would "sign off" on it. When the first MMWR article was published on April 7, and the word "epidemic" was used in the title, there were concerns expressed about the political ramifications of using the word "epidemic" rather than "outbreak." Thus, I had to explain the scientific difference between epidemic and outbreak and why we used the word epidemic.

One example of these policies involved mass gatherings. The First National Special Olympics were to be held in central Iowa on a college campus in the summer of 2006, and our public health department was asked for their advice. After discussion, our policy was that persons traveling to Iowa for events like this were advised not to change their plans but instead to ensure that they were fully vaccinated against mumps prior to arrival. This policy was then placed on our website (see http://www.idph.state.ia.us/adper/common/pdf/mumps/mass_gathering_041806.pdf).

The mass vaccination program occurred in three stages: the first stage was vaccination of young adults ages 18 to 22 years, which was expanded the next week to ages 18 to 25 years, and 2 weeks later, the ages were expanded to 18 to 46 years. We found it difficult to get college students to go and get vaccinated, and in the end only about 10,000 doses of vaccine were used in Iowa's 99 counties. (The remaining vaccine did not go to waste as large quantities of vaccine were sent to the East Coast a couple months later in response to an outbreak of measles.)

Between the mass vaccination program, college spring semesters ending, and the natural decrease of mumps in late spring, the epidemic began to slow down in late April and early May. By late May, we were saying that the epidemic was waning, and on June 2, it was publicly announced that the epidemic was contained.

Over the summer, we continued to encourage vaccination and recommended that all students planning on attending college that fall ensure that they had two doses of MMR. There was concern that mumps would re-emerge during the next school year, causing new outbreaks. Fortunately, Iowa had no further outbreaks of mumps, but unfortunately, several college campuses in other states were not as lucky.

We never did figure out how mumps got started in Iowa, although we looked hard for the index case. Our best guess is that it was brought in from the United Kingdom, probably in a college student(s). This outbreak tested Iowa's public health system and cost us over 1 million dollars. The many lessons learned will be put to use in our next public health emergency. Today, Iowans are better vaccinated, public health is better prepared, and the medical community is more aware that these vaccine-preventable diseases can come back; in addition, the role of public health is better understood. It is unlikely that this large a mumps outbreak will ever happen again in Iowa.

This mumps epidemic also served as a "natural experiment," and consequently, research into mumps occurred with many issues being better understood (Exhibit 20-8).

This was the largest epidemic that I had ever been involved with. Fortunately, mumps is typically a mild disease and one for which we had a relatively effective vaccine. Only one death occurred in Iowa (in someone with other more serious medical problems), and very few people needed hospitalization. There were reports of temporary deafness, but it appears that most, if not all, have regained their hearing. Had this been a disease such as measles or SARS, the outcome could have been devastating.

Exhibit 20-8   Mumps Research

Several studies were performed during this mumps epidemic and some of these have been published:

1. A study of transmissibility of the mumps virus among college students, found that two dose vaccine efficacy was only 76% to 80% among college students (most vaccinated >10 years prior).[3]

2. A study of transmission of mumps among airplane passengers found that mumps does not spread to any significant degree on planes. Thus, today when passengers infectious with mumps are found to have traveled on an airline, the other passengers are NOT notified. (see http://www.cdc.gov/mmwr/preview/mmwrhtml/mm5514a6.htm)

3. An economic impact study was done, which determined that this epidemic cost over 1 million dollars to Iowa's public health system alone.

4. A small health care worker study found that although over 80% of health care workers who thought that they were immune to mumps were immune, approximately 20% were not.

5. A study was done on viral shedding by the UHL and the University of Iowa, which found that patients continued to shed the virus for up to 9 days, but the most significant shedding occurred during the 5 days after onset of symptoms.[4]

6. Laboratory-based studies:
    a. The method for the new PCR test was developed by UHL during this epidemic.[5]
    b. A model was developed to predict the duration of viral shedding (http://www.idsociety.org/WorkArea/showcontent.aspx?id=8412).
    c. An analysis of the geospacial relationship of the spread of mumps was performed (see http://www.cdc.gov/eid/content/14/3/ICEID2008.pdf).

7. National recommendations of use of vaccine were changed by the Advisory Committee on Immunization Practices, particularly for all health care workers to be vaccinated with one to two doses of MMR (unless proved immune) (http://www.cdc.gov/mmwr/preview/mmwrhtml/mm5522a4.htm).

In the end, we learned a lot about how to respond to biologic emergencies and used this experience to improve our response system. I believe that should Iowa be faced with a similar biologic emergency situation in the future, we will be better prepared because of this mumps epidemic and have a more effective response.

REFERENCES

1. Hersh BS, Fine PE, Kent WK, et al. Mumps outbreak in a highly vaccinated population. *J Pediatr* 1991;119:187–193.

2. Dayan G, Quinlisk P, Parker AA, et al. Recent resurgence of mumps in the United States. *N Engl J Med* 2008;358:1580–1589. Available from http://content.nejm.org/cgi/content/short/358/15/1580.

3. Marin M, Quinlisk P, Shimabukaro T, et al. Mumps vaccination coverage and vaccine effectiveness in a large outbreak among college students—Iowa, 2006. *Vaccine* 2008;26:3601–3607.

4. Polgreen PM, Bohnett LC, Cavanaugh JE, et al. The duration of virus shedding after the onset of symptoms. *Clin Infect Dis* 2008;46:1447–1449.

5. Boddicker JD, Rota PA, Kreman T, et al. Real-time reverse transcription-PCR assay for detection of mumps virus RNA in clinical specimens. *J Clin Microbiol* 2007;45:2902–2908.

Note: MMWR weeks roughly correspond to months of the year such as weeks 1 to 4 refers to January, 5 to 8 refers to February, and so on.

Index

445